A *Jerry Baker* Good Health Book

The NEW HEALING FOODS

www.jerrybaker.com

A *Jerry Baker* Good Health Book

The New Healing Foods

1,404 Refrigerator Remedies, Countertop Cures, and Miracle Menus That Fight Everything from Arthritis, High Blood Pressure, and High Cholesterol to Diabetes, Heart Disease, and a Cranky Gut!

Colleen Pierre, M.S., R.D.

Published by American Master Products, Inc./Jerry Baker

A Jerry Baker Good Health Book and a Blackberry Cottage Production
Editorial: Ellen Michaud,
Blackberry Cottage Productions, Ltd.
Author: Colleen Pierre, M.S., R.D.
Contributing Authors: Rick Chillot, Karen Cicero, Marcia Holman

Design: Nest Publishing Resources
Book Composition: Wayne F. Michaud
Illustrator: Wayne F. Michaud
Copy Editor: Jane Sherman

Kim Adam Gasior, Publisher

Printed in the United States of America

Illustrations copyright © 2005 by Wayne F. Michaud

Publisher's Cataloging-in-Publication

Pierre, Colleen.
   Jerry Baker's the new healing foods / [Colleen Pierre].
   p. cm.
   Includes index.
   "1,404 refrigerator remedies, countertop cures, and miracle menus that fight everything from arthritis, high blood pressure, and high cholesterol to diabetes, heart disease, and a cranky gut!"
   ISBN 978-0–922433–62–9

   1. Diet Therapy—Popular works.   2. Functional foods.
3. Naturopathy.   I. Baker, Jerry.   II. Title.   III. Title: New healing foods.

RM216.P59 2005   615.8'54
                                QB104-200520

14 16 17 15   hardcover

CONTENTS

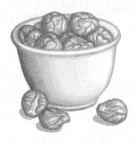

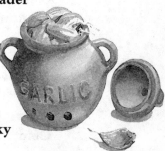

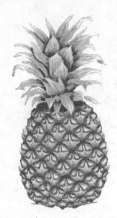

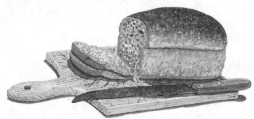

Part Two

The Healthy Heart:
Beat Ticker Shock

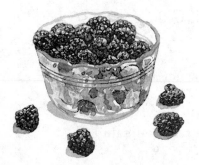

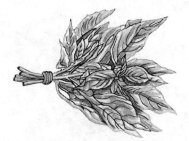

Part Four

Ahead of the Game: Face the Future with a Smile

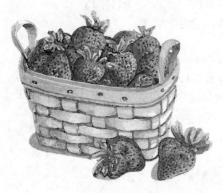

Part Five

Girl Talk: Harness Your
Raging Hormones

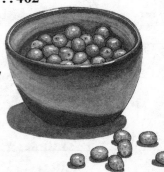

INTRODUCTION

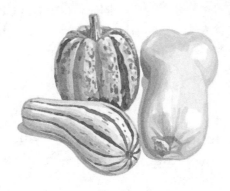

As a registered dietitian, I've spent more than 25 years counseling people about how to eat better to prevent or manage life-threatening diseases. I have to admit that I get pretty excited when clients dig into lifestyle changes that lower their cholesterol, blood pressure, and blood sugar. Yes, they really do work!

High cholesterol, high blood pressure, and diabetes are just the tip of the iceberg when it comes to the healing power of food. The world of nutrition research has exploded since I was a young R.D., creating a roller coaster ride through parts of our bodies that we never would have imagined were affected by what we eat. Memory loss, vision problems, joint pain, menstrual woes, tummy trouble, and more respond to our daily fare for good or ill, depending on our choices. In short, we have the power!

I'm also thrilled by the growing scientific evidence that shows natural, supportive strategies such as massage therapy (my all-time favorite!), herbal medicine, meditation, and even a healing touch can work wonders to provide soothing comfort and gentle healing. Better still, most of these therapies do it without the side effects of many prescription medicines.

Now don't get me wrong; I think modern medicine is tops. On many occasions, nothing less than the right prescription or life-saving surgery will do. That said, we often opt for pills or the knife when eating better, getting a little exercise, or trying some simple, all-natural remedies would do the trick—cheaper and with fewer side effects.

In this book, I've gathered gentle, healing remedies (some from my bestselling *Kitchen Counter Cures)* for 16 health conditions that threaten us all, plus 98 healing foods that work wonders to prevent or manage those ailments. Each section includes discussions of related conditions, followed by information on foods that have been shown by research to be key players in preventing or treating each one. What's really remarkable about the foods, though, is that all of them are good for more than one condition! They're all multitaskers. Apricots, for instance, are discussed with cancer, but check them out. They also play a part in fighting heart disease, high blood pressure, high cholesterol, stroke, and even yeast infections. *Amazing!*

This consistent crossover gives you a little peek at the reasons that real food—not the processed kind that's had all its important parts removed—does such a bang-up job of battling would-be health enemies and keeping us in tiptop condition. There is synergy here (you know, one plus one equals three), so the total effect is greater than the sum of the parts. And that's the best news since the introduction of whole wheat bread!

Sure, there are times when individual vitamins and minerals from a pill can really work wonders. Women who may become pregnant, for instance, should take multivitamins that include folic acid to reduce the risk of birth defects, and adults over 50 should get vitamin D from supplements to protect their bones. But modern research has revealed that although vitamins and minerals were among the first nutrients to get our attention, other compounds in food play an equal or greater role in keeping us vigorous and strong and fending off cancer, heart disease, diabetes, and a host of other ills, including the common cold. There's no way you could fit all those ingredients into a pill—and the good news is, you don't have to. Mother Nature delivers the goods in crisp, juicy apples; sweet, luscious blueberries; tangy yogurt; and brilliant bell peppers. Yum, yum!

So if you're ready to ease your aches and pains, stave off disease, and please your palate in the process, you've come to the right place. Read on, my friends, and I'll show you how to turn your kitchen into a healthy, healing place with the new healing foods!

COLLEEN

Colleen Pierre, M.S., R.D.

Part One

TACKLE THE BIG THREE

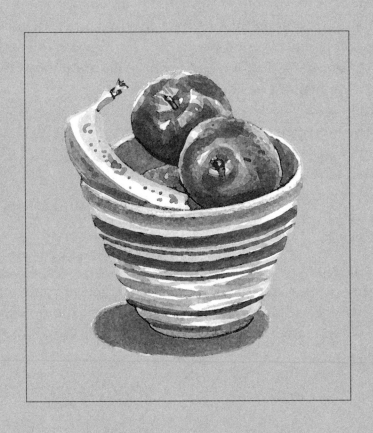

Eat to Beat Arthritis, Cancer, and Diabetes

I don't know about you, but I just don't have time to get sick or give in to aches and pains. I don't care whether the problem is something as small as a cold or the flu or as big as arthritis, cancer, or diabetes. I'd rather be out playing and having fun than draggin' around feeling crummy.

Especially now that we're living so much longer (and have so much more playtime), lifestyle diseases have more time to sneak up on us and spoil our fun. How do we fight back? With fabulous foods to keep up our defenses against troublemaking carcinogens, smother our bodies' tendency to set fire to our joints, and decrease our resistance to our abundant supply of insulin.

Thus, the first part of this book is devoted to beating the big three: arthritis, cancer, and diabetes. We'll take a closer look at each of these conditions and at strategies for managing them, then tackle them with foods guaranteed to deliver the array of vitamins, minerals, and newly discovered natural ingredients that will beat them back.

ARTHRITIS

Make No Bones about It

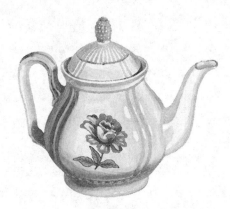

My friend Marcia has an intricate lace tablecloth that amazes her—not simply because it's so lovely but also because her grandmother somehow managed to stitch it when her fingers were stiff and sore from osteoarthritis (OA). So far, Marcia's fingers are still pliable, but her neck often gets so stiff that she wishes she could drip some WD-40 into its joints.

There are a lot of us working stiffs out there. In fact, OA is the most common form of arthritis (there are more than 100 different types) and affects a third of all adults, most of them women.

COMMON CAUSE

By age 40 or 50, many of us begin to notice some tightness in the hinges of our fingers, necks, hips, or knees because the spongy cartilage that covers and protects the bones of our joints becomes thinner due to age and daily wear and tear. At the same time, our cartilage-rebuilding cells start to slack off.

Without their protective cushioning, bones may start to grind against each other, which can damage the tissue surrounding the joint. The body's immune system attempts to come to the rescue, but instead, white blood cells overreact and release inflammatory proteins. The proteins cause swelling, pain, and further damage to the tissue. Joints become stiff and sore, although not all of them at the same time and maybe never more than a few. But the diagnosis is still the same: osteoarthritis.

EASE YOUR WAY

If your pain is severe, you'll certainly check in with your doctor for pain-relieving medication, but there are other things you can do to stymie OA. As Todd Nelson, N.D., a naturopathic physician in Denver, puts it, your joints will respond if you "shift away from the things that promote inflammation and tear down cartilage and move toward things that shore up cartilage." Try these drug-free ways to do just that—with your physician's okay, of course.

Fabulous Fill-In!

Trout, salmon, and other cold-water fish contain an abundance of omega-3 essential fatty acids (EFAs), which ease swollen, stiff joints by reducing both inflammation and cartilage destruction, says Michael E. Weinblatt, M.D. Not a fish fan? Just pop three 1-gram fish-oil capsules twice a day with meals. If you'd rather avoid fish altogether, try flaxseed oil, which also contains EFAs. You can mix 1 to 3 tablespoons with maple syrup to drizzle over waffles, or use it in place of butter on your steamed veggies. Both oils can thin your blood, so avoid them if you take aspirin, other NSAIDs, or prescription blood thinners.

Go for glucosamine. One of the most effective treatments for OA is glucosamine sulfate, a naturally occurring amino sugar that, in supplement form, is produced from shellfish. Not only does it provide pain relief as effectively as or better than nonsteroidal anti-inflammatory drugs (NSAIDs) such as aspirin, without the pesky side effects, it also combats cartilage-destroying enzymes and halts cartilage loss in the knee and hip. What's more, it's sold over the counter, so you can find it in any drugstore. Sounds way too good to be true, right? It's not—but it's also not very fast.

"You start with 500 milligrams three times a day, and it takes two to four weeks to get relief from pain—and twice that long to ease functioning in your joint," says Dr. Nelson. Also, since glucosamine is made from shellfish, you should avoid it if you're allergic to seafood.

Wager on willow. White willow bark contains salicin, which the body converts to salicylic acid to relieve pain. Comb your health food store for a supplement and take two 200- to 400-milligram capsules three times a day between meals, says Dr. Nelson. Just one caveat: Salicin is closely related to the substance found in aspirin, so check with your doctor first if you're already taking aspirin or other blood thinners.

Cap the pain. The hot

A SIMPLE SOLUTION

The next time hip pain flares, sit comfortably, close your eyes, and slow your breathing. Imagine you're running a marathon or doing the rumba with pain-free, swaying hips. Notice the expression on your face and the flower in your hair. Take the time to fully conjure the vision and savor the sensations it creates in your mind. Do it again the next day, and the next. "Repeatedly visualizing such scenarios can help reduce discomfort and may even improve mobility," explains Michael E. Weinblatt, M.D.

ingredient in red pepper is capsaicin, which helps stop production of substance P, an inflammatory prostaglandin that's present in arthritic joints. Check your supermarket or drugstore for capsaicin cream and apply it directly to inflamed joints three or four times a day for a week. Be careful not to get it in your eyes or on any areas of broken skin, and wash your hands after using it.

Confine caffeine. If you drink more than four cups of coffee a day, you're doubling your risk of developing arthritis, warns Dr. Nelson. Caffeine not only alters the mineral balance that's needed to make cartilage, it can also dry up the fluid required to keep cartilage and joints lubricated. So instead of a mocha cappuccino, reach for a mug of water—or many, as the case may be. You need to drink ½ ounce of water per pound of body weight per day (and double that when you're exercising). If you weigh 150 pounds, that's nearly 10 cups of water a day!

Sip soothing tea. Like some arthritis drugs, ginger is a COX-2 inhibitor, meaning that it blocks a pain-causing substance called cyclooxygenase-2 enzyme. Stir 1

9 1 1

If your joints are so swollen and painfully stiff that you can barely climb out of your car, and you're popping aspirin or ibuprofen tablets as if they were breath mints, it's time for a doctor visit. Standard treatments for osteoarthritis include anti-inflammatory medications, antibiotics to slow the erosion of cartilage, and injections to reduce the swelling. These treatments can be expensive, but they all work well—actually, sometimes too well. A corticosteroid shot, for instance, can mask discomfort so effectively that you keep doing the very activities that injured your joints in the first place.

FOOD NEWS

Raisins, pears, apples, and other fruits, as well as nuts and beans, all contain the trace element boron, which can relieve joint pain and stiffness and actually appears to protect against arthritis, says Michael E. Weinblatt, M.D. If you don't eat fruit on a regular basis or don't live in a particularly arid area, where concentrations of boron in the soil and water are highest, consider taking a daily multivitamin supplement that provides 1 to 3 milligrams of the mineral.

teaspoon of grated fresh ginger into a cup of boiling water, steep for 10 to 15 minutes, and strain. Sweeten with honey and down two cups a day. Your knees may soon begin to feel as nimble as that other famous Ginger's.

Take a synovial stroll. When you sit still, the synovial fluid within your joints can become as stiff as molasses in a Maine winter. Although you may not feel like walking when your joints are stiff, it's actually the ideal way to keep the synovial fluid warm and flowing—and your weight in check so you don't overload your joints.

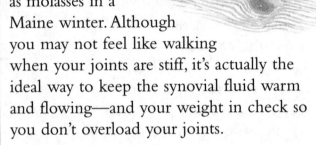

Strengthen your support system. "Strengthening the thigh muscles that support the knee is one of the best ways to control the progression of OA there," says Michael E. Weinblatt, M.D., codirector of clinical rheumatology at Harvard's Brigham and Women's Hospital in Boston. One of the best non-weight-bearing ways to build your thigh muscles is to bicycle regularly. Bike buried too deeply in the basement to retrieve? Try squats. To do them, simply stand with your legs apart and your knees slightly bent. Slowly lower your butt as if you're about to sit on a chair. Pause when your thighs are parallel (or nearly parallel) to the floor, then slowly straighten up. Repeat three to five times a day.

Access acupuncture. Research directed by the National Institutes of Health indicates that people with OA of the knee who receive acupuncture have less pain and better function than people who receive standard care—even weeks after the treatment. Ask your doctor to recommend a reputable acupuncturist near you.

Manage with magnets. Although scientists aren't sure why, studies show that wearing knee wraps embedded with magnets may help you get out of a chair more easily and walk faster and less stiffly. Look for a wrap with a "unipolar" magnet, then place the positive end of the magnet directly over your sore knee, suggests Martha Hinman, Ph.D., associate professor of physical therapy at the University of Texas Medical Branch in Galveston. You should feel relief within 30 minutes.

Trim your tummy. The next time your bathroom scale sneaks up a hair, don't fret about your fanny—it's your knees that deserve your pity! Every time you gain a single pound of body fat, experts say it'll feel like four times as much weight on your knees. The strain is especially hard on your muscles and tendons—your built-in shock absorbers. The good news is that studies show that if you lose 11 pounds, you can reduce stiffness and pain in your knees by half.

Get down in your heels. Skinny stilettos are murder on your knees—but they're not the only culprits. In fact, high, wide-heeled pumps may predispose you to osteoarthritis of the knee, too. The problem, it seems, isn't the stability of the platform but the height of the heel. Any woman who regularly wears heels higher than 2 inches is twice as likely to develop OA as women who don't, says Dr. Weinblatt. Heels shift your body weight away from your ankles and onto your hips and the inner part of your knee joints, often resulting in arthritis of the knee.

CHERRIES

A Cheery Antidote

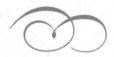

LIFE WITHOUT CHERRIES WOULD BE THE PITS. IT'S TRUE! While their nutritional profile has never seemed outstanding when it comes to vitamins or minerals, the good news about cherries is finally leaking out: They're packed with powerful disease-fighting nutrients! What's more, some of them may help relieve the pain of arthritis. Recent laboratory research at Michigan State University in East Lansing has shown that at least in the test tube, tart cherry juice is 10 times better than aspirin at reducing pain and swelling—and it won't irritate tender tummies as aspirin can. So check out cherries. While you're indulging in their juicy goodness, you'll also harvest a big bowl of other health benefits.

Dark red cherries, both sweet and sour, are packed with flavonoids called antho-cyanins. These natural plant chemicals cre-

---

...Just the facts

Cherries (10 fresh)
Calories: 49
Fat: 1 g
Saturated fat: 0 g
Cholesterol: 0 mg
Sodium: 0 mg
Total carbohydrates: 11 g
Dietary fiber: 2 g
Protein: 1 g
Vitamin C: 5% of Daily Value

---

ate the blue, pink, red, mauve, and violet colors that help flowers attract insects for pollination. Later, when fruits and vegetables are growing, anthocyanins defend them against attacks from invading germs and hungry bugs.

In your body, these flavonoids seem to act as antioxidants that protect against cancer and heart disease. The bad news is that because our record for eating fruits and veggies is the pits, Americans consume only an estimated 200 milligrams of anthocyanins a day—probably nowhere near enough. Chomping on cherries will double your protection as well as your pleasure, though, since eating just six of the juicy, dark red fruits a day will deliver an additional 200 milligrams of anthocyanins.

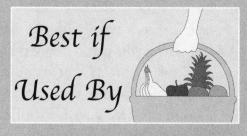

Best if Used By

Store your cherries in a covered container and eat them within a few days. (As if we need to tell you that. At my house, we wash and eat them while we're unpacking the rest of the groceries!)

A CHERRY A DAY?

Cherries are just quivering with quercetin, another flavonoid that fights cancer and heart disease. How much do they provide? As much as apples, which are tops when it comes to fruits that deliver the goods. The best news is that processed cherries, the kind you get in cans and as prepared pie filling, deliver double the quercetin of fresh cherries. That means you can get cherry-good protection all year long.

Cherries are good sources of perillyl alcohol, which has been shown to prevent the development of breast and pancreatic cancer in rats. They're also packed with the mineral boron, which seems to be important for bone health.

GET A BETTER BOWL OF CHERRIES

Fresh sweet cherries have a very short season, so grab them when you can. They won't last long! When selecting cherries, look for fruits that are shiny, plump, and firm enough to pop when you bite them and that still have their stems. Stemless cherries are ripe for spoilage—and besides, it's more fun to eat these little beauties from the stem! Avoid cherries that are underripe, soft, cut, or moldy.

Once you have your cherries, here's how to serve 'em up.

Muffin-ize them. Substitute freeze-dried cherries in any muffin or quick bread recipe that calls for raisins.

Frost 'em. Toss frozen or canned cherries and a ripe banana into your blender with a little fat-free milk and a few ice cubes for a frosty cherry cooler.

Chug. Buy all-natural sour cherry juice at a health food store or from the Internet. Drink it plain or mix it with other favorite fruit juices. For instance, mix your own orange-cherry, grape-cherry, or cranberry-cherry blend. You can also use it instead of water in your next cup of hot chocolate.

FLAXSEED

A Fishy Fix

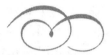

WHEN WE GOT MARRIED JUST A FEW YEARS AGO, MY husband, Ted, and I ended up with lots of kitchen doubles—silverware, dishes, pots, pans, popcorn poppers, and even coffee grinders. A major yard sale restored order. We got rid of all our doubles—except for those coffee grinders. I refused to sell either one. Why? I use one to grind fresh coffee beans for that one perfect cup each morning. The other is for grinding the flaxseed I add to the turkey burgers that help tame my arthritis.

Flaxseed? Yep, the seed of the flax plant. Admittedly, it's an oddball food, but the reason for recommending flaxseed is that it contains a special type of oil that most Americans don't get enough of in their diets.

Public health officials have been

> ### ...Just the facts
>
> Flaxseed (1 Tbsp)
> Calories: 42
> Fat: 4 g
> Saturated fat: 1 g
> Cholesterol: 0 mg
> Sodium: 4 mg
> Total carbohydrates: 2 g
> Dietary fiber: 2 g
> Protein: 2 g
> Calcium: 2% of Daily Value
> Iron: 5%

haranguing us for a good 30 years to cut down on saturated fat from burgers, cheese, butter, and ice cream so we'll cut our risk of heart disease, the number one killer of men and women. A lot of us did, so that should be the end of the problem, right? Wrong! Now another fat problem is rearing its ugly head: polyunsaturated fat imbalance.

KEEP YOUR BALANCE

It turns out that there are two kinds of fat that we need to eat (yes, we do have to eat some fat!) because our bodies can't make them. They're called essential fatty acids. The type called omega-6 comes from the vegetable oils in fried foods, cookies and cakes, and highly processed foods. As you can probably guess, we get way too much of it. The other type, omega-3, comes mostly from fish—and, of course, we get too little of that.

This imbalance—too much of one, too little of the other—creates problems with blood clotting, constricted arteries, and irregular heart rhythm. Some studies also suggest that it sets us up for arthritis, autoimmune disorders, and cancer. That's why the American Heart Association and the USDA recommend that we eat two servings of fish each week.

THE SUB WITH ATTITUDE

So what does this have to do with flaxseed? It's loaded with alpha-linolenic acid, which your body can turn into the same kind of essential fat that's supplied by fish.

Are we sure flaxseed is as good as fish? Studies on this are just beginning, so a lot more research needs to be done before we have an absolute yes. But in a University of Toronto study of nine healthy women, their total cholesterol dropped by 9 percent and their "bad" low-density lipoprotein (LDL) cholesterol plummeted by 18 percent when they ate 2 ounces of flaxseed daily for just four weeks. That's a great way to protect your heart.

Omega-3 fatty acids are also critical to brain and vision development, both before and just after babies are born. Mothers who eat plenty of fish, flaxseed, and walnuts deliver these brain builders through the placenta and through breast milk.

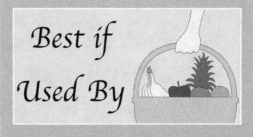

Best if Used By

Flaxseed products are a bit fragile, so after you've gone out of your way to get them, you'll want to take good care of them. Here's how.

• Store whole flaxseed in the pantry at room temperature. It will last for up to a year.

• Keep milled flaxseed in an airtight container in the fridge for up to 30 days.

• Keep flaxseed oil, which is cold pressed from the seeds and filtered, in a lightproof bottle in the refrigerator. Then use it up fast, because it doesn't keep long.

FISH WITH A DIFFERENCE

Beyond its fishlike oil, flaxseed contains up to 800 times more lignans than any other plant food. These plant compounds act like weak estrogens and have been shown to tie up the body's estrogen receptors, similar to the way telemarketers tie up your phone line. By doing this, they prevent human estrogen from being absorbed, which may prevent breast, prostate, and endometrial cancers from getting started. Flaxseed is also rich in insoluble fiber, the roughage that keeps you going and prevents constipation.

FANTASTIC FLAX

A flaxseed is a shiny, red-brown, flat oval with a pointed tip and is a little bigger than a sesame seed. The seeds are hard and chewy but add an enjoyable light, nutty taste to foods. Unfortunately, you probably won't find flaxseed in your supermarket, so you'll have to make a trip to your favorite health food store—but that's okay, since it's worth going out of your way for. You can buy whole flaxseed, milled flaxseed flour to use in baked goods, or flaxseed oil.

Here's how to make flaxseed a delicious part of your life.

Make better bread. Toss flaxseed into quick-bread or muffin dough before baking. Or brush yeast bread with egg white and top with flaxseed instead of sesame or poppy seeds before baking.

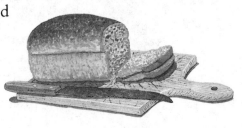

Power up cookies. Stir flaxseed into oatmeal cookie batter for a nutty crunch.

Have an oil change. Replace oil or shortening with milled flaxseed in your baked goods. Add 3 tablespoons for each tablespoon of fat you're replacing.

TEA

Bag Joint Pain

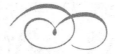

WHAT COULD BE BETTER ON A RAW, RAINY AFTERNOON than sharing a pot of tea by a cozy fire? Tea has long been my great soother, a balm for troubled times, and an elixir for pain and worries. It's also been the libation of celebration in times of joy. Often, it's simply the symbol of togetherness and family warmth, the "campfire" around which my family gathers. Now we're thrilled to discover that tea may fend off arthritis, too.

LAB LESSONS

Although tea has been soothing souls since prehistoric times, research into its possible benefits is only a few years old, but it looks oh, so promising! Researchers at Case Western Reserve University in Cleveland have been feeding green tea

> ## ...Just the facts
>
> Tea (1 cup)
> Calories: 2
> Fat: 0 g
> Saturated fat: 0 g
> Cholesterol: 0 mg
> Sodium: 7 mg
> Total carbohydrates: Less than 1 g
> Dietary fiber: 0 g
> Protein: 0 g
> Folate: 3% of Daily Value
> Riboflavin (vitamin B_2): 2%
> Magnesium: 2%
> Potassium: 2%

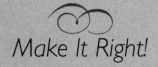
(the kind you get at Chinese restaurants) to mice, and they suspect that its polyphenols delay the beginning of arthritis as well as dampening its severity. In Austria, scientists have uncovered clues suggesting that catechins from green tea may slow arthritis inflammation, and their research may lead to an arthritis treatment.

TESTING, TESTING…

A while back, epidemiologists, the scientists who compare health risks from one big group of people to another, noticed that in countries where people drink lots of green tea, folks rarely get certain kinds of cancer. When they started plying mice with green tea, they found that it protected the rodents against cancers of the skin, lung, esophagus, stomach, small intestine, colon, bladder, liver, pancreas, prostate, and mammary glands. Whew! That covers a lot of territory!

Mind you, their research doesn't prove that green tea can prevent cancer in humans. The researchers, after all, substituted green tea for every single drop of fluid that the mice usually drank. They were also able to control the mice's genetic backgrounds and other health factors. Much is left to be done before we know for sure whether tea's benefits apply to people, but what is it about tea that makes us think they would?

ANTIOXIDANT TOP DOG

It turns out that tea is packed with antioxidants—more, in fact, than even the top fruits and veggies. One of its richest compounds, epigallocatechin-3 gallate (EGCG, for short), has been shown in laboratory tests to block the action of urokinase, an enzyme needed by cancer cells so they can do their dirty work. Without urokinase, cancer cells stop invading healthy cells and sometimes just fizzle out and disappear.

Recent research suggests that green tea and the black tea that most Americans drink have similar anticancer effects. (The two types come from the same plant; the difference is that black tea is fermented and green tea isn't.)

HALF-HEARTED RISK

Again, there is no absolute proof, but in a Dutch study, the one-third of participants who drank the most tea were the least likely to die from heart disease or have strokes. And a Boston study found that people who drank one or more cups of black tea daily had half the risk of having a heart attack compared with those who were tea teetotalers. Scientists speculate that tea's powerful antioxidant package may help keep cholesterol in your blood from gunking up your arteries.

Other preliminary studies suggest that tea is good for your body in other ways. Both mice and men seem to get a metabolic boost from green tea, indicating that it may help with weight control.

Other research suggests that tea may help keep bones strong, perhaps because of its fluoride or phytoestrogens (estrogen-like plant compounds). In studies of rodents, tea also appeared to fight strep bacteria, heal ulcers, and protect teeth. It may also protect against cataracts and rev up your immune system to fight colds and flu. So while you wait for more research and the final answers, sip some tea.

BECOME A TEA-TOTALER

Many types of tea are available. Take your pick of these.

• *Tea bags and loose leaves.* Whether you buy your tea in bags or loose, you'll get plenty of antioxidant punch, although (surprise!) the biggest boost comes from the tea bag. (And you thought that healthy eating would be harder!) That's because the crushed tea offers more exposed surfaces during brewing. Dunking your bag helps, too.

• *Caffeine-free tea.* More good news: Decaffeinating tea doesn't disturb its antioxidants, so make it tea-sy on yourself. Choose the style and brand you like best, then drink up!

• *Iced tea.* Bottled iced-tea drinks work, too. In tests of several brands and flavors, a few were as potent as a cup of brewed tea, while the rest delivered at least half the number of antioxidants of brewed tea—making any bottled tea more antioxidant-rich than any soft drink! But beware: Many bottled teas are loaded with up to 200 calories from sugar, which offers no health benefits, can raise your risk of weight gain, and can ruin your appetite for healthier foods.

CANCER AND ITS TREATMENT

Outwit a Killer

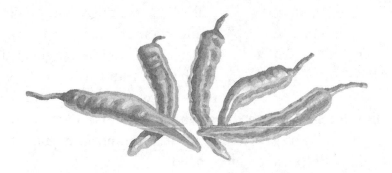

IF GETTING CANCER IS ONE OF THE GREATER, MORE TERrifying blows in life, being treated for it is like being hit when you're down. "The diagnosis was scary enough," says a friend who recently endured radiation therapy for adrenal cancer, "but when I was getting radiation, I had this equally strong fear that I was poisoning my body."

If you're among the more than one million Americans diagnosed with cancer each year, using a variety of resources to get you through the one-two punch of the disease and its treatment is vital. "First, you're zapped by the systemic effects of the cancer itself," explains Karen Lawson, M.D., director of integrative and clinical services at the Center for Spirituality and Healing at the University of Minnesota in Minneapolis. Then, whether or not you have surgery, your illness is likely to be compounded by the use of chemotherapy and radiation to treat the disease.

SURVIVING THE CURE

The drugs used in chemotherapy (the process of infusing the body with a toxin that destroys rapidly reproducing cells) affect healthy cells as well as cancer cells. As a result, if you're undergoing chemotherapy, you may experience extreme fatigue, nausea, hair loss, and concentration problems as side effects. You may also develop mouth sores, which can discourage you from eating—and getting the wealth of healing nutrients your embattled body so desperately needs.

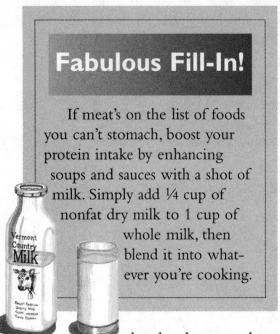

Fabulous Fill-In!

If meat's on the list of foods you can't stomach, boost your protein intake by enhancing soups and sauces with a shot of milk. Simply add ¼ cup of nonfat dry milk to 1 cup of whole milk, then blend it into whatever you're cooking.

Radiation therapy, which focuses a beam of radiation on the cancer site, is also used to kill cancer cells, and like chemo, it destroys some healthy ones as well. Nausea and extreme fatigue are often the results.

The good news is that after the treatment ends and your healthy cells have a chance to grow again, most of the side effects of cancer therapy fade. The bad news is that they can be pretty awful while they last.

If your side effects are debilitating, your doctor may prescribe a prescription anti-nausea drug such as ondansetron (Zofran), which can settle your stomach—but can also cost up to $16 per pill. The doctor may also prescribe megestrol (Megace), which mimics the hormone progesterone, to jump-start your appetite. The trouble is, Megace can also jump-start hot flashes and other annoying symptoms. And when you're already grappling with serious side effects, you don't need any more.

HEALING THE WHOLE SELF

Complementary therapies, while not cure-alls, can often help ease queasiness, fatigue, and other debilitating effects of chemo and radiation. Plus, nondrug therapies such as meditation have another edge: In addition to boosting your immune system, they may help heal the emotional and spiritual damage caused by the stress and anxiety that accompany the disease and its treatments. "Stress relief is a major consideration in your ability to heal," says Dr. Lawson. "The less stressed you are, the better you heal in the aftermath of cancer, and the better your quality of life will be." Here's a rundown of the methods that will help you get the nutrition, serenity, and rest your body needs to rebuild and continue the healing process. They will also help keep cancer from recurring.

Color-code your plate. The more nutrients you receive during treatment, the stronger and less prone to infections you'll be. "Relying strictly on supplements can place too much stress on the immune system," says Cynthia Thompson, R.D., Ph.D., assistant professor of nutritional sciences at the Arizona Cancer Center in Tucson. She suggests loading your lunch plate with a spectrum of red, yellow, and green foods to

A SIMPLE SOLUTION

Both peppermint and ginger teas, which you can find prepackaged at a health food store, have been shown to decrease nausea. Just avoid sweetening them with sugar, which can dampen your immune system and increase your risk of infection. Instead, try a grain-derived sweetener, such as rice syrup or barley malt, or an herbal sweetener, such as stevia.

get the most cancer-fighting nutrients possible. For instance, on a bed of dark leafy greens, such as spinach or kale, toss some red peppers (for vitamin C), carrots (for beta-carotene), and several cruciferous veggies, such as broccoli or cauliflower (for isothiocynates, which are potent cancer-fighting compounds).

Make mustard a must. The brown variety that contains horseradish is a great way to get isothiocynates, says Dr. Thompson, especially when you don't feel up to eating broccoli.

Drink your veggies. "When even the sight of a fruit or vegetable makes you gag," says Dr. Thompson, "juicing these nutrient powerhouses into a drinkable pulp is a great way to get a high concentration of antioxidants and chlorophyll, both of which may help neutralize toxins from chemotherapy or radiation." Toss some sweet strawberries in with a few beta-carotene–rich carrots for a nutrient-dense alternative to O.J. Or opt for tomato juice, which is a super source of the antioxidant lycopene.

Sip on soup. If keeping solid foods down is a problem, sip clear, salty vegetable broths or miso soup, made with a salty soybean paste. Soups high in sodium, as most canned soups are, can help replenish the electrolytes (minerals necessary for normal heart rhythm, muscle contraction, and a whole host of other regular body functions) you lose when you vomit.

Take tea and see. Green tea leaves are rich in polyphenols, special cancer-battling compounds that help cancer drugs attack bad cells and spare healthy ones, says Paul Riley, N.D., a naturopathic physician at the Seattle Cancer Treatment and Wellness Center. Plus, green tea protects the liver so it's able to function optimally as your body's detox center. Try to drink three to five cups daily, he suggests.

Try a peck of pectin. The pulpy white membrane on orange and tangerine wedges provides pectin, which may help reduce the spread of cancer, says Dr. Riley. If mouth sores make eating citrus impossible, you can buy pectin in powdered form at a health food store. Swirl a teaspoon or two into applesauce and eat it once a day until your mouth is better and you can savor citrus again.

Pick a peck of pepper. Early studies indicate that lozenges made with capsaicin—the ingredient in red pepper that provides its bite—may help soothe chemotherapy-related mouth sores. It seems that capsaicin not only numbs inflamed sores in the same way that benzocaine or other topical anesthetics might, but it may also draw white blood cells to the site to heal them. Another plus: Capsaicin has antioxidant properties that may help combat nitrosamine, a cancer-causing agent. Look for the lozenges in any drugstore.

Relax with flax. Flaxseed turns into a soothing, protective gel in your digestive tract, which helps promote intestinal function with none of the harshness of bran or other insoluble fiber—making it a great pre- or post-chemo addition to your diet. Plus, flax provides omega-3 essential fatty acids to help squelch the inflammation that results from chemotherapy. Stir a few teaspoons of ground flaxseed (available at health food stores) into your morning smoothie or yogurt, and your taste buds won't have a clue that you're getting your daily quota of roughage.

Enjoy the breath of life. Cancer is nothing if not scary. But in one of life's crueler catch-22s, when you're frightened, your body releases stress hormones that can depress your immune system. To relieve your anxiety, lower levels of stress hormones, and bring yourself to a healing state, breathe slowly and fully from your lower abdomen. Keep your shoulders still and expand your lungs fully so your belly bulges out as far as it can, then exhale slowly. Your heart rate will slow, your anxiety will fade, and your feelings of control may increase. "When I was facing surgery and later radiation, I inhaled the word *let* and exhaled the word *go*," my friend Laura told me. "This really helped my state of mind."

Mend with massage. In one study, more than half of a group of people with cancer who received regular massages experienced increased immune function. Both their white blood cell counts and their natural killer cell activity went up! Plus, massage after surgery can help drain off fluids that build up in the lymphatic system. Ask your cancer specialist for the name of a massage therapist near you who specializes in lymphatic drain massage, or contact the American Massage Therapy Association at 888-843-2682 for a referral.

See yourself better. Picture this: A noninvasive way to reduce not only your nausea and anxiety but also the amount of pain medication you need—by half! That's exactly the promise of guided imagery, "a profound form of stress relief that can help lessen pain from cancer treatment," says Dr. Lawson.

Here's how it works: With either a tape or a practitioner to guide you, you learn breathing exercises and how to develop mental images that suggest relaxation or safety and invoke all five senses, which help you gradually gain control of your mood and decrease your feelings of anxiety. Studies prove that in the process, you'll reduce pain and boost immune function. To find out more, talk to your doctor.

Quiet queasiness. Research from the University of Rochester Cancer Center in New York indicates that those acupressure wristbands sold to fishermen to stave off seasickness may also ease chemotherapy-related queasiness. The bands (also called acustimulation wristbands) have a button that pushes on an acupressure point called P6, which lies on the inside of the wrist along what acupuncturists refer to as the body's anti-nausea meridian. The wristbands are available in many drugstores.

Use an ancient herb. The mucous membrane in the gastrointestinal tract, which starts in the mouth, is very vulnerable to chemotherapy drugs, which can cause acutely painful canker

Two Good!

To improve your appetite and corral a host of cancer-fighting nutrients from your meal, enjoy some wine before dinner. Not only can it help stimulate your appetite, but the anthocyanins (pigments that give red wine its color) in wine act as antioxidants that battle cancer and may help to correct an imbalance of B vitamins, which can be a result of cancer treatments and may contribute to mouth irritation, anemia, and nerve problems, says Cynthia Thompson, R.D., Ph.D.

Red wine also contains an antifungal compound that's converted by the body into a powerful cancer-fighting agent. If you have breast cancer, you should avoid alcohol altogether because it may boost estrogen levels and fuel cancer. Eating red grapes, though, is a good choice for anyone.

sores. But there is an ancient solution: myrrh, the herb carried to Bethlehem by one of the biblical Wise Men. Long prized for its astringent properties, myrrh soothes sore mouth tissues and works as a fluoride alternative. Look for it in mouthwashes and toothpastes at a health food store or buy an extract and make your own rinse by mixing 20 drops in ¼ cup of water.

Try milk thistle. This spiny, purple-flowered herb protects the liver from damage, including damage from toxins infused during chemotherapy. As a result, it may minimize chemotherapy-related nausea, fatigue, and flu-like aches. The recommended dose is 250 milligrams of standardized extract (which you can get at a health food store) three times a day. Check with your doctor before taking it.

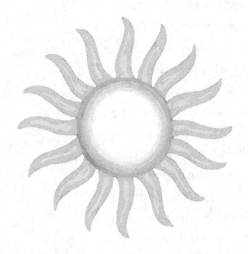

APRICOTS

A+ Cancer Protection

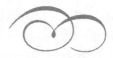

HAVE YOU BEEN FOLLOWING THE NEWS? BETA-CAROTENE drifts in and out of the spotlight because research continues to reveal its amazing array of health benefits. True, megadose supplements were all the rage for a while, but then researchers discovered that supplement overload could actually increase a smoker's chance of getting cancer. And all the while, delicious fruits and vegetables were safely on hand for the taking! To take advantage of nature's bounty, you'll want to stock your refrigerator with all the right stuff. Apricots are a smart start.

When you think of beta-carotene sources, you usually think of orange veggies—especially carrots, pumpkins, and sweet potatoes—right away. And that's right. But here's a news flash: Some sweet, luscious fruits deliver the goods, too. In

> ## ...Just the facts
>
> Apricots (3 fresh)
> Calories: 48
> Fat: 0 g
> Saturated fat: 0 g
> Cholesterol: 0 mg
> Sodium: 1 mg
> Total carbohydrates: 11 g
> Dietary fiber: 2 g
> Protein: 1 g
> Vitamin A: 52% of Daily
>   Value
> Vitamin C: 17%

fact, lovely yellow-orange apricots were recently named to the University of California, Berkeley, Wellness Letter's list of top 10 beta-carotene sources. As it turns out, just three apricots supply more than half of the vitamin A you need daily. (Your body converts beta-carotene to vitamin A.)

While beta-carotene supplements may have limited—if any—benefits, getting plenty of the nutrient through foods makes big things happen. What's the difference? Beta-carotene has hundreds of lesser-known cousins that are present in foods but not added to supplements. Scientists speculate that beta-carotene and its family members—collectively called carotenoids—work together to stave off illnesses.

CANCER-FIGHTING COMBO

Beta-carotene and its clan have amazing synergy. Each family member attacks cancer in a different way, creating far more cancer-killing power than any one of them working alone. (The other five active carotenoids are alpha-carotene, lycopene, cryptoxanthin, lutein, and zeaxanthin.)

For instance, beta-carotene gobbles up free radicals, substances that cause cell damage, from fluids located inside and outside the body's fats. Lycopene, which is also found in apricots, may arrest the growth of tumor cells. Still other carotenoids may stimulate an enzyme in your immune system that breaks down carcinogens.

"A diet rich in beta-carotene from plenty of fruits and vegetables may reduce the risk of breast cancer recurrence by one-third," says Cheryl Rock, R.D., Ph.D., associate professor of family and preventive medicine at the University of California, San Diego. So bring on the apricots for women's health—and men's health. A National Cancer Institute review of 156 studies found that a diet packed with fruits and veggies cuts the risk of most cancers—including bladder, cervical, lung, and stomach—by about half.

A HEFTY BONUS

Beta-carotene and company don't just fight cancer. They also stave off the leading killer of men and women in the United States—heart disease. Beta-carotene and lycopene fight a process that makes "bad" low-density lipoprotein (LDL) cholesterol even more likely to contribute to plaque formation on artery walls. A study of more than 85,000 nurses showed that a diet rich in beta-carotene reduced the risk of heart disease by a whopping 22 percent!

BETTER THAN BANANAS

Besides providing beta-carotene, apricots—particularly the dried variety—pack potassium, a nutrient that helps lower blood pressure and reduce the risk of stroke. In a Harvard study of more than 40,000 men, those who got the most potassium had about 40 percent less chance of having strokes than those who consumed the least.

Fabulous Fill-In!

Can't get your hands on fresh apricots? Try these great alternatives.

• *Canned apricots.* These account for more than 80 percent of U.S. apricots and can substitute for the fresh fruits in most recipes. Buy them packed in juice to cut calories.

• *Dried apricots.* Weight watchers, be warned: Ounce for ounce, the dried fruit has three times the beta-carotene but five times the calories of its fresh counterpart.

To enjoy your apricots at the peak of their flavor, try these tips.

• Place ripe apricots in a plastic bag and refrigerate them. Eat them within three to seven days.

• Place partially ripe apricots in a brown paper bag and store them at room temperature, away from direct sunlight, until they're ready to eat, usually within a day or two. Then transfer them to the fridge.

How much potassium do these golden fruits offer? A 3½-ounce serving of dried apricots gives you close to 1,400 milligrams—three times the amount found in a banana!

APRICOT APPRECIATION

Depending on when you'd like to buy fresh apricots, they may be as difficult to find as a comfy pair of sandals. More than 95 percent of the U.S. crop comes from California and is available only between mid-May and late June. In August, your supermarket may carry apricots from Oregon and Washington, while Chilean imports usually appear from late November to April.

Whenever you buy them, look for apricots with smooth skins. The fruits should be soft if you want to use them immediately or somewhat firm if you'd like to keep them for a few days. Avoid apricots that have a greenish hue or are hard, because they may never fully ripen.

Once you introduce apricots to your kitchen, you'll find plenty of ways to use them. Start with these.

Fold 'em. Fold ½ cup of diced fresh, canned, or dried apricots into your batter for muffins or pancakes. They'll create quite a stir in your family!

Blend 'em. In a blender, combine two pitted fresh apricots with 2 tablespoons of white wine vinegar and 1 table-spoon of sugar. Slowly add ¼ cup of canola oil. Blend until thick and smooth, then stir in 2 tablespoons of chopped fresh basil. Pour the dressing over a salad made of dark green lettuce, carrots, cucumbers, raisins, and feta cheese and toss to coat. You can also use the dressing as a marinade for chicken.

Dice 'em. Create this easy-to-make apricot salsa: In a medium bowl, combine 2 tablespoons of lemon juice, 2 tablespoons of canola oil, ⅛ teaspoon of coarsely ground black pepper, six diced fresh apricots, ½ cup of diced red onion, and ⅓ cup of diced red bell pepper. Break out the tortilla chips!

Prepack 'em. Instead of hitting the vending machine when you're hungry at work, pull some homemade trail mix from your purse or desk drawer. To make it, mix ¼ cup each of dried apricots, mini pretzels, peanuts, raisins, and whole grain cereal, such as Wheat Chex or Cheerios, in a self-sealing plastic bag. Crunch away!

BLACKBERRIES

Shield against Invaders

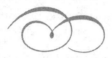

ARE YOU STUCK IN A FRUIT RUT? YOU KNOW, APPLES, bananas, and oranges—with an occasional handful of strawberries thrown in? Then it's time to perk up your palate and give your taste buds a treat. Blackberries taste scrumptious enough to liven up breakfast cereal, fruit salads, muffins, and pancakes, but there's more! New research suggests that these berries are a treasure trove of compounds that rush to your defense against the health risks you fear most: cancer and heart disease.

FRESH DEFENDERS

Blackberries are brimming with two recently discovered compounds, catechin and epicatechin. Ounce for ounce, blackberries have about 50 percent more catechin and three times more epicatechin

...Just the facts

Blackberries (1 cup fresh)
Calories: 75
Fat: 1 g
Saturated fat: 0 g
Cholesterol: 0 mg
Sodium: 0 mg
Total carbohydrates: 18 g
Dietary fiber: 7 g
Protein: 1 g
Folate: 12% of Daily Value
Vitamin A: 5%
Vitamin C: 50%
Calcium: 5%

← *Berry Bonanza* →

This chart shows how your favorite berries stack up nutritionally. The values for each are based on a 3½-ounce serving. (The equivalent in cups is listed next to each type of berry.)

Berry	Calories	Fiber (g)	Folate (mcg)	Vitamin C (mg)	Potassium (mg)
Blackberries (⅔ cup)	52	4	34	21	196
Blueberries (⅔ cup)	56	3	6	13	89
Raspberries (¾ cup)	49	4	26	25	152
Strawberries (⅔ cup)	30	2	18	57	166

than red raspberries do. Research has shown that these compounds can help:

• *Prevent cancer.* Catechin and epicatechin neutralize free radicals, substances that damage cells' genetic material and provoke cancer-causing mutations in DNA. Although scientists aren't sure exactly how these two compounds work their cancer-fighting magic, experts speculate that they may inhibit an enzyme that's associated with the reproduction of free radicals.

• *Head off heart disease.* What's more, a Japanese study has shown that catechins help lower cholesterol levels, especially levels of low-density lipoprotein (LDL) cholesterol—the bad kind. Better cholesterol numbers mean a lower risk of heart disease.

ALLERGY ENEMY

In addition to catechins, blackberries contain another compound, called quercetin. In fact, they boast at least four times as much quercetin as raspberries (and raspberries pack plenty). Like catechins, quercetin dampens the production of free radicals and helps prevent bad cholesterol from damaging blood vessels.

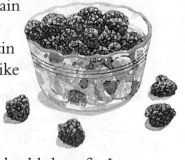

Quercetin has a very surprising additional health benefit: It halts the production of histamine, the substance that makes allergy sufferers sneeze, wheeze, and generally feel miserable. Isn't it wonderful that blackberries ripen just as the hay fever season starts?

FIBER FILLER

While scientists are studying these newly discovered nutrients, we shouldn't forget about an old standby—fiber. Blackberries pack a whopping 7 grams of the good stuff in a single cup—one-third of the amount you need for the entire day! Fiber fills you up so you feel satisfied with fewer calories. It also prevents constipation, helps reduce your risk of heart disease, and may lower your chances of developing colon cancer. Not too shabby, huh?

PICK OF THE PATCH

During some months, fresh blackberries are so pricey that

Best if Used By

Once you find the cream of the crop, refrigerate your berries immediately. You'll have just two or three days to enjoy them before they start to spoil. Just before eating them, place the berries in a shallow pan lined with paper towels, carefully wash them, and pat them dry with additional paper towels.

you may have to stop by the ATM for extra cash. Preserve your investment by buying only the best. Look for berries that are shiny and black, not dull or reddish. Avoid any that look a little wet, because moisture speeds decay, and those that appear to have been squeezed or flattened. And pass up berries that are dripping juice—a telltale sign that they're past their peak.

Once you've found the best blackberries, see how they can add excitement to everyday dishes.

Don't waffle. Instead of maple syrup, sprinkle your griddle cakes with fresh blackberries and top with a dollop of whipped cream.

Add sparkle. Stir blackberries into lemon or vanilla pudding that you make from an instant mix. Try doing the same with yogurt.

BROCCOLI SPROUTS

Mighty Mini Cancer Fighters

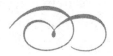

MAMA ALWAYS SAID, "AN OUNCE OF PREVENTION IS worth a pound of cure." And that's really the cancer-fighting strategy of Paul Talalay, M.D., the researcher at Johns Hopkins University in Baltimore who tapped into the chemoprotective power first of broccoli and then of broccoli sprouts.

Why wait until you have a dread disease, such as breast cancer, Dr. Talalay reasoned, to try to do something about it? So he went to work with test tubes and laboratory mice to figure out how to use real, live foods to turn on the body's natural defense mechanisms.

AMP UP YOUR DEFENSES

Researchers have long known that people who eat the most cruciferous (cabbage family) vegetables have very low

---

...Just the facts

Broccoli sprouts (½ cup raw)
Calories: 5
Fat: 0 g
Saturated fat: 0 g
Cholesterol: 0 mg
Sodium: 1 mg
Total carbohydrates: 1 g
Dietary fiber: 0 g
Protein: 1 g
Vitamin C: 2% of Daily Value
Manganese: 2%

---

rates of certain cancers. But the "why" remained to be seen—so Dr. Talalay went hunting.

What he found was a natural chemical called sulforaphane that hampered the growth of breast cancer cells in petri dishes in the lab. Digging further, he discovered that all cabbage family vegetables pack sulforaphane, but broccoli delivers the biggest dose. It was an interesting finding that started an amazing chain of events.

The goal of cancer prevention is to cut down on our exposure to carcinogens, cancer-causing agents such as cigarette smoke, air pollution, radiation, and alcohol, so that they can't attack our cells and make them sick. The hang-up here is that you need to know that a substance is a carcinogen in order to avoid it.

Dr. Talalay's strategy is to find foods that make the body's defenses stronger so that it can fight off carcinogens, both known and unknown. The cool thing about this approach, called chemoprotection, is that you don't have to know what you're fending off. It's like building a fortress and a moat so that no matter which marauders attack, you have everything covered. Thus, even though Dr. Talalay is working with breast cancer cells, the protection stirred up by broccoli's sulforaphane should defend against other cancers as well.

GIANT-SIZE SPROUTS

Cells produce a family of enzymes that neutralize carcinogens before they can attack your DNA and start cancer cells growing. When Dr. Talalay moved from test tubes to mice, he learned that sulforaphane was dynamite for increasing the activity of detoxification enzymes. Among animals simultaneously infected with potent carcinogens and fed sulforaphane,

A Word to the Wise

Thoroughly wash any sprouts you buy, especially if you plan to eat them raw, since some sprouts are contaminated with *E. coli* bacteria. For safety and guaranteed sulforaphane levels, look for trademarked BroccoSprouts, which are grown from sterilized seeds; tested weekly for contamination; and then cleaned, packed, refrigerated, and subjected to surprise inspections.

- The number of animals that developed tumors decreased by 60 percent.

- In each animal that did develop tumors, the number dropped by 80 percent.

- The tumors were 75 percent smaller.

- They showed up later and grew more slowly.

Now tests are being done on women to see if sulforaphane stimulates human detoxification enzymes.

Dr. Talalay also learned that the amount of sulforaphane was 10 times higher in some types of broccoli than in others. In trying to grow his own standardized broccoli, he stumbled onto the fact that ounce for ounce, three-day-old broccoli sprouts packed 20 to 50 times more sulforaphane than mature broccoli, but the sprouts he bought varied as much as the broccoli did.

Consequently, he developed standardized seed and a process for growing sprouts that together guarantee to deliver a high dose of sulforaphane. He calls his product BroccoSprouts. You can get them at a supermarket.

SPRING FOR THE FRESHEST

Broccoli sprouts are available in the produce section of most supermarkets, but choose carefully! Search for perky-looking sprouts that are just bursting to get out of their container. Pass up any that appear shriveled or weak.

When you're ready to add a spicy bite to ho-hum foods, try these top-notch ideas.

Go for bold flavors. Toss arugula, watercress, and spinach leaves with broccoli sprouts. Sweeten with light Catalina dressing.

Startle your soup. Swirl a handful of broccoli sprouts into your favorite soup—from tomato to vegetable to classic chicken noodle.

Pile it high. On a hearty slice of seven-grain bread, stack romaine lettuce, turkey, sweet red and green pepper rings, a pile of broccoli sprouts, slivers of onion, and a slice of avocado. You'll have to attack it with a knife and fork because you'll never get your mouth around it!

Wrap it up. Fill a tortilla with tuna salad, grated carrots, sliced celery, red leaf lettuce, and a handful of broccoli sprouts. Wrap the bottom of the tortilla over the middle, then roll up the rest.

BRUSSELS SPROUTS

Always on Alert

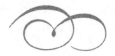

CONTRARY TO POPULAR BELIEF, BRUSSELS SPROUTS DON'T taste all that bad. Just season them with a little oil or butter and some bread crumbs, and they're good to go. Unfortunately, many of you probably don't share even a tiny bit of our enthusiasm for this widely (and wrongly) maligned vegetable. That's a shame, because brussels sprouts offer plenty of protection against big-time diseases—namely, cancer, osteoporosis, and heart trouble.

DON'T CELL YOURSELF SHORT

Consider brussels sprouts as security guards that help protect your DNA from cancer-causing villains. When researchers gave people 10½ ounces of cooked brussels sprouts daily for three weeks (really,

...Just the facts

Brussels sprouts (½ cup cooked)
Calories: 30
Fat: 0 g
Saturated fat: 0 g
Cholesterol: 0 mg
Sodium: 16 mg
Total carbohydrates: 7 g
Dietary fiber: 4 g
Protein: 2 g
Folate: 12% of Daily Value
Vitamin A: 11%
Vitamin C: 80%
Iron: 5%

this wasn't torture), they noted a 28 percent drop in DNA damage as measured by a compound excreted in the participants' urine.

Then they went a step further and examined the effect of the sprouts on cancer-fighting enzymes in the colon-rectal area. Their findings: The little green globes supersized levels of these enzymes, indicating that they may be able to prevent colon cancer.

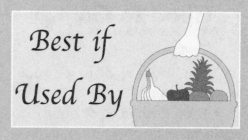

Best if Used By

When storing brussels sprouts, place them in a plastic bag in the refrigerator right away. They'll stay fresh for three to five days. At room temperature, they'll turn yellow fast.

Other studies suggest that brussels sprouts may stave off bladder and prostate cancers, too.

• Harvard researchers studied nearly 48,000 men and found that those who consumed five servings of cruciferous veggies a week—namely, brussels sprouts, broccoli, cabbage, and cauliflower—were half as likely to develop bladder cancer as those who ate only one serving per week or less. It didn't matter how many other veggies the men consumed overall.

• At the Fred Hutchinson Cancer Research Center in Seattle, researchers showed that men who consumed three or more servings of veggies daily—especially the cruciferous kind—could lower their risk of prostate cancer by nearly 50 percent.

BONE-DEEP SECURITY

If you're feeling a little left out with all this talk about cancer in men, say no more. Brussels sprouts may help protect women from osteoporosis—a bone disease that

When you're ready to use your brussels sprouts:

• Drop them in a pot of luke-warm water for about 10 minutes to roust any insects that may be hidden in the leaves.

• Trim the stem ends, but not quite flush with the bottoms, or the outer leaves will fall off during cooking.

• Use a sharp knife to cut a shallow X in the base so the core cooks as fast as the leaves.

• You can steam, boil, or microwave your sprouts—each method will take about 6 to 10 minutes. You can test for doneness by poking the base of each sprout with the tip of a knife; they're ready when the bases are slightly tender but the sprouts are still a bit firm, like al dente pasta.

plagues more than three times as many women as men.

They don't help in the way you might suspect, though, by supplying calcium. Instead, they offer vitamin K. A Harvard study suggests that women who consume at least 109 micrograms of vitamin K daily—that's less than the amount in a 3-ounce serving of brussels sprouts—can reduce their chances of a hip fracture by 30 percent.

Brussels sprouts also supply other essential vitamins. Just ½ cup of cooked sprouts packs nearly all the vitamin C (great for your heart and immune system) that you need daily, along with about 12 percent of the daily requirement for folate (another heart helper that's also essential for reducing birth defects).

If your doctor tells you that you're at high risk for a stroke (or if you have high blood pressure, which ups your odds), start incorporating cruciferous veggies into your diet. A recent study showed that eating at least five servings of fruits and veggies daily, especially citrus fruits and members of the cabbage family (we hate to nag you, but that means brussels sprouts), can lower your chance of stroke by about 30 percent. So eat up!

SASSY SPROUTS

You'll find brussels sprouts in your supermarket all year long, although they're most plentiful in November and December. If you've never bought them before, don't worry—they're a cinch to select. Choose firm, bright green sprouts; avoid any that look yellow, are wilted, or feel soft. Buy them loose rather than packed in a tub, so you can choose sprouts of the same size. They'll cook more evenly.

To bring out their very best, kiss your sprouts with herbs and spices. Here's how.

Break out the bulb. In a nonstick pan, sauté minced garlic and red onion slices, then toss your sprouts with a bit of olive oil and the sautéed mixture.

Dip into dill. Season sprouts with dill, toasted sesame seeds, and a teeny bit of canola oil.

Count on a classic. Toss sprouts with lemon juice and nutmeg—it's a traditional favorite.

CABBAGE

The Sweet Smell of Success

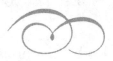

POOR, POOR CABBAGE; IT'S SO MISUNDERSTOOD. HERE'S a vegetable that is chock-full of cancer fighters, heaping with heart menders, and brimming with bone builders, and no one wants to cook it because they're afraid it will smell—okay, really reek.

Well, here's a news flash for all of you who can't stand the smell: Cabbage offends your nose only when you cook it too long! Just take it out of the pot in a jiffy, and you'll get the good stuff without the bad aroma.

ONE OF MOTHER NATURE'S HELPERS

Along with broccoli and brussels sprouts, cabbage is a cruciferous vegetable.

...Just the facts

Red cabbage (1 cup shredded)
Calories: 20
Fat: 0 g
Saturated fat: 0 g
Cholesterol: 0 mg
Sodium: 30 mg
Total carbohydrates: 8 g
Dietary fiber: 1 g
Protein: 4 g
Vitamin C: 70% of Daily Value
Calcium: 4%

While broccoli has gotten all the glory, scientists have consistently found that cabbage is every bit as healthy—if not more so!

"Cabbage contains at least 11 of the 15 families of vegetable-related compounds found to prevent cancer," says Wendy Demark, R.D., Ph.D., a researcher at the Duke University Comprehensive Cancer Center in Durham, North Carolina.

Foremost among those compounds are indoles, which scientists believe can destroy carcinogens before they trigger cancer or can stop the process in its tracks.

At Rockefeller University Hospital in New York City, researchers extracted a specific indole from cabbage and gave it to men and women for one to eight weeks. The compound lowered their levels of estrogen, a hormone thought to play a role in breast and prostate cancers. And scientists from the University of Illinois in Urbana found that indoles protected mice exposed to a carcinogen from developing breast and skin tumors.

Meanwhile, in a study of more than 47,000 men, researchers at Harvard determined that those who ate just one ½-cup serving of cabbage or two ½-cup servings of broccoli once a week lowered their risk of bladder cancer by

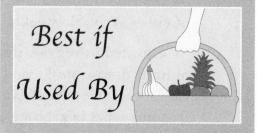

Best if Used By

Here's how to be sure your cabbage is king.

• Store cabbage in a plastic bag in the fridge so that it retains its vitamin C. Most kinds of cabbage will keep for about two weeks, but Savoy lasts just a week or so.

• Wash cabbage in cold water after you've chopped it.

• Sprinkle the unused portion of the head with lemon juice to prevent browning, then cover with plastic wrap. Use the leftovers within a few days.

44 percent compared with those who ate less than one serving of either vegetable weekly.

Cruciferous veggies, studies show, may also reduce your risk of heart disease, stroke, and cataracts. And here's one more plus for cabbage: Compared with other veggies in the crucifer family, some types of cabbage are high in calcium, boosting your bone density. So, what do you say? Want to give cabbage another chance?

HEADY ADVICE

Sizing up fresh cabbage is a snap. Look for solid, well-trimmed heads with no more than three or four outer leaves, which should be free of worm damage. (Worms can penetrate the interior.) Check for crisp leaves and a dry stem. Avoid heads with yellow leaves, which are a sure sign that the cab-

← Of Cabbages and Kings →

All cabbages contribute plenty of vitamin C, but some varieties kick in more vitamin A and calcium than others do. See how 1-cup servings of different cabbages stack up against each other and against America's second favorite hot-dog topping, canned sauerkraut. The bottom line: They're all winners!

Cabbage	Calories	Folate (mcg)	Vitamin A (RE)	Vitamin C (mg)	Calcium (mg)
Bok choy	9	46	210	31	73
Green	18	30	9	22	32
Red	19	15	3	19	36
Savoy	19	56	70	21	24
Sauerkraut, canned	44	56	4	35	70

bage has been hanging around too long.

Here are some ways to get more delicious cabbage in your life.

Think fast. In general, most people cook cabbage way too long, which is why it gives off an unpleasant odor. Endless cooking also destroys its vitamin C—so cook it quickly.

Stir-fry it. In a large nonstick skillet or wok, heat 1 tablespoon of canola oil and ¼ cup of chopped scallions. Add 3 cups of shredded cabbage and 2 tablespoons of sesame seeds. Sauté over medium heat for 8 to 10 minutes, or until the cabbage begins to wilt.

Dog it. Traditional hot dogs pack a wad of calories and fat, but they're oh-so-good with sauerkraut. Make this favorite healthier by using low-fat beef franks: Cook a few, slice them into small pieces, and add to warmed kraut.

Pump up pasta. Slice cabbage into long, thin strips and stir them into your favorite pasta sauce. Serve with fettuccine.

Toss fruit salad. You don't have to make coleslaw with creamy dressing. Instead, toss shredded cabbage with apple or pear wedges and citrus vinaigrette.

CARROTS

Cancer Crunchers

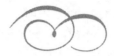

I PRACTICALLY GREW UP ON HORSEBACK, AND I LOVED the chomping and crunching of my favorite mount sharing my handful of carrots, but now I keep those carrots all to myself. "Let 'em eat grass!" I say. Why have I become so reluctant to share? Well, we now know that carrots are loaded with beta-carotene, making them one of the leading vegetable contenders for the title of cancer-fighting champ.

Just one 7-inch carrot packs four days' worth of beta-carotene. When I'm too pooped to peel, I snag a bag of babies. A generous handful of these golden nuggets nets me three days' quota of beta-carotene.

Researchers have long known that people who eat the most fruits and veg-

...Just the facts

Baby carrots (10 raw)
Calories: 38
Fat: Less than 1 g
Saturated fat: 0 g
Cholesterol: 0 mg
Sodium: 35 mg
Total carbohydrates: 8 g
Dietary fiber: 2 g
Protein: 1 g
Vitamin A: 300% of Daily
   Value

etables rich in beta-carotene have the lowest risk of lung cancer. The research continues, trying to pin down exactly why. Is it the beta? One of its relatives? Or is it the interplay of the entire nutrient mix in a beta-rich whole food that gets to wear the winner's crown?

5-ALARM CARROTS

One recent study of nonsmokers gave the nod to vegetables—tomatoes, lettuce, and carrots—and suggested that eating more of these and other vegetables may lower lung cancer risk by 25 percent for nonsmokers. Another study, in Italy, found that among people who had never smoked, eating more fruits and carrots, along with reducing alcohol and saturated fat intake, may cut the risk of cancers of the mouth and pharynx.

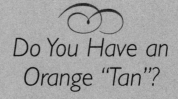

Do You Have an Orange "Tan"?

Maybe! It's true that you can take on an orange hue when you eat lots of carrots, because the same pigments that color the carrots can settle in your skin. Not to worry, though. The condition, called carotenemia, is harmless, and the color will start to fade the minute you cut back on carrots. If the whites of your eyes turn yellow, though, you could be jaundiced, and you need to check in with your doctor.

Also, 16 years into the Nurses' Health Study, researchers have learned that eating more vegetables, especially carrots, may significantly lower lung cancer risk, even in women who smoke. Don't get me wrong: Eating better is no substitute for quitting smoking, but eating more carrots while you're quitting looks like a plus.

24-CARROT BONES

Carrots are tops among vegetables for delivering beta-carotene. Since beta-carotene, more than any of its 500-plus carotenoid cousins, stands ready to convert to vitamin A as the need arises, carrots should get called on a lot.

Bone building is a case in point. When children's bones are trying to grow, remodeling is in order. Just as you would tear down part of your house to attach an addition, vitamin A tears down the finished ends of bones so that additional bone can be added. Remodeling goes on all the time in adults, too—not to make bones longer, but to make them stronger—as calcium is constantly subtracted from and added to existing structures.

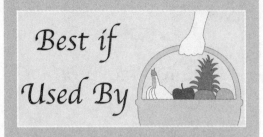

Best if Used By

Want your carrots to be tender and sweet? Here's what to do.

• Keep carrots fresh by twisting off the tops. Otherwise, they'll just keep growing and sucking up their own sugars.

• Keep them in the refrigerator so they'll stay fresh and tasty until you put them in the pot or munch them as a snack.

• In the fridge, keep them away from your apples. Apples produce ethylene gas, which helps other fruits ripen but prompts carrots to produce isocoumarin, a bitter-tasting chemical that keeps bugs from biting carrots in the field—and may stop you from biting them, too.

A PILL IS JUST A PILL

Beta-carotene is a powerful antioxidant that may help deter cancer. Should you boost your protection by taking a hefty supplement? Not a good idea. A Finnish study found that lung cancer actually increased among 29,000 smokers taking high-dose beta-carotene supplements. And in a study of 22,000 male American doctors, researchers found that scarfing down 50-milligram supplements every other day had absolutely no effect, good or bad, on the men's risk of cancer, heart disease, or death from any cause.

The lesson here is that you should focus on plant foods instead of pills. Orange, yellow, and red fruits and vegetables, such as carrots, butternut squash, cantaloupe, and apricots, are packed with beta-carotene, so it's easy to get all you need from them. They're also loaded with fiber, fluids, and an array of carotenoids and other newly discovered (and possibly undiscovered) elements that work together for better health.

BUGS BUNNY'S GOLDEN BEST

Most of the carrots we buy come packaged in plastic bags with tricky, fine orange lines that make the carrots look better and black borders that hide the freshness clues the carrot tops can give us. Try to wiggle the bag around to get a better look inside.

When selecting carrots, look for those that are bright orange, with no little root hairs growing out of them. Choose ones with narrow "shoulders," signaling a thinner core and sweeter flavor. If the shoulders are a little green, that's okay, although the green part is bitter, so you may want to trim it off before eating.

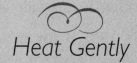

Heat Gently

Almost everyone thinks that vegetables are best eaten raw, but occasionally, everyone can be wrong. It turns out that the same plant materials that give carrots and other veggies their crisp, crunchy texture also imprison their sugars and carotenes. Light cooking, just to the crisp-tender stage, actually releases the beta-carotene so you can absorb more of it. But don't overcook carrots. If you cook them too long—say, 20 minutes—all their food value ends up in the cooking water, and the carrots end up tasting terrible.

Try these delicious ways to add carrots to your diet.

Make liquid gold. Puree cooked carrots and onions to use as a thickener for soups and sauces. It makes great fat-free "gravy" for Yankee pot roast, grilled pork tenderloin, or baked chicken, too.

Sliver for slaw. To create colorful slaw, shred both green and red cabbage, then toss in long slivers of carrot.

Simmer souper carrots. Gently boil fresh carrot slices with onions in low-sodium chicken broth, then puree to make the sweetest carrot soup ever. Pureed carrots make a great thickener all by themselves, so no cream is needed. If you want thinner soup, add a little fat-free milk.

Shred for salads. Of course, you add celery to tuna, chicken, and shrimp salad. Now pump up the nutritional volume with shredded carrots, too.

CAULIFLOWER

Crusader Cousin

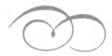

HAVE YOU EVER NOTICED THAT WHENEVER THERE'S A vegetable tray at parties, cauliflower is, well, a wallflower? For this book, I asked a friend why she eats broccoli but not cauliflower. Her answer: Broccoli is supposed to be really good for you, while cauliflower is nothing special.

Well, my friend is half right. Broccoli is an incredible disease fighter, but cauliflower is every bit as good. Both are members of the cruciferous family of vegetables, a clan of anticancer crusaders that share a lot of the same traits.

THE WARRIOR TRIBE

You know that most vegetables contain cancer-fighting compounds with hard-to-pronounce names, but study after study

> ## ...Just the facts
>
> Cauliflower (½ cup cooked)
> Calories: 14
> Fat: 0 g
> Saturated fat: 0 g
> Cholesterol: 0 mg
> Sodium: 9 mg
> Total carbohydrates: 3 g
> Dietary fiber: 1 g
> Protein: 1 g
> Folate: 7% of Daily Value
> Vitamin C: 46%

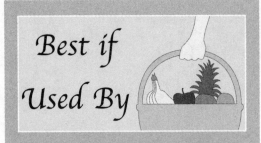

Best if Used By

Once you bring your cauliflower home, store it in a plastic bag in the crisper of your fridge, where it'll keep for up to a week. Wash it when you're ready to use it.

suggests that the compounds in cruciferous veggies pack the heaviest punch. Let's look at some of the scientific evidence.

• In studying prostate cancer, researchers at the Fred Hutchinson Cancer Research Center in Seattle found that men who ate three or more servings of vegetables daily—especially the cruciferous kind—had about half the risk of prostate cancer of those who didn't "do" veggies.

• Scientists at Harvard couldn't link overall vegetable consumption with a lower chance of developing bladder cancer, but they did find a connection with cruciferous veggies. The study's authors discovered that nonsmoking men who consumed five or more servings of cruciferous veggies per week had a 51 percent reduction in their risk of bladder cancer compared with men who ate just one serving per week.

• New findings on breast cancer prevention show that cruciferous veggies aren't just good for guys. Researchers at the University of Buffalo think that cauliflower, broccoli, and the rest of the family may be able to lower a woman's risk of breast cancer, especially before she reaches menopause.

Exactly how these vegetables work their magic in preventing breast cancer is a little complicated, but here are the basics: Your body can break down the hormone estrogen in a number of ways. If it produces estrogen by-products with little biological activity, the researchers found, your risk of breast cancer may drop by 40 percent. Cruciferous veggies make your estrogen by-products less active.

STROKE SPECIALIST

The latest stroke research shows that cruciferous vegetables also lower your risk of having a stroke. In a study of more than 75,000 women, researchers found that those who ate the most produce, especially crucifers, had a 30 percent lower chance of suffering a stroke than those who consumed the least produce.

FLOWER POWER

In addition to being part of a family rich in cancer- and stroke-fighting compounds, cauliflower offers big helpings of vitamin C and folate. Vitamin C helps protect your heart by gobbling up free radicals, compounds that play a role in the development of heart disease. Folate may also safeguard your heart by lowering your levels of the amino acid homocysteine, which increases the risk of ticker trouble. Plus, a diet rich in folate (and its synthetic version, folic acid) keeps unborn babies from developing neural tube birth defects, such as spina bifida.

Women shouldn't wait until they're pregnant to make sure that they get enough folate, though. These birth defects can occur early in pregnancy—often before a woman knows that she's in the pink (or blue). Researchers therefore suggest that all women who are capable of having children, regardless of whether they're trying to conceive, eat a diet rich in this B vitamin. Since cauliflower can

FOOD NEWS

Plagued by a parade of colds? Maybe you're not getting enough vitamin C. Don't run out for a supplement, though; just eat more foods that are rich in the nutrient. Cauliflower, perhaps unexpectedly, is loaded with it.

lose a lot of its folate when it's boiled, you should sometimes eat it raw.

CHOOSE AND USE

You can find cauliflower year-round, although its availability usually peaks in the spring and fall. Choose heads that are firm, heavy, and white or creamy white, with no brown spots. Look for leaves that are fresh and green.

Cauliflower tastes great both raw and cooked. If you're cooking it, squeeze a little lemon juice into the water so the cauliflower retains its white color. Ready for some serving ideas? Here you go.

Dip it. Cauliflower's mild flavor is perfectly matched with hummus, that wonderful chickpea spread.

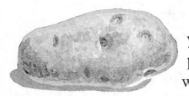

Hide it. Mix chopped cauliflower florets into your family's mashed potatoes. Spuds are the perfect camouflage—kids, big or small, won't know the cauliflower is there.

Bake it. Toss cooked cauliflower in a little olive oil, sprinkle some bread crumbs on top, and bake until the crumbs are light brown.

Stir it. Swirl cooked cauliflower pieces into canned tomato soup for the ultimate prostate cancer–fighting duo.

Mound it. Skip the pepperoni; instead, top your pizza with cauliflower and broccoli florets.

GARLIC

The Anticancer Clove

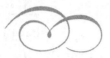

BELIEVE IT OR NOT, SAN FRANCISCO PROUDLY BOASTS Garlic World, a market that carries every product in the world that's made from garlic—including garlic ice cream and garlic jelly. Sound pretty wild? Maybe, but what's not wild is garlic's amazing ability to keep us well, including its protective effect against cancer.

In one analysis of medical studies, for instance, researchers from the University of North Carolina in Chapel Hill found that people who consumed six or more garlic cloves per week had a 30 percent lower risk of colon cancer and a 50 percent lower risk of stomach cancer than those who ate a clove or less weekly. Other studies have hinted that garlic staves off breast and prostate cancers, too, but the evidence is still preliminary.

> ## ...Just the facts
>
> Garlic (5 cloves)
> Calories: 22
> Fat: 0 g
> Saturated fat: 0 g
> Cholesterol: 0 mg
> Sodium: 3 mg
> Total carbohydrates: 5 g
> Dietary fiber: 0 g
> Protein: 1 g
> Vitamin C: 8% of Daily
>   Value

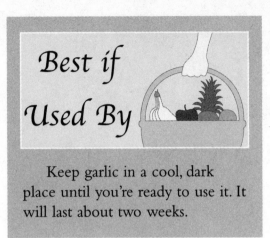

Best if Used By

Keep garlic in a cool, dark place until you're ready to use it. It will last about two weeks.

How does garlic ground cancer? It contains allicin, a cancer-fighting sulfur compound. Garlic supplements, by the way, don't seem to have an effect on cancer because they have only trace amounts of allicin, according to the researchers.

BRING ON THE BULB!

People have used garlic since ancient times to help ward off dozens of health problems. The Greeks actually ate garlic before running races to get a competitive advantage (maybe no one wanted to be near them!).

Scientists haven't checked out the validity of every use, but besides fighting cancer, garlic seems to help in these five areas.

• *Heart disease.* A review of studies found that consuming one-half to one clove of garlic daily lowers total cholesterol levels by about 9 percent, reducing the risk of heart disease by about 20 percent.

• *Immune function.* Garlic is loaded with compounds that may be able to kill some bacteria and viruses. A study at Brigham Young University in Provo, Utah, reported that crushed garlic in oil killed rhinovirus type 2 (a common cause of colds), two forms of herpesvirus, and several other common viruses.

• *Mood.* We're not kidding here. A recent study found that when garlic is served at a meal, families are more likely to be nice to each other. A possible explanation is that garlic evokes positive childhood memories, making people chill out.

• *Weight control.* Plain old steamed broccoli, cooked carrots, and other vegetables come alive when you add some minced garlic. The more you like your veggies, the more likely you will be to eat them—and that's good news for your hips and your heart.

• *Athlete's foot.* It's the ultimate irony: You may be able to end athlete's foot with none other than the "stinking rose." Just soak your feet in a basin of warm water with a few crushed garlic cloves and a splash of rubbing alcohol, suggests James Duke, Ph.D., retired USDA researcher and author of *The Green Pharmacy.* "Because of its antifungal properties, garlic is my first choice of treatment," he says.

FOOD NEWS

Peeling garlic cloves is a cinch with this method.

• Place the cloves on a cutting board and lay the flat side of a knife on top of them.

• Tap the knife gently with your closed fist to split the peels; like magic, the cloves will pop out.

• To get rid of the odor on your hands, rub them with salt or lemon juice and wash with warm, soapy water.

GETTING GARLICKY GOODNESS

There's nothing complicated about buying any variety of garlic. Choose plump, firm bulbs and look for tightly closed cloves. Then cast your cloves on these dishes.

Add magic to mayo. Think low-fat mayo tastes blah? Mix 2 tablespoons with 1 teaspoon of minced garlic, then watch it come alive. Spread it on a veggie sandwich.

Make savory chicken. When you're roasting a chicken, tuck a few peeled garlic cloves into the cavity for extra flavor.

MUSHROOMS

Funky Fighters

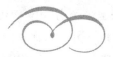

OKAY, I KNOW THAT ALICE'S ZANY adventures in Wonderland were triggered by hallucinogenic mushrooms. Those are not the kind I'm recommending! Instead, I can suggest an increasing variety of fabulous fungi, including the popular buttons, meaty portobellos, cancer-fighting shiitakes, and more. Let's take a look at a few varieties and see just why they are so good for you.

MUSHROOM EXPLOSION

The past few years have seen mushroom varieties, well, mushroom. This is good news. The amazing array of shapes, colors, and sizes makes you wonder what Mother Nature was nibbling when she invented mushrooms (way to go, Mom!).

...Just the facts

Shiitake mushrooms (½ cup cooked)
Calories: 40
Fat: 0 g
Saturated fat: 0 g
Cholesterol: 0 mg
Sodium: 0 mg
Total carbohydrates: 10 g
Dietary fiber: 2 g
Protein: 1 g
Riboflavin (vitamin B_2): 7% of Daily Value
Niacin (vitamin B_3): 5%
Vitamin B_6: 6%
Copper: 32%
Zinc: 6%

The increasing variety sure makes dinner more interesting, but even better, the more exotic mushrooms also appear to be sprouting natural chemicals with health-enhancing qualities. For example, shiitakes have a slight but definite ability to lower very low density lipoprotein (VLDL) cholesterol. (Eat them instead of a fatty burger for a double whammy!) Both shiitake and maitake mushrooms appear to boost immune system function, fight cancer, and lower blood pressure. Mushroom extracts are also being studied for their cancer-curing potential.

Best if Used By

Once you get your mushrooms home, bag them twice: first in a paper bag and then in plastic, says food physiologist Brian Patterson in his book *Fresh*. The paper bag will absorb moisture so they don't get slimy, and the plastic bag will keep them from drying out.

BUTTON UP!

We're all most familiar with the white button mushrooms that spill out of produce bins. They're really low in calories, and despite their mild taste, they're powerful flavor enhancers for just about any food you mix them with. And they have some pretty special qualities.

• *Great tasting!* Why do mushrooms turn a good meal into a great one? It's because they serve up a nice dose of glutamic acid, the good-for-you part of monosodium glutamate (MSG) that's also known as the fifth taste. Along with sweet, sour, salty, and bitter, experts now recognize the "umami," or meaty, taste.

You've probably noticed that when you cook mushrooms, they nearly vanish. That's because they're like little sacks of water that leak when heated—and that's okay. It makes for tasty broth, and it concentrates the nutrients in the 'shrooms so you get more per forkful.

• *More filling!* Even though they have so few calories, mushrooms make a wonderful bulking agent for salads, soups, and sauces. They help you fill up without filling out! (Don't sauté them in butter, though, or they'll soak up a ton of fat and calories!)

• *Good for you!* Buttons are a good source of niacin and riboflavin, two of the B vitamins that act like converters as you metabolize your meals, turning your food into stuff your body uses for energy and to fight disease. They're also laced with copper, an important mineral for healthy blood and sturdy bones.

← Fungal Fantasia →

Once upon a time, there were only buttons. Now, fabulous fresh mushrooms abound. Check out the differences in these fantastic fungi.

Mushroom	Looks Like	Color	Taste
Button	Smooth, white button	White or off-white	Mild
Chanterelle	Frilly trumpet	Brown-gold to yellow-orange	Like apricots
Enoki	Long, skinny bouquet	Creamy white	Sweet
Oyster	Oyster clusters	Off-white or gray-brown	Meaty
Portobello	Burger patty	Dark brown	Meaty
Shiitake	Open umbrella	Brown-black	Rich
Wood ear	Flat plate	Grayish white	Mild

MESMERIZED BY MUSHROOMS

Mushrooms are available in all seasons. Regardless of which kind you choose, they should look pretty chipper—smooth, dry, and firm, without cuts or bruises. Pass up 'shrooms that look limp, dried out, wrinkled, leathery, or slimy. Choose those that smell fresh and nutty, like bread, and avoid any with a moldy scent. Also, check out the gills under the cap. Closed gills mean the mushroom is young; open gills are a sign of aging.

Good to Go

Don't wash your mushrooms! They're like sponges when they get wet. Instead, clean them gently by dusting them off with a fine, soft mushroom brush or a soft paper towel. Most mushrooms are grown in sterilized compost, so they're really very safe to eat when handled this way.

Now make room for mushrooms in your meals. Here are some ideas.

Streamline pasta. Substitute a can of sliced mushrooms for the usual meat in your spaghetti sauce. You'll cut calories while boosting flavor.

Sauce your salmon. Sauté sliced fresh shiitake mushrooms, 1 sliced yellow onion, and 2 cloves of finely diced fresh garlic in a few drops of olive oil. Season with a pinch of dried basil or oregano and serve over grilled salmon.

Surprise your bun. Fill it with a grilled portobello mushroom instead of a burger.

Stock up. Save fresh mushroom stems to make stock for yummy mushroom soup.

Savor the flavor. Keep dehydrated exotic mushrooms on hand to create sensational dishes on a moment's notice.

OKRA

Power Pods

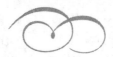

ALL YOU SOUTHERNERS WILL PROBABLY LAUGH AT A Northern woman trying to talk about okra. You most likely grew up on the stuff. But, for the benefit of Northern folks, give me a break and let me explain. Okra is a small, green (although some varieties are white), ribbed pod that's shaped like a tube. It has an unusual texture and a unique flavor that has been described as somewhere between eggplant and asparagus, and it goes well when mixed with other veggies.

IT KEEPS YOU SMILING

Why should you bother trying it? Okra contains glutathione, a compound that shows potential to stave off cancer by preventing cancer-causing chemicals from wreaking havoc with DNA.

...Just the facts

Okra (½ cup cooked)
Calories: 27
Fat: 0 g
Saturated fat: 0 g
Cholesterol: 0 mg
Sodium: 4 mg
Total carbohydrates: 6 g
Dietary fiber: 2 g
Protein: 2 g
Folate: 9% of Daily Value
Vitamin C: 22%
Magnesium: 11%

In a study of more than 1,800 people at Emory University in Atlanta, researchers found that those who had the highest intake of foods rich in this compound were half as likely to develop oral and throat cancers as those who had the lowest intake.

PERFECT PODS

If you live in the South, you can probably buy fresh okra year-round, but most other folks will just have to settle for it in the spring and fall. Look for pods that are bruise-free and tender but not mushy. Make sure they're no longer than 3 to 4 inches. Avoid pods that are longer or are blackish or brownish, because they won't be as tender.

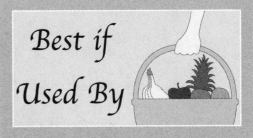

Best if Used By

For great okra that will make you glad you gave it a try:
- Store it in a plastic bag in the refrigerator. It will keep for three to five days.
- Don't wash it until you're ready to use it, or the pods will get slimy.

Here are some Southern-style suggestions for enjoying okra.

Stir it fast. Toss okra into any of your favorite stir-fries—it makes a fine substitute for green beans.

Make it thick. Gumbo soup is traditionally made with okra, and while we rarely whip up a batch from scratch, we do like Healthy Choice Gumbo Soup. You can stir okra into any soup, really—it'll even thicken the broth a bit.

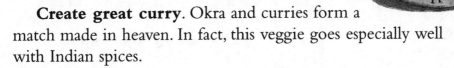

Create great curry. Okra and curries form a match made in heaven. In fact, this veggie goes especially well with Indian spices.

PAPAYA

Gift-Wrapped Goodness

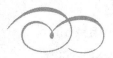

DURING FEBRUARY, NOTHING IS FINER THAN MUNCHING on a bit of papaya. Its sunny colors and voluptuous flavor will brighten winter days better than a trip to the Bahamas. (Well, maybe not that much, but it helps.) And papaya is packed with carotenoids that build your defenses against cancer and help fight off colds and flu until spring's warm weather returns.

It's this simple: Carotenoids can boost your immune system and protect you from just about anything that can kill you, including cancer. Of course, they work only when they're in your bloodstream, not when they're merely on your plate.

PACKAGING MATTERS

If you checked the stats and compared the amount of beta-carotene in a papaya

...Just the facts

Papaya (½ large)
Calories: 59
Fat: 0 g
Saturated fat: 0 g
Cholesterol: 0 mg
Sodium: 6 mg
Total carbohydrates: 19 g
Dietary fiber: 3 g
Protein: 1 g
Folate: 18% of Daily Value
Vitamin A: 11%
Vitamin C: 130%
Vitamin E: 14%
Calcium: 5%

(60 micrograms) with the amount in a bowl of spinach (9,200 micrograms), you'd say, "No-brainer! Spinach wins hands down." But hold on for an amazing revelation.

In its new dietary reference book about carotenoids, the Institute of Medicine in Washington, D.C. (the group that publishes the Recommended Dietary Allowances, or RDAs) has disclosed that packaging counts. In fact, packaging is critical to how much beta-carotene your body can extract from the green and orange foods you eat and how much is delivered to your blood.

Guess what? Fruits, especially papaya, lead the parade of foods that easily release their beta-carotene, while spinach and other green vegetables bring up the rear, so papaya is more potent than it first appears. And here's a bonus: Papaya is loaded with cryptoxanthin, another carotenoid that can help beat vitamin A deficiency and its threats to your vision and skin.

Good to Go →

When you're ready to indulge in papaya, wash the outside under running water and pat dry. Place the papaya on a cutting board and slice in half lengthwise. You'll find a yellow-pink, fleshy interior and a hollow filled with sparkling black seeds. Beautiful! Scoop out the seeds, and it's ready to eat!

FRIENDS COUNT

You'll get even more carotenoids if you serve your papaya (and your spinach) with a little fat. Nuts, olive oil, and canola oil are especially good choices. In fact, why not warm some papaya chunks and serve them on a bed of steamed spinach tossed with olive oil and sprinkled with toasted pine nuts? Talk about carotene heaven!

A SIMPLE SOLUTION

Annoyed by hiccups, belching, or bloating? Eat papaya. Its digestive enzymes may help relieve your distress.

BENEFITS ABOUND

If minimizing heart disease and reducing high blood pressure are on your list of things to do today, have a papaya. It's packed with these nutrients.

• *Potassium.* This mineral is important for lowering blood pressure—and there's more in a papaya than in a banana.

• *Folate.* This is the B vitamin that tames homocysteine so it can't trigger a heart attack and helps prevent some birth defects.

• *Vitamin C.* It may help prevent "bad" low-density lipoprotein (LDL) cholesterol from clogging your arteries and may help heal surgical wounds. A papaya offers more C than an 8-ounce glass of orange juice.

So get happy. Have a papaya!

GET A TASTE OF THE TROPICS

Papaya is a tropical treat that's available all year long, although you'll probably find the biggest piles of this fruit in late spring/early summer and then again in early fall. A papaya looks like a large, fat, greenish yellow pear. Choose fresh papayas that are about half yellow. As they ripen, they'll begin to glow with a beautiful yellow-orange color. Skip fruits that are all green,

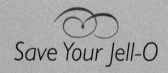

Save Your Jell-O

Don't put uncooked papaya in gelatin. Like fresh pineapple, it contains an enzyme that disrupts protein and turns gelatin to water.

because they've been picked too early and may never ripen.

Here's how to enjoy your papaya.

Take a mini vacation. When you just can't take the snow anymore and need a bit of sunshine, grab a papaya. Stuff it with seafood salad made with crab, shrimp, and scallops. Sit by a sunny window and eat your fill.

Grill a tropical treat. Line up fresh papaya quarters alongside your chicken or skewer papaya cubes and shrimp for kebabs.

Wet your whistle. Have a cup of papaya nectar as an afternoon snack.

Have a Mexican smoothie. Add fresh papaya chunks, along with a banana, to your next smoothie.

Improve on trail mix. Stash chunks of dried papaya in your fanny pack when you go hiking. They're great for an energy boost along the way.

Enjoy saucy meat. Replace high-fat gravy with pureed papaya. It works great on chicken, pork, or fish.

Best if Used By

Here's how to handle your papaya just right.

• Speed ripening by putting your papayas in a paper bag with a banana. (Yes, bananas produce ethylene gas just like apples do!)

• When the fruits are about three-quarters golden, they'll give slightly when pressed near the stem. If they feel soft and mushy, you've waited too long.

• Once they're ripe, put them in the refrigerator (if you can wait!), where they'll last about a week. Better yet, eat them right away, before the flavor starts to fade.

PINEAPPLE

Lei It On!

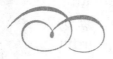

THIS FRUIT CONJURES VISIONS OF HAWAII—YOU KNOW, glorious days filled with swimming, sightseeing, and, yes, eating lots of pineapple. In a word: paradise. Well, if you can't make it over there, do the next best thing—pick up some pineapple at your local supermarket. Sure, it isn't exactly the same, but you'll love it nonetheless. And pineapple is as good for you as it is good-tasting, giving you a sweet head start in beating cancer.

"C" CHANGE

Depending on the variety of pineapple you select, one 4-ounce serving contains 25 to 150 percent of the vitamin C you need for the day. As you probably know, vitamin C is an antioxidant, gobbling up those free radical bad guys that cause cell damage that can lead to cancer and heart

...Just the facts

Pineapple (4 oz; two 3-in slices)
Calories: 65
Fat: 0 g
Saturated fat: 0 g
Cholesterol: 0 mg
Sodium: 10 mg
Total carbohydrates: 16 g
Dietary fiber: 1 g
Protein: 1 g
Vitamin C: 25–150% of Daily Value

disease. It also revs up your immune system so it can ward off colds, flu, and other infections that make you feel miserable.

Besides vitamin C, pineapple is packed with additional compounds that may fend off cancer. Chief among them is bromelain, an enzyme that may help halt the spread of tumors. Animal studies suggest that bromelain holds promise in fighting lung cancer and leukemia especially, but more tests need to be done. In the meantime, it certainly won't hurt to add luscious pineapple to your list of anticancer foods.

Bromelain also gives you the more immediate benefit of aiding your digestion, so if a bowl of five-alarm chili has your stomach in knots, have a few chunks of pineapple or a glass of pineapple juice. It may supply the relief you need without the side effects of antacids.

TIPTOE THROUGH THE PINEAPPLE

Buying a pineapple is pretty much a no-brainer because you're rarely—if ever—going to see one that isn't ripe. That's because, unlike many other fruits, pineapple is picked only when it's ripe

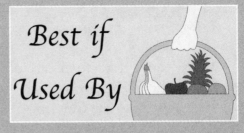

Best if Used By

To keep that island-hopping taste, wrap the pineapple loosely in plastic and refrigerate it for as long as five days.

A SIMPLE SOLUTION

To soften a callus, apply a piece of pineapple rind and cover it with an adhesive bandage overnight, suggests James Duke, Ph.D., retired USDA researcher and author of *The Green Pharmacy*. An enzyme in the rind does the trick.

When you're ready for a taste of paradise, twist off the crown, cut the shell away from the fruit, and slice. Cut pineapple lasts up to three days in the fridge if you store it in a sealed container.

To make chunks:

• Cut the pineapple into quarters lengthwise.

• Trim each end, then cut away the center core strip.

• Cut the quartered fruit into bite-size pieces, and that's it!

and then shipped to supermarkets. Look for fruits that have dark green leaves and avoid those with bruises or soft spots. (Myth alert: The color of the pineapple's outer shell is no indication of its quality or ripeness.) Also check the variety. All varieties pack vitamin C, but the fairly new Del Monte Gold offers four times more than traditional types—all the vitamin C (and then some) that you need for a day in a single serving.

Try these simple suggestions to get the delicious benefits of pineapple.

Go tropical for breakfast. Stir fresh or dried pineapple pieces into your morning yogurt. Warm fresh or canned pineapple slices and top your waffles with them. Or follow the Hawaiians' lead: Just slice one up and eat it plain.

Think paradise for dessert. Grill pineapple slices on both sides just until warmed. Top with vanilla frozen yogurt for a decadent dessert.

Get luscious for lunch. Tuck a pineapple slice into your next ham and cheese sandwich.

RADISHES

Red-Hot Protection

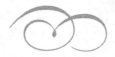

WHEN MY HUSBAND AND I THROW A PARTY (BIG OR small) for friends or relatives, we always have a vegetable platter. To us, it's just as essential as buying a good bottle of wine or making a memorable dessert. What's on that platter? Usually carrot sticks, red bell pepper strips, celery slices, and slivers of radish. Most people think the radish is there just for a little extra color, but we really want our guests to eat it. Its slightly peppery taste is a welcome contrast to blander veggies—plus, it's loaded with compounds that fight cancer. Is there a better gift we can give someone?

A FIERY BONUS

Like broccoli, brussels sprouts, and cauliflower, radishes are cruciferous vegetables. Compounds in this type of vegetable can reduce the risk of cancer—especially

---

...Just the facts

Red radishes (8)
Calories: 6
Fat: 0 g
Saturated fat: 0 g
Cholesterol: 0 mg
Sodium: 9 mg
Total carbohydrates: 1 g
Dietary fiber: 1 g
Protein: 0 g
Vitamin C: 14% of Daily
  Value

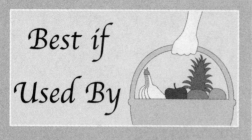

Best if Used By

When storing your radishes:
• Remove any attached leaves.
• Store in a plastic bag in the fridge. Just perforate the bag so they remain dry.
• Red radishes and daikons will keep for about a week; black radishes may stay fresh for months.

prostate, colon, bladder, and stomach cancers. In a study of nearly 1,500 people, researchers in Germany found that radishes and onions significantly lowered the participants' chances of developing stomach cancer, while sausage, not surprisingly, increased them.

Sure, you're probably never going to eat as many radishes as you will broccoli florets and other members of the cruciferous clan, but every little bit helps. Just by sticking some slivered radishes in your sandwiches or salads, you can rack up an extra serving or two of veggies every week for barely any calories—and that may be just the edge you need to avoid cancer in the long run.

CALORIE BURNER

When you're trying to lose weight, you're probably always hungry. That's because your stomach is used to having a larger volume of food in it. You can trick your tummy into thinking it's full by filling it with low-calorie, high-volume foods such as radishes. Eight radishes have just 6—that's not a typo; I really mean just 6—calories. Crunch on them plain or dunk them in a little low-fat yogurt dip. Or come to my house for a party— I'll have some on the vegetable platter.

RAVISHING RADISHES

Some supermarkets carry a few different kinds of radishes. They offer red radishes (the kind you've seen all your life), daikons (large, carrot-shaped radishes), and black radishes (with dark brown or dull black skin and a white interior). Chances are, you'll want to pick up the red radishes, but just in case you're feeling adventurous, we'll give you the lowdown on the other kinds, too.

When selecting red radishes, choose those that are smooth, firm, well formed, and brightly colored. Skip any that are large (you won't like the taste), cracked, or spotted.

Look for daikons that are firm and evenly shaped, with glossy skin. The best black radishes are solid, heavy, and free of cracks.

Here's a rule that applies to all three: If you're buying radishes with the tops attached (they're sold with and without), make sure the leaves look fresh.

Now use your radishes in these tasty ways.

Kick up crudités. Slice red radishes, along with carrots, celery, and other veggies, and serve with a low-fat dip, such as ranch.

Color slaw. Add ½ cup of slivered red or black radishes to your favorite coleslaw. What a color contrast!

Add sizzle to sandwiches. Mix chopped radishes into egg, tuna, or chicken salad or tuck radish slices into your veggie pita pocket or turkey club.

Good to Go

Ready to crunch into your radishes? Here's what to do.
- Trim off the stem ends and tips.
- Wash the radishes carefully.
- Don't peel any type of radish except black ones that have developed a thick skin.

ROSEMARY

Scented Sentry

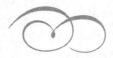

LAST YEAR, I WAS ASTONISHED TO SEE A 3-FOOT-TALL "Christmas tree" that was actually a large rosemary plant trimmed to shape. What a great kitchen gift for a favorite friend! When those postholiday blues strike, she'll still have pine-scented rosemary for comfort and cooking. And along the way she'll get protection from cancer, and—wait until you hear this—skin damage!

BODY, MIND, AND SPIRIT

Rosemary is packed with carnosol, a phenolic compound that fights cancer by interrupting inflammation so those evil cells can't get a toehold in your body and grow. Carnosol also appears to boost the liver's production of several cancer-fighting substances, including one called glu-

...Just the facts

Rosemary (1 Tbsp dried)
Calories: 2
Fat: 0 g
Saturated fat: 0 g
Cholesterol: 0 mg
Sodium: 0 mg
Total carbohydrates: Less than 1 g
Dietary fiber: Less than 1 g
Protein: 0 g
Vitamin A: 1% of Daily Value
Calcium: 1%
Iron: 1%

tathione-S-transferase. In addition, rosemary may protect against foodborne illness, since various studies suggest that it fights fungi, viruses, and bacteria. (To be really safe, though, always keep cold foods below 40°F and hot foods above 140°F.)

As an added benefit, when you flavor with rosemary instead of lots of butter or sour cream, you protect your heart from saturated fat and your waistline from excess pounds.

Rosemary is also being explored for its ability to relax you when its aroma is inhaled—so always breathe deeply when cooking with rosemary.

A SIMPLE SOLUTION

Feeling a little dizzy? Make your own smelling salts by placing 1 to 4 drops of rosemary essential oil on a tissue, then wave it under your nose. Rubbing the oil on your temples also helps.

This works because the oil stimulates both olfactory and trigeminal nerve endings, causing a reflex that improves breathing and circulation, according to *Rational Phytotherapy: A Physician's Guide to Herbal Medicine* by Volker Schulz, Rudolf Hänsel, and Varro E. Tyler.

LET'S FACE IT!

While no one is advocating skipping your sunscreen, there's been some pretty exciting face-saving research focused on rosemary. It turns out that your skin is just as vulnerable to oxygen damage as your heart is, and maybe even more so, because it's constantly exposed to air, sun, and pollution.

Preliminary laboratory and human studies have shown that consuming an extract of antioxidant-packed rosemary can help prevent damaging changes

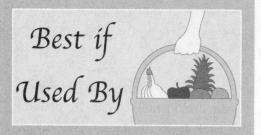

Best if Used By

When you get your fresh rosemary home, wash it, pat it dry, wrap it in paper towels, and store it in a plastic bag. Or put it in a plastic container designed to allow air circulation. It should last about a week.

to skin by protecting the fat in skin cells. Much more study is needed, of course, but you'd better believe that we're cooking with rosemary!

REACHING FOR ROSEMARY

In some supermarkets, you'll find fresh rosemary tied in hand-size bunches. In others, you'll see a few little sprigs sealed in tiny plastic containers. Which size to buy depends on how much you need, although overabundance is rarely a problem. When selecting this piney-looking herb, it should appear every bit as fresh as you'd want your Christmas tree to be. The needles should be deep green on top with whitish-looking undersides, without mold or dark or wet spots.

Perk up your palate with these ideas for using this timeless herb.

Sprig it. To infuse meat with flavor, place a rosemary branch on pork, chicken, or beef while it's cooking—and savor the aroma!

Grind it. Sprinkle ground rosemary on salmon or tuna steaks before grilling.

Soup it up. Stir ground rosemary into canned minestrone soup for authentic Italian flavor.

Sprinkle it. Shake a little ground rosemary on your next pizza—it'll add some pizzazz.

SWEET POTATOES

Top Taters

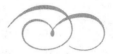

THANKSGIVING DINNER JUST WOULDN'T BE THE SAME without warm, melt-in-your-mouth sweet potatoes. Mmm, can't you almost taste them now? It's hard to fathom why then, if they're so good, most people eat white potatoes most of the time and reserve the sweetest spuds for holiday meals. This is even more of a mystery since besides having remarkable flavor, sweet potatoes stuff our bodies with beta-carotene, a powerful antioxidant and cancer fighter.

ALL-STAR SPUDS

When it comes to vitamins and minerals, sweet potatoes shine. The Center for Science in the Public Interest, a nutrition advocacy group in Washington, D.C., recently ranked vegetables by adding up

...Just the facts

Sweet potato (1 medium cooked)
Calories: 117
Fat: 0 g
Saturated fat: 0 g
Cholesterol: 0 mg
Sodium: 11 mg
Total carbohydrates: 28 g
Dietary fiber: 4 g
Protein: 2 g
Vitamin A: 498% of Daily Value
Vitamin C: 47%

If you wake in the middle of the night with painful leg cramps, you may not be eating enough foods rich in potassium. Add more sweet potatoes, bananas, or orange juice to your diet to boost your stores of this important mineral.

their percentages of daily requirements for six important nutrients: folate, vitamin A, vitamin C, calcium, copper, and iron. Largely because of their vitamin A content, sweet potatoes came out on top, scoring 582 points. (Carrots, incidentally, ranked second, with 434 points.)

This contest, a Veggie Bowl of sorts, would mean nothing if the sweet potato's track record in research studies weren't so impressive, but here are some phenomenal findings.

• A Swedish study suggests that women who take in about 3.7 milligrams of beta-carotene each day from foods—the amount in about one-third of a single sweet potato—are up to 68 percent less likely to develop breast cancer than those who eat the least beta-carotene.

• Researchers from the Netherlands followed the diets and medical histories of nearly 5,000 people ages 55 to 95 for four years. They found that those who got the most beta-carotene had a 45 percent lower risk of heart disease than those who consumed the least.

• Closer to home, a study at Tufts University in Boston showed that older people who consumed at least 15 milligrams of beta-carotene daily—the amount in one sweet potato and ⅔ cup of baby carrots—bolstered their immune systems to ward off all kinds of bugs.

• Research from Albert Einstein

College of Medicine in New York City suggests that a diet rich in beta-carotene may help prevent yeast infections.

The list could go on and on. Dozens of studies have shown a link between beta-carotene and lower risks of cancer, heart disease, and other heavyweight health problems.

GIVE THANKS

Before you're tempted to take a supplement instead of having a serving of sweet potatoes, consider this: Beta-carotene from foods seems to offer protection, but beta-carotene supple-

---

← A Sweet by Any Other Name →

What's in a name? Plenty, if you're trying to find sweet potatoes. Many supermarkets and canned-good manufacturers mislabel sweet potatoes—especially the darker-skinned varieties—as yams. True yams are hard to find, and if you do run across them, they're usually sold in chunks sealed in plastic wrap. Here's a rundown of the differences between the two.

Characteristic	Sweet Potato	Yam
Beta-carotene content	Very high	None
Appearance	Smooth, thin skin	Rough, scaly skin
Skin color	Light yellow to dark orange	Brown or black
Flesh color	Pale yellow to bright orange	Off-white, purple, or red
Size	About ¼–½ pound each	Can grow up to 150 pounds each
Taste	Moist	Dry
Preparation	Can be used raw or cooked	Toxic if eaten raw
Where grown	In the United States	In the Caribbean

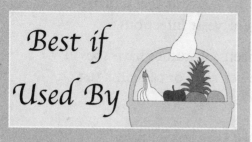

Best if Used By

Here's how to keep your all-star sweets in tiptop condition.
- Store fresh spuds in a dark, cool, dry place. They'll be good for one to two weeks.
- Unless they're cooked, don't put them in the fridge; the cold will sap their sweetness.

ments are iffy at best. In fact, supplements may even increase the risk of lung cancer in smokers. So here's some good advice: Have Thanksgiving—at least the sweet potato part of it—every Thursday of the year!

SENSATIONAL SWEETS

For the sweetest flavor, select and store with care. Look for fresh tubers with tight, unwrinkled, unblemished skin. Avoid bruised sweet potatoes. They deteriorate quickly, and the flavor of the entire potato is compromised. When buying canned sweets, compare sodium content and calories among brands. Some may have added sugar.

Once you've selected the best potatoes, you could make candied sweets, but why not try one of these healthier but equally delicious options?

Make a super sub. Substitute sweet potatoes for white in your mashed potato recipe. Season with ground cinnamon and nutmeg instead of salt and pepper.

Bake a special treat. Bake sweet potatoes at 400°F for 40 to 50 minutes. Top with a touch of maple syrup, ground ginger, and chopped pecans instead of butter or sour cream. Tempt your kids by tossing on a few mini marshmallows.

Have a sweet good morning. Try Bruce's Sweet Potato Pancake Mix for breakfast (visit www.brucefoods.com).

TOMATOES

Sauce for the Gander

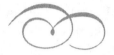

ROVER MAY BE A GUY'S MOST FAITHFUL COMPANION, BUT a gorgeous tomato is his true best friend. A growing pile of research shows that a compound found in tomatoes and tomato products, such as spaghetti sauce, can cut your risk of certain cancers by up to 40 percent. Isn't life sweet?

PIZZA PARTY

Red tomatoes and all the yummy foods that you make with them—even pizza—are teeming with lycopene, an antioxidant that caught the attention of scientists in 1995. That's when Harvard researchers released the results of a study involving 47,000 men ages 40 to 75.

During the six-year project, doctors diagnosed 812 cases of prostate cancer

...Just the facts

Tomato (1 medium)
Calories: 35
Fat: Less than 1 g
Saturated fat: 0 g
Cholesterol: 0 mg
Sodium: 5 mg
Total carbohydrates: 7 g
Dietary fiber: 1 g
Protein: 1 g
Vitamin A: 20% of Daily
    Value
Vitamin C: 40%

among the study participants. The researchers wanted to see if there were differences between the diets of the men who developed this all-too-common cancer and those who remained healthy.

Of the more than 40 foods examined, they found that only 4 protected against prostate cancer. Of those, 3 were good sources of lycopene—tomato sauce, tomatoes, and pizza. (Strawberries were the other beneficial food.) Eating tomatoes or tomato products twice a week, the researchers concluded, could lower prostate cancer risk by 20 to 40 percent.

A SAUCE FOR ALL REASONS

Four years later, the Harvard researchers analyzed 72 studies that dealt with the relationship between lycopene and preven-

← Hit the Sauce →

Some tomato products pack more cancer-fighting lycopene than the fruit itself does. Use this chart to calculate how to get your 30 milligrams of lycopene daily, the amount suggested by many researchers.

Tomato Treat	Lycopene (mg)
Tomato sauce (½ cup)	21.9
Tomato juice (¾ cup)	19.8
Tomato paste (2 tablespoons)	18.2
Vegetable juice cocktail (¾ cup)	17.6
Tomato puree (¼ cup)	10.4
Chopped raw tomato (½ cup)	8.3
Ketchup (2 tablespoons)	5.2

tion of any type of cancer. A whopping 57 of those studies found that frequently eating tomatoes and tomato products reduced the risk of cancer, especially prostate, lung, and stomach cancers. Lycopene may also help ward off breast, cervical, and colon cancers, the researchers found.

In fact, another group of researchers is now trying to determine whether eating more tomato products will improve the outcomes for breast cancer patients or those who are at high risk for the disease because of genetic susceptibility.

The Harvard researchers are also examining whether having one or two servings of tomato products daily can keep heart disease at bay, since preliminary research suggests that lycopene may lower "bad" low-density lipoprotein (LDL) cholesterol.

Best if Used By

To keep that "just-picked" quality:

- Store ripe tomatoes at room temperature, out of direct sunlight, to preserve their flavor.
- Place partially ripe tomatoes in a paper bag with an apple or a banana to speed ripening; keep the bag out of direct sunlight,
- Refrigerate only when you need to extend their shelf life.

YOUR DAILY DOSE

How much lycopene do you need to consume to get these health benefits? "We're not exactly sure, but getting 30 milligrams a day seems to offer protection," says A.V. Rao, Ph.D., professor of nutrition at the University of Toronto.

That's a cinch to do: Just have ¾ cup of tomato juice, a single tomato or a bowl of pasta with tomato sauce, and a few tablespoons of ketchup.

TUNE IN TO TOMATOES

There's nothing like a tomato picked fresh from your garden, and I'm counting the days until ours ripen! If you don't have garden-grown tomatoes, be choosy about supermarket or farmers' market fare. Look for those that are smooth, plump, firm, and fragrant. Aroma is important; if you can't smell a thing, the tomatoes are immature and probably will never ripen. If you want to use your tomatoes in the next day or two, select ripe fruits that yield to your touch. Not planning on using them until later in the week? Then opt for those that are partially ripe. They'll be light pink.

Now try these tempting treats.

Make them the main attraction. Sure, you put tomatoes in your green salad, but then they're just the supporting cast. To give them top billing, make tomato-cucumber salad (⅔ cup of chopped tomatoes and ⅓ cup of chopped cucumbers tossed in Italian dressing) or tomato-basil salad (1 cup of chopped tomatoes and ¼ cup of chopped basil leaves drizzled with balsamic vinaigrette).

Make 60-second sauce. Try this recipe, courtesy of the California Tomato Commission. Coarsely chop three or four medium tomatoes. In a large saucepan, make the pasta of your choice according to the package directions. While it's cooking, combine the tomatoes, 1 tablespoon of olive oil, ¾ teaspoon of sugar, ½ teaspoon of black pepper, 2 teaspoons of balsamic vinaigrette, and 2 tablespoons of chopped parsley in a food processor or blender, then puree. Drain the pasta and return it to the pot, add the sauce, and heat on low.

WATERMELON

Cancer Chiller

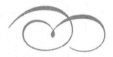

CLEARLY, THE VERY BEST WAY TO EAT WATERMELON IS TO sit with your legs dangling over the edge of a pier and spit the seeds into the water. You should be wearing your bathing suit, and the juice should be dripping off your chin and elbows. There should be plenty of kids around to compete to see who can spit the seeds the farthest. And when you're done, you should dive into the water to clean up and cool off. Barring that, second place goes to the more civilized plate, knife, and fork method of indulging in this sweetest of all cancer fighters.

GET THE RED OUT

Red watermelon is rich in lycopene, one of the six active carotenoids that create the red, orange, and yellow colors in

...Just the facts

Watermelon (1 cup cubed)
Calories: 49
Fat: 1 g
Saturated fat: 0 g
Cholesterol: 0 mg
Sodium: 3 mg
Total carbohydrates: 11 g
Dietary fiber: 1 g
Protein: 1 g
Vitamin A: 11% of Daily
    Value
Vitamin B$_6$: 11%
Vitamin C: 16%

Wash any dirt off the watermelon rind before you cut it so you don't drag soil and bacteria through the melon with the first slice. Cover cut surfaces with plastic wrap or store chunks in airtight containers. Once the melon is cut, its quality can deteriorate quickly, so go ahead and eat it.

foods and are now being scrutinized for their power to prevent various cancers.

At least two studies have shown that lycopene is tops when it comes to gobbling up a dangerous type of oxygen before it can damage your cells and start them on the road to becoming cancer. Both studies found that men who ate the most lycopene-rich foods had the least chance of developing prostate cancer. Although the men got most of their lycopene from tomatoes, analyses show that watermelon delivers one-third more of this carotenoid than fresh tomatoes do.

A POWERFUL PICK-ME-UP

Absolutely nothing tastes as good as a big chunk of ice-cold watermelon after a game of tennis or a long, hot afternoon of yard work. Watermelon is, after all, more than 90 percent water, so it goes a long way toward quenching your thirst.

What's more, watermelon's natural sugars are refreshing! They'll boost your energy and get your blood sugar (your brain's only food) back to normal, so you'll be physically coordinated and able to think straight. And like most commercial sports drinks, watermelon packs potassium, which is especially important for maintaining normal heart rate in people who take diuretics.

STRAIGHT TO THE HEART

Scrimping on potassium can also open the door to rising blood pressure, a major risk factor for heart attack and stroke.

Getting plenty of vegetables and fruit, such as watermelon, has been shown to lower high blood pressure. Also on the heart front, most of the fiber in watermelon is the soluble kind that ties up cholesterol in your intestinal tract so you don't reabsorb it, and that helps lower your total blood cholesterol. What a sweet, wonderful way to a healthy heart!

SOLVING THE WATERMELON MYSTERY

Want wonderful watermelon? Be choosy! Remember: A whole watermelon gives very few clues as to what's inside. Unlike cantaloupe or honeydew, with watermelon, the fragrance won't guide you. And the "thump" test turns out to be bogus (although it's still fun).

Fortunately, most places that sell whole watermelons also provide cut pieces, which may give clues to the quality of their whole melons. Always check out the pieces to be sure that most of them look red, ripe, and juicy and that the flesh looks dense and firm. If so, it's probably safe to buy a whole watermelon, following these directions from the National Watermelon Promotion Board, which says that choosing is as easy as 1, 2, 3.

1. *Look it over.* Choose one that's firm, symmetrical, and free of bruises, cuts, and dents.

2. *Lift it up.* The melon should be heavy for its size. Watermelon is 92 percent water, which accounts for most of its weight.

3. *Check the bottom.* On the

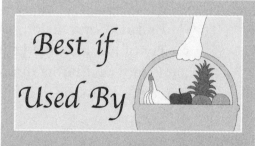

Watermelon ripens on the vine, not on your kitchen counter, so basically, what you buy is what you get. To keep your melon at the peak of flavor, chill it promptly. A whole melon will keep for about a week in the refrigerator.

underside of the watermelon, there should be a creamy yellow spot that formed as it sat on the ground and ripened in the sun. If the melon's underbelly is still green or white, it's probably immature.

Here are a few fun and festive ways to serve watermelon.

Freeze it. Remove the seeds (or use a seedless variety), cut the melon into chunks, and puree it in your blender. Freeze the juice in ice-cube trays, adding little sticks for tasty pops.

Shape it. Thinly slice seedless watermelon or watermelon heart. Using cookie cutters, cut the slices into festive shapes to match the occasion.

Ball it. Get a melon baller with two sizes. Scoop out a variety of big and little balls to add to fruit salad, then shape the empty rind into a disposable serving basket for the salad. Puree the odd-shaped leftovers for ice pops (see above).

Layer it. Alternate thin slices of lean ham and watermelon on a bed of dark green lettuce for a cool, no-cook luncheon salad.

Cheese it. Surround a serving of calcium-enriched cottage cheese with watermelon cubes. Dust with ground cinnamon and garnish with a mint sprig.

DIABETES

Lower Your Insulin Resistance

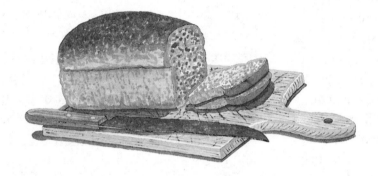

SOME CONDITIONS ANNOUNCE THEMSELVES WITH OB-vious symptoms—a sharp pain in the chest, difficulty breathing, or stiffness in the joints. Not so with diabetes. It's stealthy, which is why many of us are walking around with the beginnings of the disease and don't even know it.

For example, the only clue Evie had that something might be out of whack was that she was always running to the store for creams to treat repeated yeast infections. Her doctor eventually tested her blood and found that her blood sugar (glucose) level was high—a hallmark of diabetes. When you think about it, the link makes sense, because yeast infections thrive in high-sugar environments, which is exactly what diabetes creates.

When you eat, the food is converted to blood sugar. Your

pancreas then secretes the hormone insulin, which whisks the glucose from your bloodstream and plunks it into your cells for energy. Any leftover glucose in the bloodstream is stored in your liver as glycogen. If your insulin level drops too low, the liver releases glycogen into the bloodstream so you always have a ready supply for energy.

In diabetes, however, this tidy system for controlling blood sugar goes awry. In the rarer type 1 diabetes, the pancreas makes little or no insulin. People typically develop this type as kids or young adults and must take injections of insulin for the rest of their lives to keep their blood sugar stable.

In type 2 diabetes—which accounts for 90 percent of cases and can develop in people of any age—the body makes adequate or even high amounts of insulin, yet the cells are unable to use it because they've become insulin resistant. The result? Blood sugar isn't absorbed into the cells and is left to wander around the bloodstream, where it can wreak havoc. It not only feeds yeast infections but also damages major organs and sets the stage for a heart attack, stroke, or other serious diseases.

GOOD CARBS VS. BAD CARBS

Type 2 diabetes is about lifestyle. "We were not meant to gorge on huge quantities of simple sugars, like soft drinks, or starches, like potatoes, and then just sit around," says Richard K.

Bernstein, M.D., who specializes in diabetes and obesity in Mamaroneck, New York. Whole grains are digested slowly, but refined grains and sugar—fast-acting carbs, as Dr. Bernstein calls them—literally flood the system with glucose. If you don't immediately burn off the glucose (and, honestly, how many of us go off for a sprint after wolfing down a Cinnabon?), the pancreas sends out a surge of insulin to get the sugar out of circulation. Over time, the pancreas poops out on producing insulin, the cells become insulin resistant, and blood sugar takes over.

Beyond flooding your system with glucose, those fast-acting carbohydrates also just make you fat—often around the midsection, which is another contributing factor for diabetes. Carbs from your Cap'n Crunch breakfast quickly spike your blood sugar, but a crash soon follows. You become hungry again, so you eat more— and you gain weight. Today, a third more Americans have diabetes than eight years ago, and this expanded figure is directly related to our expanding waistlines.

STAY ON AN EVEN KEEL

If you are 20 pounds above your ideal weight, have a spare tire around your middle, or have other risk factors (such as a

FOOD NEWS

Here's how to lower the glycemic index of your favorite foods.

• Choose bananas that are bit underripe—that is, still a little green at the tip. They produce half the glycemic response of ripe bananas and are less likely to spike your blood sugar, says Thomas Wolever, Ph.D.

• Gram for gram, potatoes are converted to blood sugar faster than any other food—including sugar sprinkled on cereal. If you're a spud lover, you could opt for potato salad made with unpeeled potatoes and vinaigrette dressing. The acid in the dressing will reduce the effect on your blood sugar. To do the same with French fries, simply eat them the British way—doused with vinegar.

family history of diabetes; Hispanic, African American, or Native American heritage; or high blood pressure), two tests—the fasting plasma glucose test and the glucose tolerance test—could help you head off diabetes. They can determine if you have prediabetes, meaning that your glucose levels are higher than is healthy but too low to be diagnosed as diabetes.

Whether the tests reveal diabetes or prediabetes—or neither—all of us would benefit from steadying our bouncing blood sugar levels, and there are myriad ways to do just that. Even the smallest changes in your diet and activity level can lower your glucose to healthier levels—and, if you're taking medication to control blood sugar, you may be able to cut back on or even eliminate your doses. Here's where to start—with your doctor's approval, of course.

Choose low GI foods. Those Cinnabons, along with ice cream, potatoes, and even corn and carrots, rank high on the GI, or glycemic index, which is basically a list of foods ranked by how much they boost your blood sugar after eating them. By eating foods lower on the GI scale at every meal for a month—for example, trading Cheerios for rice bran, having rye bread instead of a Kaiser roll, and eating more legumes and whole, unpeeled veggies—you may reduce your blood sugar and insulin by a third, according to research conducted by Thomas Wolever, Ph.D., professor of nutritional science and medicine at the University of Toronto. Be sure to bypass packaged, processed foods as well, since they're all rated super-high on the GI.

Fill up on fiber. Getting 50 grams of fiber daily—double the amount normally recommended—may lower insulin resistance, studies show. Those fiber-rich psyllium powders sold in drugstores and supermarkets could help you meet that goal, but select brands without sugars or laxatives, follow the package directions, and consult your doctor before using them.

Find grassy cows. Compared with milk produced by grain-fed cows, milk from grass-fed cows contains twice as much conjugated linoleic acid (CLA), which, in supplement form, has been found to decrease blood sugar levels fivefold in people with diabetes. While CLA looks promising for reversing insulin resistance, says Diane Guthrie, Ph.D., a nurse practitioner with the Mid-American Diabetes Association in Wichita, it's not clear how much you need in order to benefit. "I suggest you make sure you get CLA from food sources," she says. Besides milk, these include beef, lamb, eggs, and turkey.

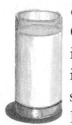

Beware of hidden sugar. A high intake of high-fructose corn syrup—now the leading sweetener in packaged foods— may put you on the road to insulin resistance. "Stay away from foods that have ingredients ending in '-ose' at the top of the list," advises Dr. Bernstein. And don't be conned into thinking that brown sugar, raw sugar, or any other sugar is "healthy." To your body, sugar is sugar.

A SIMPLE SOLUTION

Who said controlling your blood sugar has to be hard? According to a small study at the University of Colorado Health Sciences Center in Loveland, taking a 30-minute soak in a hot tub six days a week for one month may inch down your glucose level enough for you to reduce your insulin dose. The hot water may simulate exercise by increasing the blood flow to muscles, thus reducing insulin resistance. Talk to your doctor before trying hot-tub therapy, though; if you have nerve damage or impaired circulation, it may not be right for you.

Cold-water fish such as tuna and salmon are the prime source of omega-3 essential fatty acids, which appear to help cells become less resistant to insulin. If you're not much of a fish eater, consider supplementing with 1 to 2 grams of fish oil in capsule form or 1 to 2 tablespoons of flaxseed oil a day for the same effect. Both are available in health food stores and some drugstores. *Note:* If you already have diabetes, fish oil may have no effect. Also, people taking aspirin or prescription blood thinners should not take fish oil or flaxseed oil.

Hit the sack. It'll not only enhance your beauty, it will also help your blood sugar. In fact, studies show that if you're short-changing yourself by as little as 2½ hours of sleep a night, you may be 40 percent less sensitive to insulin than you would be if you got your full 8 hours.

Cancel your sweet tooth. Ever feel helpless to resist the lure of a candy bar? Well, help is here, in the form of an Indian herb called gymnema, which means "sugar destroyer" in Sanskrit. When the leaf is chewed, it decreases the ability of the taste buds to detect sweet flavors. Gymnema capsules, which you can find at health food stores, also make sugar distasteful, says Dr. Guthrie. "I suggest taking 200 milligrams twice a day, about a half hour before breakfast and then again before supper." Just one caveat: Gymnema can lower blood sugar too much, so consult your doctor before you take it.

Find fenugreek. Nutty, maple-flavored fenugreek seeds are used to flavor Indian curries, but they may do more than provide taste: They may also lower blood sugar, says Kathi Head, N.D., a naturopathic physician

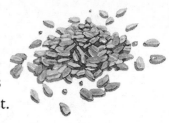

in Sandpoint, Idaho. To get enough, she suggests adding about 2 tablespoons of defatted fenugreek powder (available in health food stores) to yogurt or a smoothie once a day. If you're taking diabetes medications, however, check with your doctor first.

Assess another risk. If you have polycystic ovary syndrome (POS), as 10 percent of American women of childbearing age do, you should be tested for diabetes. Having POS puts you at seven times the normal risk of getting diabetes, although it's unclear why. One theory is that because the ovaries are part of the endocrine system, which regulates not only when you get your period but also your insulin output, a glitch in one may cause a glitch in the other.

BARLEY

Pearls of Wisdom

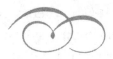

A LOT OF NUTRITION INFORMATION IS DELIVERED WITH caveats, and you've probably heard them all: "More research is needed," "these are preliminary findings," and so forth. Well, here's a fact: Barley is beneficial for your blood sugar and your heart.

Some recent research findings show how barley helps control type 2 diabetes. In one study, at the University of California, Davis, researchers gave men meals made with regular pasta or pasta with barley flour. The guys who chowed down on the barley pasta didn't produce as much insulin (the hormone that plays a major role in diabetes) as those who ate the other pasta.

Also, a Harvard study of women suggests that eating whole grains such as barley low-

...Just the facts

Pearl barley (1 cup cooked)
Calories: 193
Fat: 1 g
Saturated fat: 0 g
Cholesterol: 0 mg
Sodium: 5 mg
Total carbohydrates: 44 g
Dietary fiber: 6 g
Protein: 4 g
Folate: 7% of Daily Value
Niacin (vitamin B$_3$): 16%
Iron: 11%
Magnesium: 9%
Phosphorus: 9%
Zinc: 8%

ers the risk of type 2 diabetes, so it makes sense to add a little barley to your soups, salads, and side dishes.

AND THE BEAT GOES ON

Sadly, people with diabetes are more likely than others to have early heart disease. That's why the latest scoop on barley's secret ingredients will make your heart go pitter-pat.

Researchers at Texas A&M University in College Station tested the effect of barley bran flour, barley oil capsules, and wheat flour on men and women with high cholesterol levels. All the participants followed a low-fat diet for about a month. The result: Those who used either kind of barley significantly lowered their cholesterol levels and their blood pressure.

So what's the magic ingredient? Researchers think that several compounds in barley work together to keep your ticker trouble-free. First, barley contains beta-glucan, a type of fiber that study after study has shown to lower cholesterol. (By the way, it's also what gives barley its creamy texture.) Beta-glucan traps some fat and cholesterol from the foods you eat and ushers them out of your body before they can be absorbed.

Barley also boasts tocotrienol, which triggers a series of events that tell your liver to produce less artery-clogging low-density lipoprotein (LDL) cholesterol. Researchers are also testing a few other hard-to-pronounce substances in barley to see if they play a role. Stay tuned.

Also, if you're having trouble with constipation, you may not be getting the 25 to 30 grams of fiber you need daily. Just 1 cup of cooked barley can provide 6 to 14 grams of fiber. That's sure to get things moving in a hurry!

BARLEY BEST-BUYS

The next time you wander down the rice aisle at your supermarket, look for barley, which is sold in a variety of forms. Here's what's available.

• *Pearl barley.* When barley is pearled, the husk is removed and the kernel is polished. Although this process strips the grain of at least one-third of its fiber, pearl barley still packs a sizable amount.

• *Hulled barley.* Here you get the whole grain. A cup of cooked hulled barley offers 14 grams of fiber—half of what you need for the entire day.

• *Quick-cooking barley.* This variety can be fully cooked in just 10 to 12 minutes, while pearl and hulled types generally take 45 and 95 minutes, respectively.

After you've chosen your barley, try these stylish serving suggestions.

Simmer a side dish. In a large skillet, sauté ½ cup of sliced fresh mushrooms in 2 teaspoons of olive oil. Add 1 cup of pearl barley, 3 cups of low-sodium chicken or vegetable broth, ¼ teaspoon of dried rosemary, and 2 tablespoons of minced onion. Bring to a boil. Cover and cook for 45 minutes, or until the barley is tender and the liquid is absorbed.

Stir it into soup. Add cooked barley to your canned or homemade favorites. Mmm!

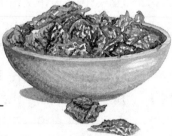

Add it to salads. Have some leftover cold barley? Stir it into your favorite salad along with a little tuna or chicken for a complete meal in a bowl.

BEETS

Keep Sugar on the Level

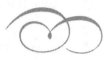

WAY BACK WHEN, ONE OF MY CHILDHOOD PLAYMATES proudly gave me a handful of fresh beets she had grown in her own backyard garden. I went running home, eager to have my mom cook them up for dinner. Unfortunately, their earthy taste was a bit much for me then. (New research says kids need to taste a new food 15 times before they consider it edible!) So I abandoned beets.

That didn't seem like much of a problem, though, since nutritionists stuck beets on the back burner. After all, they offered only trivial amounts of the "big" vitamins, such as A and C. (Who knew about phytochemicals then?)

Later, the authors of those high-pro-

...Just the facts

Beets (1 cup fresh, cooked)
Calories: 75
Fat: 0 g
Saturated fat: 0 g
Cholesterol: 0 mg
Sodium: 484 mg
Total carbohydrates: 17 g
Protein: 3 g
Dietary fiber: 3 g
Folate: 34% of Daily Value
Vitamin A: 1%
Vitamin C: 7%
Calcium: 3%
Iron: 7%

Here's how to serve the best beets ever.

• Before cooking, scrub beets well but gently, trying not to break the skins. Leave the short stems and taproots on for color containment.

• After cooking, peel, slice, and dice. Add vinegar or lemon juice to preserve the crimson color.

tein, low-carbohydrate diet books started bashing beets. Somehow, they got the idea that beets are loaded with sweet ingredients that raise blood sugar and insulin production and cause insulin resistance and even diabetes. They were wrong. Today, beets are starting to look better, now that the facts are finally becoming known.

TAME BLOOD SUGAR

Here's why beets got a bad rap for raising blood sugar levels. When you eat carbohydrates, they become blood sugar, also known as glucose. In your blood, glucose pairs up with insulin, which coaxes your cells to open up and let the glucose in so it can be used for fuel.

Some people's cells are reluctant to cooperate; that is, they're insulin resistant. Insulin resistance has been linked to heart disease, high blood pressure, and diabetes. Some carbohydrate foods raise blood sugar slowly, making it easier for resistant cells to accept it, while others raise it rapidly, which aggravates the problem.

Beets were thought to be in the second category, but it turns out that their effect is merely moderate. In fact, a full cup of cooked beets packs about the same amount of carbohydrates as a slice of whole wheat bread—and raises your blood sugar even more slowly. So eat your beets.

DELIVER TLC

Beets are beneficial in many other ways, too. How many can you think of? Here are just a few.

• Beets are shaped like little hearts for a reason: Just 1 cup of fresh beets delivers one-third of your folate requirement for the day. That's the B vitamin noted for keeping homocysteine in check so that it can't trigger a heart attack. (Getting enough folate also dramatically reduces neural tube birth defects.)

• Then, of course, there's cancer. Betacyanin, the phytochemical that gives beets their deep red color, may be a cancer fighter. Research done in Russia suggests that beet juice may help inhibit normal, healthy cells from mutating into cancer cells.

• Beets are also a good source of fiber, delivering about 3 grams in each cupful. Most Americans get only half of the recommended 25 to 30 grams of fiber needed daily for good bowel function. Constipation makes you feel tired and cranky, so who needs it? Have a glass of water, eat your beets, and get moving!

• Finally, if you need an edible red dye, forget artificial food coloring and use beet juice instead. Tests show that, unlike some synthetic dyes, beet juice is safe because it doesn't trigger liver cancer cell growth.

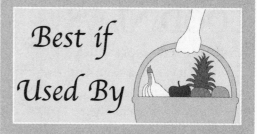

Best if Used By

Protect your fresh beets, and they'll protect you. Here's what to do.

• Before storing, trim any leaves to ½ inch long. If they've already been clipped, be sure there's at least ½ inch of stem.

• Leave about 2 inches of taproot, too, to keep the beets from bleeding all over everything.

• Store fresh beets in a plastic bag in the refrigerator, where they'll keep for up to three weeks.

GET READY FOR BEET TREATS

Fresh beets come in a range of sizes, from radish-size babies to 2½-inch-diameter giants. The babies are gourmet fare and

FOOD NEWS

Beets' red color comes from betacyanin, a pigment some folks can't process very well, so it turns their urine and feces red or pink. Don't be alarmed if this happens to you; it's completely harmless.

may be expensive, and the giants may be woody and tough, so shoot for the mid-size beets, about 1½ inches in diameter. These young beets are perfect for most uses. Look for smooth, hard, round, deep red beets with thin taproots. Any attached leaves should be small, fresh, and green.

Now, head for your kitchen and try out some colorful dishes!

Roast. For the most intense, earthy flavor, scrub whole beets, brush them with olive oil, and place them on a baking sheet in a 375°F oven. Bake the beets for 35 to 60 minutes (depending on their size) until they can be pierced easily with a sharp knife. You can roast potatoes and carrots at the same time for a colorful root-vegetable side dish.

Grate. For an unusual salad, cover a lettuce leaf with a pile of grated carrot, a mound of grated fresh beets, and a heap of thinly sliced cucumber.

Chill. Keep a can of baby beets in the fridge. Toss them into winter salads for cheery color and to balance the taste of bitter greens.

BROWN RICE

The Living Color

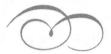

CHANCES ARE, YOU LOVE RICE; MOST of us eat about 25 pounds of it each year. Unfortunately, it's usually the white kind. This is too bad because, as our friend Ellen keeps saying, brown rice overshadows its paler cousin in nearly every vitamin and mineral. Even more to the point, brown rice is the *whole* grain, and that's important for fending off diabetes.

"Did you know that all rice actually starts out brown?" Ellen asks with an admonishing wag of her finger. The grain is harvested in its hull, a hard, inedible covering that protects whole brown kernels. To make rice look shiny and white, manufacturers remove the kernels' husk, bran, and germ—refine it, in other words. Yet, researchers have found that these are

...Just the facts

Brown rice (⅔ cup cooked)
Calories: 170
Fat: 1.5 g
Saturated fat: 0 g
Cholesterol: 0 mg
Sodium: 10 mg
Total carbohydrates: 34 g
Dietary fiber: 2 g
Protein: 4 g
Niacin (vitamin B_3): 8% of Daily Value
Copper: 4%
Iron: 2%
Magnesium: 15%
Zinc: 6%

the parts that store a vast array of vitamins, minerals, and disease-fighting phytochemicals. Happily, these components, and the nutrients they contain, remain intact in brown rice.

THE BENEFITS OF BROWN

So what are all those nutrients going to do for you? Take a look at this.

• *Diminish the danger of diabetes.* A study of more than 65,000 nurses revealed that those who ate large amounts of refined grains had twice the risk of developing diabetes as those who consumed mostly unrefined carbohydrates, such as whole grains. Now, a group of researchers at Harvard is examining why brown rice and other whole grains seem to protect you from type 2 diabetes. "Your pancreas needs to quickly secrete a lot of insulin for your body to absorb refined carbohydrates," explains Walter Willett, M.D., chairperson of Harvard's department of nutrition. "Over time, your pancreas may slow down insulin production, triggering diabetes."

• *Hinder heart disease.* A study conducted at Columbia University in New York City suggests that women who eat

← *The Rice Cook-Off* →

Which is healthier—brown or white rice? Here are the facts; you can tally up the score.

Rice (½ cup cooked)	Fiber (g)	Vitamin E (mg)	Phosphorus (mg)
Brown	1.60	2	79
White	0.03	0	34

three daily servings of whole grains, such as brown rice, have a 27 percent lower risk of developing heart disease than those who eat only refined grains, such as white rice.

Another study found that eating two servings of whole grains daily can reduce the risk of dying from a heart attack by about 30 percent. "We're now trying to determine what exactly it is in whole grains that seems to be protective—the fiber, the vitamins and minerals, the phytochemicals, or the entire package," says Lawrence Kushi, Sc.D., professor of human nutrition at Columbia. In the meantime, feel free to chow down on brown rice and other whole grains!

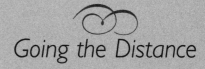

Going the Distance

If you choose regular rice, you'll need to decide on the length of grain you'd like.

• Medium grain is considered the all-purpose length. Instant rice almost always comes in a medium grain.

• Short grain works best in puddings and stuffings.

• Long grain is ideal for pilafs, salads, and stir-fries.

TAKE YOUR CHOICE

You'll find a couple of different types of brown rice at your local supermarket.

• *Regular brown rice.* If you're not racing to beat the clock, opt for regular brown rice because it has better flavor and consistency than the instant version. You can also speed the cooking process for regular rice by using a rice cooker or by soaking the rice in water for 2 to 3 hours beforehand.

• *Instant brown rice.* For those days when you don't have a second to spare in the kitchen, try a package of instant brown rice. It'll be ready to eat in just 10 minutes—a far cry from the

30 to 45 minutes that traditional brown rice takes.

You can use brown rice in virtually any dish that calls for white rice. It'll add a slightly nutty flavor and heartier texture. Try these brown rice treats.

Take a slow boat to China. Use whole grain brown rice in your favorite Chinese dishes, such as moo shu chicken. You can even ask Chinese restaurants to substitute it for the sticky white rice they usually deliver.

Ride an elephant to Thailand. You'll think you're in Bangkok when you fix brown rice with a spicy seafood stir-fry.

Vacation at home. What's as American as Mom's apple pie? How about chicken and (brown) rice soup?

CURRY POWDER

Sugar and Spice

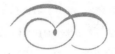

DON'T YOU LOVE TO EAT AT LITTLE NEIGHBORHOOD Indian restaurants? Besides not having to wash the dishes, you get that wonderful curry flavor. Curry powder, made from as many as 20 different spices, including cinnamon, coriander, nutmeg, and turmeric, plays a starring role on the menu at all Indian restaurants. What's more, this dynamic quartet plays a surprising role in helping to control blood sugar.

SOAK UP SUGAR

I don't mean to scare you, but people are getting type 2 diabetes earlier and earlier. It used to appear in folks in their forties and fifties; now it's showing up in people in their twenties. This type of diabetes can be the result of your bad habits—too much high-calorie, high-fat food and not enough exercise—catching

> ### ...Just the facts
>
> Curry powder (1 tsp)
> Calories: 7
> Fat: 0 g
> Saturated fat: 0 g
> Cholesterol: 0 mg
> Sodium: 1 mg
> Total carbohydrates: 1 g
> Dietary fiber: 1 g
> Protein: 0 g

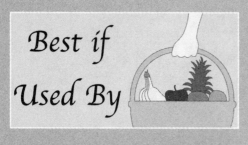

Best if Used By

Store curry powder in a cool, dry, dark place. If you reseal it after each use, it'll last for a few months before losing its kick.

up with you. But with a better diet, regular exercise, and perhaps a few spices, you may be able to ward off this condition, or at least diminish its severity.

When you have diabetes, your body either doesn't make enough insulin, the hormone that delivers glucose (blood sugar) to your cells, or is unable to use it properly. Turmeric, along with bay leaves, cinnamon, and cloves, can help regulate your insulin levels. In lab studies, this foursome spice creation tripled the ability of insulin to metabolize glucose. More research is under way, but in the meantime, it can't hurt to be, well, a little spicy.

KILL CANCER

Turmeric, the spice that lends curry powder its distinctive yellow color, is probably a potent cancer crusader. Preliminary studies from India suggest that two compounds in the spice—curcumin I and II—possess cancer-fighting properties and boost the immune system. Researchers around the world are trying to pin down the details. Here's what they've learned so far.

• A British study found that turmeric may inhibit production of an enzyme found in high levels in people with certain cancers, including those of the bowel and colon.

• Research at Columbia University College of Physicians and Surgeons in New York City suggests that turmeric may help in the fight against prostate cancer, too.

Stay tuned. You'll probably hear about more studies on the

news soon. Meanwhile, if heartburn has its evil spell on you, sprinkle a little curry powder on your food. Turmeric stimulates the flow of digestive juices, which helps stave off the buildup of heartburn-provoking acid.

GO EXOTIC

There are up to 20 different spices in traditional curry powder, so unless you have a big budget and a lot of time, buy the prepackaged spice instead of making your own.

Curry powder is readily available in your supermarket. Almost every spice manufacturer makes it—although some with more success than others. When staffers at the *Seattle Times* taste-tested several brands of curry powder, they found that these two were tops.

• *Spice Islands Curry Powder.* The testers described it as having a "smooth quality and soft golden color."

• *Trikona Mild Curry Powder.* This brand was touted for its "rich golden color and deep, spicy flavor."

Now, here are some all-American approaches to using this traditional Indian flavor.

Add zip to dips. Stir a teaspoon or two of curry powder into a cup of low-fat plain yogurt. Serve with baked tortilla chips or warm pita bread.

Garnish garbanzos. Mix a can of drained, rinsed chickpeas with a couple of teaspoons of curry powder and bake at 375°F for 12 to 15 minutes.

Make snazzy snacks. Sprinkle curry powder on air-popped popcorn or even low-fat chips. It'll give them a shot of flavor!

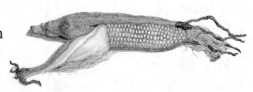

PEAS

Starch Blockers

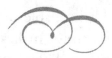

...Just the facts

Green peas (½ cup cooked)
Calories: 67
Fat: 0 g
Saturated fat: 0 g
Cholesterol: 0 mg
Sodium: 2 mg
Total carbohydrates: 13 g
Dietary fiber: 4 g
Protein: 4 g
Folate: 13% of Daily Value
Calcium: 2%
Copper: 7%
Iron: 7%
Zinc: 6%

WHEN MY KIDS WERE LITTLE, I LIKED TO TAKE THEM TO "pick-your-own" farms so they'd know where food really comes from. It was a real eye-opener finding out that not only did early spring peas grow on vines, but they also tasted completely different from their frozen or canned cousins. In fact, those fresh peas were so sweet and delicious that on the way home, the kids ate half of what they'd picked! And that was good news for their blood sugar, weight control, and just about any nutritional concern.

WHAT COLOR ARE YOUR PEAS?

Sometimes it's hard to figure out just where peas fit in the overall scheme of nutrition. Technically, they're green vegetables, but when dietitians talk about greens, they're usually referring to leafy vegetables. Peas are starchy little things, not fibrous veggies packed with vitamins A and C.

Maybe you're thinking that because peas are starchy, they'll make you fat. Think again; peas make a great weapon against weight gain, and here's why. While the starch in peas is pure carbohydrate, it's the slow-moving kind, with a low glycemic index (GI). Unlike high-GI carbs (the kind found in white bread and potatoes) that get sucked into your bloodstream in a rush, the carbs in peas dillydally while being digested. Their energy is released slowly, and that keeps you from getting hungry again too soon.

Two Good!

Worried about high cholesterol? If you replace cold-cut sandwiches with pea soup for lunch, you'll get a double benefit: You'll cut out saturated fat that raises cholesterol and add the soluble fiber that lowers it!

In fact, five out of five studies show that dieters eat fewer snacks after a low-GI meal, says Susan Roberts, Ph.D., director of the energy metabolism laboratory at Tufts University in Boston. If you have diabetes or insulin resistance, a modest portion of peas can also help control the rise of blood sugar and allow time for insulin to work better.

A FAMILY AFFAIR

What about snow peas? Yes! These are more like the traditional "greens" loved by nutritionists. They're immature versions of peas in the pod, so you can eat them whole. Indeed, 1 cup of cooked snow peas packs more vitamin C than you'd get from a cup of cooked spinach or even from an orange—a full day's worth—and more fiber, too. It also provides a little vitamin A, about 4 percent of what you need for the day, so snow peas are great for building and protecting skin and for keeping your bowels working, too. Color snow peas green.

MEAT IN A POD

Okay, if peas aren't a green vegetable, what are they? Try "meat substitute," only better. Here's what they offer.

• *Powerful protein.* One cup of fresh, frozen, or canned green peas provides as much protein as an egg or an ounce of lean beef—without the fat! In fact, 1 cup of peas, plus a cup of fat-free milk, provides more than one-third of your protein for the day. The protein is complete, like the protein in meat, so it's great for building muscle, repairing tissue, boosting your immune system, and bolstering every cell, enzyme, and hormone in your body.

• *Fabulous fiber.* As if that weren't enough, here's a bonus: Peas deliver one-third of your day's fiber—something you never get from meat!

• *Mighty meaty minerals and vitamins.* Except for zinc and vitamin B_{12}, peas match or exceed the vitamin and mineral content of a full 3-ounce serving of lean beef. Color peas powerful protein.

FOOD NEWS

Feeling fit as a fiddle and ready to work out? A bowl of pea soup before your run will fuel you steadily until you're done. Now that's powerful pottage!

PEAS, PLEASE

If you like fresh peas, be ready to rush to the farmers' markets or "pick-your-own" farms in April or May, the only time they're available. Then be ready to rush home and tenderly cook them as fast as you can. Like fresh corn, peas lose that incomparable sweetness quickly. In just 4 to 6 hours, you'll have old peas! When selecting fresh peas, choose plump, bright green pods without blemishes, spots, or yellowing.

Now that your pantry's packed with peas, here's how to get all their benefits.

Treat 'em like meat. Pile peas and a sliced hard-boiled egg on your salad for complete protein along with your veggies.

Kill three birds with one can. Take a can of pea soup for lunch at work and heat it in the microwave. It counts as carbs, protein, and veggies, and it's so easy!

Stir 'em into soup. Pour frozen peas into any soup to provide protein.

Fry 'em. Stir snow peas into a stir-fry at the very last minute for crisp nutrition.

Kiss 'em with carrots. Perk up sugar snap peas with a few cooked carrots. They add color, texture, flavor, and fiber, and the combo is a feast for your eyes!

WHOLE GRAIN CEREAL

A Bran New Day

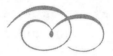

WHAT COULD BE BETTER ON A FROSTY MORNING THAN a steaming bowl of whole grain cereal to coax you into the day? And if your bowl is filled with oatmeal, your heart and all its blood vessels, from your big coronary arteries to your tiniest capillaries, will want to give you a great big hug—a hug you deserve for taking such tasty good care of yourself! And while your heart is doing backflips, your blood sugar will be calmly sending energy to your entire body. Here's why.

THE WHOLE STORY

Oatmeal and oat bran cereals were the first individual foods ever permitted to bear an FDA-approved health claim on their packages. The reason? An impressive pile of research showed that adding oats to

...Just the facts

Dry quick-cooking oats
   (½ cup cooked)
Calories: 155
Fat: 3 g
Saturated fat: 0 g
Cholesterol: 0 mg
Sodium: 2 mg
Total carbohydrates: 27 g
Dietary fiber: 4 g
Protein: 6 g
Thiamin (vitamin B$_1$): 20%
   of Daily Value
Magnesium: 15%
Manganese: 74%

your diet lowers total and low-density lipoprotein (LDL) cholesterol without lowering high-density lipoprotein (HDL) cholesterol, which is just what a struggling heart needs.

Nationwide, hearts started beating louder, because the folks who benefit most from oats are those in greatest jeopardy. With a cholesterol reading of 229 or less, a drop of 2 to 3 percent is common, but at levels above 229, a whopping 4 to 7 percent drop rewards those who skip lumberjack breakfasts and start the day by eating enough oats to provide 3 grams of beta-glucan, its soluble fiber. You'll get that amount from ½ cup of dry (uncooked) oats.

A SIMPLE SOLUTION

Is a case of hives driving you crazy? To soothe the itchiness, soak for 10 to 15 minutes in a bathtub full of warm water and some finely ground colloidal oatmeal, an over-the-counter bath powder made by Aveeno. It stays suspended in water so it won't clog your drain—but it will fix your itch.

A REAL PAGE TURNER

Now the story gets even better. In a recent study of a 500,000-member HMO group, 50 percent of people who were taking blood pressure drugs were able to stop taking them after eating 5 grams of soluble fiber from oatmeal and oatmeal squares every day for four weeks. Another 20 percent were able to cut their doses in half. (*Warning:* Don't try this on your own. Always consult your doctor before making changes in your medication.)

In addition, the patients' total and LDL cholesterol levels dropped, and the side effects of taking blood pressure medication—such as low blood potassium, muscle cramps, sexual dysfunction, and bad moods—vanished.

Researchers speculate that all this has to do with a complex array of interactions that affect insulin resistance, but the details aren't clear yet. Soluble fiber slows the movement of partially digested food through your intestines, trapping cholesterol and bile so your body can't reabsorb them. What's more, that slow-moving digestive mix gradually releases food energy, spurring a

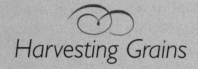

Harvesting Grains

There are plenty of whole grain hot cereals out there, each with its own benefits. Check them out.

• *Oat bran.* Made from the finely ground outer layer of oats, just ½ cup of dry oat bran packs 6 grams of fiber—3 soluble and 3 insoluble. Oat bran is also rich in thiamin, iron, magnesium, phosphorus, and zinc. It's tops for keeping cholesterol at bay.

• *Oatmeal.* This type is made from thinly sliced whole oats, and it contains everything good in the oat—bran, germ, and endosperm. Cooking time depends on the thickness of the slices. About ½ cup of dry quick-cooking oats serves up 4 grams of fiber—2 soluble and 2 insoluble.

• *Whole wheat cereal.* Wheateena and other cereals of this type are made from whole wheat kernels that have been ground. They deliver all the goodness of other whole wheat products—bran, germ, and endosperm—and are tops for maintaining regularity. Just ½ cup of dry whole wheat cereal delivers 4 grams of fiber, 1 soluble and 3 insoluble.

• *Harvest Mornings cereals.* One packet of any of these instant multi-grain cereals made from oatmeal, whole wheat, and barley flakes supplies 3 grams of fiber.

gentle rise in blood sugar that requires only a minimal amount of insulin to help the blood sugar get into cells.

BOUNTIFUL BREAKFASTS

Keep a variety of whole grain cereals on hand and do some breakfast day trading. You'll be nutritionally rich! When selecting cereal, check the "best-used-before" date and look for packages that are well sealed and undamaged.

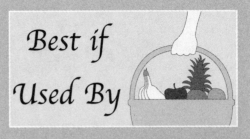

Best if Used By

Store unopened cereals in a cool, dry place. Once you've opened them, store whole grain cereals in the refrigerator. Even bugs are smart enough to go for the good stuff!

Here's how to enjoy whole grain cereal often.

Add fruit and nuts. Microwave a bowl of oat bran and stir in chopped apples, walnuts, and a dash of ground nutmeg.

Have a PBH. Microwave a bowl of whole wheat cereal, then add 1 tablespoon of peanut butter and 2 teaspoons of honey. Yummy!

Use brown bananas. Whip up a bowl of farina, then stir in a mashed overripe banana and a sprinkle of brown sugar. This is tops when your tummy's feeling funky.

Store in your drawer. Keep instant cereal packets in your desk drawer at work. Heat and eat when you need to warm up or chill out.

WHOLE WHEAT BREAD

A Grain of Truth

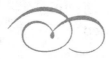

YOU MAY NOT LIVE AS LONG AS METHUSELAH, BUT there's a good chance that you'll increase your life span if you include a couple of pieces of whole wheat bread in your daily diet. That's the conclusion of the Iowa Women's Study, which compared the diets of more than 40,000 women ages 55 to 69 to see how what they ate matched up with the chronic diseases, such as diabetes, they developed over a span of nine years.

The good news: Women who ate at least one serving of whole grain foods daily were 15 percent less likely to die of heart disease, cancer, or any other chronic disease than were women who blew off whole grains and stuck with starch. Further, the study revealed that whole grains, cereal fiber, and dietary magnesium

...Just the facts

Whole wheat bread (1 slice)
Calories: 69
Fat: 1 g
Saturated fat: 0 g
Cholesterol: 0 mg
Sodium: 147 mg
Total carbohydrates: 13 g
Dietary fiber: 2 g
Protein: 3 g
Copper: 4% of Daily Value
Iron: 5%
Manganese: 32%
Zinc: 4%

appear to protect older women from developing type 2 diabetes. So please pass (up) the white and grab the wheat!

THE WHOLE TRUTH

Why is white flour so inferior, healthwise, to whole wheat? The process that turns whole wheat kernels into white flour hangs on to the powdery endosperm but dumps two important parts: the bran and the germ. These two parts are loaded with vitamins, minerals, fiber, and other functional bits and pieces, such as phytic acid, phenols, and saponins, that protect against destructive oxidation and keep your body in tiptop shape.

And it's not just a matter of life and death. Sure, wheat bran's insoluble fiber has been linked to protection against cancer, but comfort counts, too, and the rough stuff protects against embarrassing, usually unmentionable problems, such as constipation, hemorrhoids, and diverticulosis. So whole up, and get things moving!

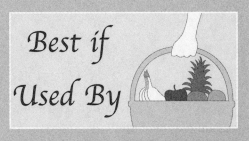

Best if Used By

If you choose 100 percent stone-ground whole wheat bread, store it in the refrigerator to prevent the natural oils from turning rancid. It will last about a week.

WHOLE GRAIN GOODNESS

Be careful in your choice of wheat bread, because there are many pitfalls. Read the ingredients list, found in small print somewhere on the packaging. (You may have to take along a magnifying glass to get the scoop!) Ingredients are listed in order of predominance by

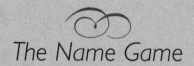

The Name Game

A rose by any other name may smell as sweet, but in the whole grain business, the name is your key to the best bread. Here's a rundown geared to guide you toward the grainiest slices.

• *100 percent stone-ground whole wheat bread.* This bread is made from flour created when wheat kernels are crushed between rolling stones without separating out the bran and germ. One possible drawback: It may turn rancid more quickly since the wheat germ oil is crushed in with the endosperm. Don't let that stop you from buying it, though; just be sure to store it in the refrigerator.

• *Whole wheat bread.* Roller milling, the process used to make flour for whole wheat bread, temporarily separates the bran and germ from the endosperm, which can be ground to the best consistency. The three parts are then reunited to make bread flour. Legally, bread must contain at least 51 percent whole wheat flour to be called whole wheat, but 100 percent is better. When bread is made from only whole wheat flour, it's nutritionally equal to 100 percent stone-ground whole wheat bread.

• *Enriched white bread.* In this case, the roller-milled flour has the bran and germ removed but never restored. Four B vitamins (folic acid, niacin, thiamin, and riboflavin) and iron are added to restore natural levels, but at least 20 other vitamins and minerals, as well as fiber, are permanently AWOL.

• *Wheat bread.* Made from a mixture of mostly white flour and some whole wheat flour, wheat bread is a step up if you're stuck on white bread, but don't stop there. You haven't really arrived yet.

weight. That means there's the most of whatever ingredient is listed first and the least of the ingredient listed last. Choose bread made with only whole wheat flour so you get the biggest nutritional bang per calorie. Some "whole wheat" breads are only 51 percent whole wheat, with white enriched flour as the second ingredient. Also check the Nutrition Facts label for fiber content—the more, the better.

Once you've found the staff of your life, lean on it like this.

Fuel up fast. Spread two slices of whole wheat bread with peanut butter, slap them together, and take off.

Fill your pockets. Pita pockets count as bread! And yes, they come in whole wheat. Toast a pocket until it puffs, let it cool, then slit the side. Fill it with tuna, shrimp, or chicken salad; leftover tossed salad and cheese chunks; or vegetarian refried beans and salsa.

Trim your toast. Cut whole wheat pita pockets into wedges, toast them, and dip in salsa, olive spread, or veggie dip.

Go halvesies. Having a hard time adjusting to the more full-bodied taste of real whole wheat bread? For a while, make your sandwiches with one slice of white and one slice of whole wheat, then bite so that the white touches your tongue.

Two Good!

To get more of two crucial minerals, try whole wheat couscous. It serves up twice as much calcium and four times as much iron as regular couscous.

Part Two

THE HEALTHY HEART

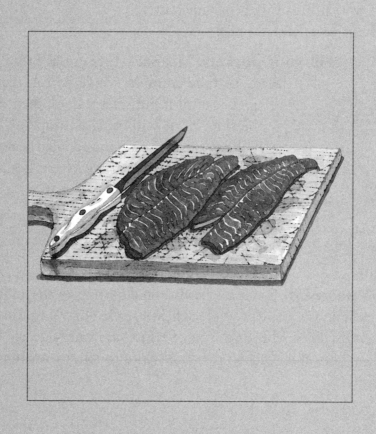

Beat Ticker Shock

Heart disease is the number one killer of both men and women in the United States, but the past 30 years have brought an amazing explosion in knowledge about the lifestyle strategies that can help your heart keep on ticking for a long, long time.

The American Heart Association notes that healthy eating habits can help you reduce three of the major risk factors for heart attack—high cholesterol, high blood pressure, and excess body weight. Also, because heart disease and high blood pressure are major risk factors for stroke, eating well will also help you avoid that threat.

Better still, all the good diet habits that are beneficial for your heart may also reduce your risk of other chronic health problems, such as type 2 diabetes, osteoporosis, and some kinds of cancer. What a bargain!

In the following chapters, we'll introduce you to some major risk factors for heart disease, toss in some lifestyle strategies known to add years to your life, and offer up bunches of healthy foods known to keep your heart ticking merrily away. So read on for a healthier, happier, longer life!

ANGINA

Get It Off Your Chest

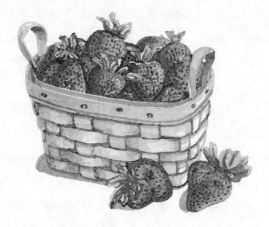

Maybe you've just had a shouting match with your spouse, a four-course meal at your mom's, or an arduous Saturday morning spent hauling bags of gravel to build a serpentine garden path. Suddenly, you feel as if someone has rolled a giant boulder onto your chest. It weighs heavily on your lungs, making it difficult to breathe. You stop what you're doing and take stock, but after a few minutes, the boulder disappears. The pressure eases. You're fine.

But are you really?

YOUR CHEATING HEART

Sudden, heavy chest pressure is a hallmark of angina—chest pain that occurs when your heart can't get enough oxygen because the arteries that deliver blood to it have narrowed.

This occurs either because fatty deposits have accumulated on the insides of the artery walls (coronary artery disease) or, much more rarely, because the arteries are simply in spasm. But angina takes many forms: Sometimes, it can be a shooting pain up your arm; at other times, it's a sharp, squeezing sensation near your shoulders. In women especially, it can even be super-subtle—say, a tiny twinge that radiates toward your neck—and therefore super-scary.

"Angina is the heart's distress call, but it's not an early warning system," says Peter Brunschwig, M.D., director of Helios Integrated Medicine in Boulder, Colorado. "By the time a person gets angina, his arteries have probably already become narrow and weak from a slow buildup of cholesterol-laden plaque." Anyone with angina, no matter how infrequent or fleeting, should consult a doctor immediately to rule out serious heart disease.

THE "FIX" VS. THE "CURE"

If you've been diagnosed with angina due to coronary heart disease, odds are that you have nitroglycerin, the drug equivalent of an American Express card—you simply don't leave home without it. Taking nitroglycerin during an angina attack quickly relaxes the arteries, opening them so oxygen-rich blood can flow easily to your heart—and that breath-sucking boulder can slip easily away. Other drugs, called beta-blockers and calcium channel blockers, do essentially the same thing.

If your angina persists, and your physician finds that the arteries to your heart are very nearly closed due to a pileup of plaque there, she may recommend angioplasty—a surgical procedure that involves inflating a balloon to force open blocked vessels—or bypass surgery to shunt blood flow around the narrowed arteries.

These treatments work in the sense that they increase blood flow to the heart, possibly preventing a heart attack, but while that's hugely significant, it's not a cure. "The very best way to control your angina," explains Dr. Brunschwig, "is to adopt a comprehensive program aimed at lowering plaque." Here are several ways to do that.

Follow Ornish. It's been more than 10 years since studies by renowned heart guru Dean Ornish, M.D., showed that people who eat a low-fat diet loaded with fruits and veggies, exercise regularly, maintain a healthy weight, and manage stress are less likely to be ambushed by angina than sedentary, overweight, stressed-out types. In fact, Dr. Ornish's regimen proved even better for reducing angina than taking cholesterol-lowering drugs. "And the evidence still holds," says Gerdi

Weidner, Ph.D., director of research at Dr. Ornish's Preventive Medicine Research Institute in Sausalito, California. "Our studies show that people who follow our program cut their angina episodes in half."

Include amino acids. The mighty amino acid arginine, much like nitroglycerin, helps relax artery walls and keep the vessels open. In fact, supplemental arginine has been shown to prolong the time people can exercise before chest pain kicks in, which is significant because exercise reduces cholesterol, blood pressure, stress, and weight—all risk factors for heart disease.

A SIMPLE SOLUTION

Sprinkle your Wheaties with wheat germ. The idea is to pad your diet with vitamin E, which is also found in nuts, seeds, olives, and spinach and other green leafy veggies. Vitamin E is an antioxidant, meaning it prevents what's called oxidative damage in cells—including those in the arteries. As a result, low blood levels of vitamin E are associated with higher rates of angina.

Arginine's cousin, carnitine, is an amino acid abundant in red meat that may help strengthen the heart muscle. Robert Bonakdar, M.D., director of pain management and heart health at the Scripps Center for Integrative Medicine in La Jolla, California, recommends that people with angina take 500 milligrams of carnitine a day, but since there's no exact dose for arginine, he suggests asking a doctor about a combination formula that's tailored to their specific condition.

Hook some fish oil. According to the American Heart Association, people with heart disease should take at least 1 gram of fish oil a day, for two reasons. First, the oil that comes from tuna, salmon, and other cold-water fish is packed with omega-3 essential fatty acids (EFAs), which can make red blood cells more slippery and improve their flow, even in tiny capillaries. Second, fish oil helps lower triglycerides—other blood fats that can clog arteries—and stabilize insulin resistance, a major factor in heart disease. Some doctors recommend taking 1 to 3 grams of fish oil in capsule form a day, but talk to your doctor first, especially if you're taking aspirin or prescription blood-thinning medication.

Take control. Some margarine-like spreads, such as Benecol and Take Control, contain plant stanols that block the absorption of cholesterol in the intestines, forcing your liver to snatch it from your bloodstream—and keep it away from your heart. In fact, studies show that people who add plant stanols to a low-fat diet can reduce plaque-building cholesterol by 10 to 24 percent. To get the benefits, you'll need three servings a day of 2 tablespoons each. Spread it on toast at breakfast, crackers at lunch, and a dinner roll at your evening meal. But don't go overboard—these spreads still contain fat.

Try CoQ$_{10}$. "This antioxidant appears to bring oxygen to the heart and may even help curb the damage caused by a lack of oxygen," says Dr. Brunschwig, who recommends taking 100 milligrams a day. You can find CoQ$_{10}$ supplements at health food stores and drugstores.

Abate anger. "People who have angina tend to be hostile," notes Dr. Bonakdar. Anger releases adrenaline, the "fight or flight" hormone that signals a bump up in blood pressure, heart rate, and blood flow away from the heart and to the muscles (so we can fight or flee). All of these physiologic responses can precipitate angina. To help manage your anger and sidestep angina, you might seek the help of a support group. To locate one in your area, contact the cardiac rehabilitation unit at your local hospital.

Turn down tasks. "The behavior that seems to make the most difference in reducing heart disease is managing stress," notes Dr. Bonakdar. "The outside pressure to, say, head another church committee is absolutely matched by the pressure inside your arteries." The best way to minimize that internal pressure? "Say no to mounting demands," he says. As a bonus, once you're not quite so overcommitted, you'll have the time for yoga, deep breathing, or other calming techniques proven to help keep a lid on angina.

Make beautiful music. Beat a drum. Blow a horn. Even pound the ivories. "Music therapy is one of the best outlets there is for stress and aggression," notes Dr. Bonakdar. The physical work of making music releases pent-up energy and emotions. Plus, it improves heart rate, blood pressure, and the ability to sleep soundly—all of which lessen the demands on your heart. Your neighbors may not love your new drum set, but your heart certainly will.

Plant oxygen. If you can muster the energy to plant just one packet of seeds, make them beet seeds. Betacyanin, the compound that gives beets their rich color, may help cells take in more oxygen, so eating fresh beets or freshly grated beetroot

911

Angina and a heart attack differ significantly. While both signal that the heart isn't receiving enough oxygen, the oxygen deprivation and pain associated with angina are temporary and don't damage the heart. The pain of a heart attack, on the other hand, doesn't go away, and the oxygen deprivation can be permanent— or lethal. Be alert to changes in your angina pattern that may signal a heart attack. Call 911 if you have chest pressure, squeezing, fullness, or pain in the center of your chest, or pain in your neck, jaw, shoulders, or arms, that lasts longer than 5 minutes, even if you take nitroglycerin.

in salads could give your heart a breath of fresh air!

See a marriage counselor. If you're a husband who feels your wife doesn't show her love, studies show you're twice as likely as husbands with more demonstrative wives to have angina. Likewise, if you're a withholding wife, anger, depression, or even garden-variety stress may have left you feeling stingy with your emotions—and predisposed to your own chest pain. Let a counselor help you sort out the affairs of the heart, and you may ease pain in your life in more ways than one.

Walk on air. "With your doctor's guidance, you should not be afraid to exercise, as long as it's not an activity where you suddenly break into a sprint," says Dr. Brunschwig. The best way to start is with slow walking. "It reduces cholesterol, blood pressure, stress, and weight," he notes. In fact, if you're overweight, daily walks combined with a low-fat diet could help you lose a pound a week, which studies show can help reduce chest pain.

Help yourself to hawthorn. "Hawthorn is one of the best heart tonics around," says Dr. Brunschwig. "It works to dilate the blood vessels, but it can also help the heart squeeze harder." In fact, studies show that people who take hawthorn can exercise for longer periods without chest pain. Follow the package directions. Just be sure to consult your doctor first; if you take digoxin for irregular heart rhythm, hawthorn may interfere with its effectiveness.

GRAPES

Purple Heart

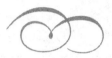

THERE'S SOMETHING SO INDULGENT ABOUT EATING A bunch of grapes. Picture yourself leaning back at your desk and popping one after another into your mouth. It calls up images of reclining Romans feasting at a bacchanal, doesn't it? Yet, while we may not enjoy grapes in such opulent luxury, we do have one thing in common with those feasting residents of ancient Rome: We reap heart health benefits and fend off cancer.

HEARD IT THROUGH THE GRAPEVINE

Purple grape juice, like red wine, is bursting with flavonoids, which are naturally occurring plant compounds that help prevent unnecessary blood platelet aggregation. (When platelets "aggregate," they

...Just the facts

Tokay, Empress, or Red
    Flame grapes (1 cup)
Calories: 114
Fat: 1 g
Saturated fat: 0 g
Cholesterol: 0 mg
Sodium: 3 mg
Total carbohydrates: 28 g
Dietary fiber: 2 g
Protein: 1 g
Thiamin (vitamin B$_1$): 10%
    of Daily Value
Vitamin C: 19%
Copper: 7%

133

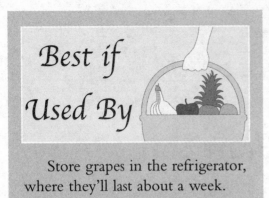

Best if Used By

Store grapes in the refrigerator, where they'll last about a week. Wash them just before eating.

form tiny blood clots that can get stuck in a clogged coronary artery, cutting off the blood supply to that part of your heart. That's a heart attack.)

A small clinical study of five men and five women showed that drinking 5 ounces of 100 percent purple grape juice every day for a week reduced platelet aggregation by 60 percent, a result even better than that brought about by taking aspirin.

Here are some additional hearty findings available through the scientific grapevine.

• Clinical studies have shown that drinking grape juice makes arteries more flexible, which can improve blood flow and in turn could reduce angina pain.

• Both purple and red grape juices have been shown to make "bad" low-density lipoprotein (LDL) cholesterol less likely to oxidize, a chemical process that makes cholesterol stick to artery walls.

ANOTHER BUNCH OF FINDINGS

On the cancer front, grape skins are the richest known source of resveratrol, a naturally occurring compound that puts the brakes on an enzyme that cancer cells need in order to grow. Not only that, resveratrol appears to interfere with the kinds of gene mutations that create cancer cells in the first place! And grapes, like other berries, are a good source of ellagic acid, a substance that is thought to protect against several kinds of cancer. They also supply a good amount of boron, a mineral that's important for healthy bones.

If you're pregnant, and morning sickness makes even drinking a glass of water send you running for the bathroom, eat a bunch of grapes first thing in the morning. They're a great fluid replacer, but they don't cause that queasy feeling, says prenatal nutrition specialist Miriam Erick, R.D., director of the National Morning Sickness Nutrition Clinic at Brigham and Women's Hospital in Boston.

THE PICK OF THE BUNCH

Grapes ripen on the vine, but the ripening process comes to a screeching halt when grapes are picked. So shop carefully, because the moment of purchase is as good as it gets. For the sweetest grapes, look for green ones that are yellow-green, red ones that are deep crimson, and purple ones that are nearly black. Choose plump grapes that seem to be bursting with goodness and have green, supple stems.

Now you can enjoy your grapes in all these delicious ways.

Have a PBJ. Want a quick lunch? Have a good old-fashioned peanut butter and purple grape jelly sandwich. The peanut butter packs the kind of fat that's heart healthy, and the jelly is loaded with flavonoids that protect against heart disease and cancer.

Sweeten salads. Seedless grapes add sweet, crispy crunch to chicken, tuna, or shrimp salad. Sprinkle on a little curry powder, too, for a spicy contrast.

Decorate with grapes. Skip the parsley and go for the grapes when you garnish the plates and platters at your next dinner party.

Get your just desserts. Serve fruit kebabs as postmeal treats. Skewer grapes, banana slices, whole strawberries, and pineapple chunks, then drizzle with honey, lime juice, and allspice and broil just until warm.

Give candy the boot. Replace that candy dish with a grape centerpiece. Combine small bunches of white, red, and purple grapes for a color extravaganza.

Have a purple cow. In a blender, whirl 1 cup of plain fat-free yogurt with ½ cup of purple grape juice for a sweet treat that will do your body good.

Chill without diluting. Wash and separate grapes, place them on a baking sheet, and freeze. Use them in place of ice cubes in cold drinks. Because they thaw but don't melt, they won't dilute the beverage. (Finish by eating the grapes, of course!)

Keep a desk-drawer emergency kit. Stash 8-ounce cans or boxes of purple grape juice in your desk. When you're desperate for a snack, get juiced up instead of running to the vending machine.

Have a juice spritzer. Combine ½ cup of grape juice, 1 cup of sparkling soda, and the juice of ½ lime in a tall glass. Fill with ice and garnish with a mint sprig.

GREENS

Leaf the Pain Behind

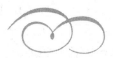

SOME GREENS ARE WALLFLOWERS: THEY JUST DON'T SEEM to attract a lot of attention. If you look a little closer, though, you'll find that they're worth your time and attention. While kale, spinach, and even bok choy are greens that most of you know, here I'm talking about another set of greens: collard, mustard, and turnip. These oft-overlooked leafies are helpful to folks with angina because they deliver substantial doses of magnesium, which helps relax the arterial spasms that cause angina pain.

What's really cool about these quiet contenders is that they're great at multi-tasking. They're loaded with beta-carotene and vitamin C, antioxidants that gobble up free radicals, those compounds that spell trouble for your heart and increase your

...Just the facts

Turnip greens (½ cup cooked)
Calories: 29
Fat: 0 g
Saturated fat: 0 g
Cholesterol: 0 mg
Sodium: 42 mg
Total carbohydrates: 6 g
Dietary fiber: 5 g
Protein: 2 g
Folate: 43% of Daily Value
Vitamin A: 79%
Vitamin C: 66%
Vitamin E: 12%
Magnesium: 8%

risk of cancer. Meanwhile, they also protect your eyes and your bones. No wonder they're so quiet: They're too busy working to make a lot of noise!

SEEING GREEN

Like kale and spinach, collard, mustard, and turnip greens are loaded with lutein and zeaxanthin, two important compounds for eye health. Two Harvard studies—one of 36,000 men, the other of 50,000 women—found that people who ate foods richest in these compounds had about a 20 percent lower chance of needing cataract surgery.

These foods help protect your vision in another way: They may help ward off age-related macular degeneration (AMD), the leading cause of blindness in people over age 65. In this disease, the macula of the eye—a small spot on the retina—starts to fizzle, making it difficult for people who have AMD to see straight ahead. As it turns out, the macula is loaded with

← Green Giants →

Relish the nutrients and flavor of these great greens.

Greens (1 cup cooked)	Flavor	Vitamin A (% of Daily Value)	Vitamin C (% DV)	Lutein & Zeaxanthin (units)
Collard	Strongly cabbage-y	42	29	8,091
Kale	Mildly cabbage-y	96	44	15,798
Mustard	Mild, peppery	43	30	N/A
Spinach	Slightly tart	147	15	7,043
Turnip	Cabbage-y	79	33	8,440

the same two compounds abundant in these leafy green vegetables.

One small study found that 13 of 14 people with AMD who ate ½ cup of cooked spinach four to seven times a week showed improvements in their vision. Collard greens, turnip greens, and kale actually have more of these compounds than spinach does.

HIP, HIP, HOORAY!

You've heard it a zillion times: Make sure you get enough calcium to prevent osteoporosis, a disease that makes your bones weak and more likely to fracture at the slightest slip. While calcium certainly is crucial, researchers are also investigating the role of another nutrient: vitamin K.

Research at Tufts University in Boston showed that vitamin K activates at least three proteins involved in bone health. And which foods are rich in vitamin K? You guessed it—greens.

KEEN GREENS

Fresh greens are available most of the year in all parts of the country, although you're sure to find them everywhere from Thanksgiving to Christmas. When you're shopping, make sure the greens have been chilled while on display. No matter which type you're buying, look for small leaves, which are more tender and have milder flavor than larger leaves. The

Good to Go

When you're ready to use your greens:
• Cut off and discard the stems, roots, and any discolored leaves.
• Swish the leaves in a large bowl of cold water, rinse, and drain. If they're very gritty, rinse them a few times.
• Dry the greens in a salad spinner or roll them in several paper towels and put them in the fridge for a few minutes.
• Whether you boil, steam, microwave, or stir-fry your greens, cook them for the least amount of time possible so they retain more of their nutrients.

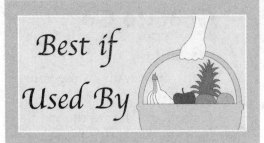

Best if Used By

Store your greens, unwashed, in a plastic bag in the coldest part of your fridge, where they'll keep for up to five days.

leaves should be fresh and green, not wilting or yellow, and they shouldn't have little holes, which are signs of insect damage.

Try these ideas for great greens your family will love.

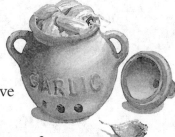

Chill out. Cook collards, then chill and serve with lemon juice, olive oil, pine nuts, and garlic.

Stack 'em. Place greens between the layers of your favorite lasagna.

Heat 'em. Sauté collards with onions, garlic, and small pieces of lean smoked ham.

Soup 'em up. Stir collards or mustard greens into your favorite soup.

OLIVE OIL

Fat for Life

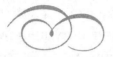

Years ago, long before meatless meals were cool, I discovered a recipe for Pesto Genovese. It was rich in olive oil and sweet basil, and it drove my husband and kids wild. Now, research has shown that all that olive oil was actually building a heart-protective shield around my family. That was quite a relief after watching my grandmother pop nitroglycerin pills to soothe her angina pain.

FAT BY ANY OTHER NAME...

Researchers became interested in olive oil in the 1960s, when they realized that people in southern Italy and Greece and on the Greek island of Crete ate whole vats of it, yet their life expectancies were the longest in the world. In addition, their rates of heart disease and some cancers were very low.

...Just the facts

Olive oil (1 Tbsp)
Calories: 120
Fat: 14 g
Saturated fat: 2 g
Monounsaturated fat: 11 g
Cholesterol: 0 mg
Sodium: 0 mg
Total carbohydrates: 0 g
Dietary fiber: 0 g
Protein: 0 g
Vitamin E: 22% of Daily Value

Americans were eating just as much fat—about 35 percent of our total calories came from fat—but we were dropping like flies. The difference? We were eating cheeseburgers, hot dogs, and French fries—all of which are loaded with heart-trashing saturated fat.

Research by Penny Kris-Etherton, R.D., Ph.D., professor of nutrition at Pennsylvania State University in University Park, explains the big fat difference. When 22 people were switched from a typical American diet to a diet high in the monounsaturated fat of olive oil, their total cholesterol dropped by 10 percent, their "bad" low-density lipoprotein (LDL) cholesterol plummeted by 14 percent, and their triglycerides fell by 13 percent—yet their beneficial high-density lipoprotein (HDL)

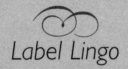

Label Lingo

The Commission of the European Communities defines the types of olive oil as follows.

• *Extra-virgin olive oil.* This is the highest-quality oil (less than 10 percent make the grade) from the first cold press. It has perfect flavor and aroma and less than 1 percent acidity, with great mouthfeel. This is the best for use on salads, dipping, or adding to foods at the table.

• *Fine virgin olive oil.* With perfect flavor and aroma, this type has less than 2 percent acidity.

• *Ordinary or semi-fine olive oil.* Although this oil may have been refined to remove unwanted flavors or odors, it has good flavor and aroma and less than 3.3 percent acidity. It's fine for frying when flavor isn't a major concern.

• *Pure olive oil.* This is a low-cost blend of refined and virgin oils and has less than 1.5 percent acidity.

cholesterol didn't drop. All told, simply substituting olive oil for saturated fat lowered their chances of having heart attacks by 25 percent! That was double the reduction achieved with the American Heart Association's very low fat Step II diet plan.

PRESSURE BEATER

As Dr. Kris-Etherton was conducting her studies in the United States, researchers in Naples, Italy, decided to see what effect olive oil might have on blood pressure, so they had 11 people with high blood pressure switch to a diet rich in extra-virgin olive oil. The result: In 8 of the participants, blood pressure dropped enough so that they could give up their blood pressure medications. (Now, adding a teaspoon of olive oil to your salad sure beats the heck out of taking a pill, but don't stop taking medication without talking to your doctor. Discontinuing any blood pressure medication can be tricky.)

CANCER CONQUEROR

Olive oil is made simply by squeezing (cold pressing) fresh olives, pits and all. Unlike other vegetable oils, it can be used fresh from the vat without heating or refining. This natural, unprocessed oil contains little bits of olive leftovers, such as phenols and squalene, that create its unique flavor, make it stable, and—best of all—may fight colon, breast, and prostate cancers.

Which is the best olive oil? Well, one market-basket analysis suggests that olive oils from the Mediterranean contain the most squalene, which preliminary studies suggest is the big gun that protects you.

Best if Used By

"Olive oil does not age like fine wine," according to the Olive Oil Source. Light and heat are its enemies, so store it in a dark cupboard, a dark glass bottle, or a tin can in a cool location (not near the stove, where cooking heat will ruin it). You can put it in the fridge, but the oil will turn almost solid, so you'll have to warm it before you use it.

BEST OF THE BARREL

You may think that the color of olive oil tells you something about its taste. Not so, says the Olive Oil Source in Greenbrae, California. Greener oils are usually pressed from greener olives earlier in the season, and some olives are greener or more golden than others.

The flavor of the oil really depends on when the olives were picked, how they were stored, how they were processed, the soil and weather conditions where they were grown, and the age of the tree. (Olive trees reach maturity at anywhere from 35 to 150 years of age and can live up to 600 years.) You'll just have to taste-test a few brands to find those you like best.

Here's how to get the most from olive oil.

Kiss with it. Stop by a kitchenware store and invest in an oil mister. Fill it with olive oil, pump up the pressure, and spray a light layer on broiled chicken or fish, oven-fried potatoes, or steamed vegetables.

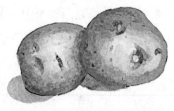

Dunk in it. Instead of butter for your bread, serve up small saucers of olive oil for dipping. Quality counts here, so choose oil with a flavor that knocks your socks off. For added zing, season with crushed garlic and chopped fresh basil.

ORANGES

Critical Care

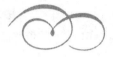

OF COURSE, YOU KNOW THAT ORANGES ARE HIGH IN vitamin C. Your mother's been telling you that practically since the day you were born. Just one large orange or a 6-ounce glass of freshly squeezed juice feeds your need for C for the whole day. (Oh, and oranges are so refreshing!) But did your mother also tell you that oranges are good for your heart? No? Well, here's something you can share with her.

IN A SERIOUS VEIN

The orange's bountiful benefits haven't all been linked to specific nutrients or phytochemicals. In one small Canadian study, for instance, women who drank orange juice daily got a big surprise: Their levels of high-density lipoprotein (HDL) cholesterol rose by 21 percent, which was

> ## ...Just the facts
>
> Orange (1 large)
> Calories: 86
> Fat: 0 g
> Saturated fat: 0 g
> Cholesterol: 0 mg
> Sodium: 0 mg
> Total carbohydrates: 22 g
> Dietary fiber: 4 g
> Protein: 2 g
> Vitamin C: 109%
> Folate: 14% of Daily Value

very unusual, since wine and chocolate are the only other foods known to raise HDL. Larger studies will be needed to confirm these results, but more HDL means more help cleaning the bad cholesterol out of your arteries, and that may mean less angina pain for you.

If you want bigger studies, there's the one in which 100,000 nurses and professional men were tracked by Harvard researchers. The scientists found that cabbage family vegetables, green leafy vegetables, and citrus fruits and juices protected against ischemic stroke, the kind that comes from a blood clot in the brain. Each daily serving of these fruits and vegetables lowered stroke risk by 6 percent.

C'S THE DAY

Okay, so your mom knew oranges were full of vitamin C. Did she know all the great things it can do for you? While it doesn't seem to prevent the common cold, maybe the C stands for "critical" when it comes to protecting your entire body in many ways.

• Vitamin C creates collagen, the protein in connective tis-

← Winter Wonderland →

Here's a mini schedule to help you find oranges at the peak of perfection.

Orange	Season
Tangelo	November to February
Navel and Clementine	November to April
Jaffa	Mid-December to mid-February
Temple	January to March
Blood orange	March to May
Valencia	March to June

sue that forms the matrix to hold calcium in your bones and teeth.

• It forms scar tissue, so it's vitamin C that helps knit your skin back together when it's been damaged by anything from a paper cut to a surgical incision.

• It helps prevent wrinkles—so stay out of the sun, don't smoke (yes, smokers do need more C), and drink your orange juice.

• Vitamin C helps you absorb iron, making it particularly important for vegetarians, teenagers, and women of childbearing age. Each of these groups is at high risk for iron-deficiency anemia.

• It's an antioxidant that prevents other vitamins and minerals from being ruined before they can perform their normal tasks.

• Vitamin C helps prevent the formation of gallstones.

Wow! All that work being done by one little round orange!

OUTSTANDING ORANGES

Consider trying the many different types of oranges. Part of the fun is to eat your way through the winter and spring, enjoying each variety at its peak. When selecting

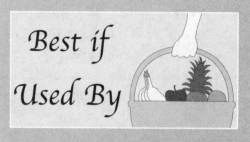

Best if Used By

Here are some inside tips on how to get the best from your oranges.

• There are some benefits to being thick skinned. A heavy covering on the outside of an orange protects the fragile vitamins on the inside, such as vitamin C and folate. You can store thick-skinned oranges equally well at room temperature or in the refrigerator. In either place, they'll stay fresh for about two weeks.

• Definitely keep your O.J. in the fridge, though. If it's freshly squeezed, it begins to lose its vitamin C in 24 hours. Chilled juice will hang on to about 90 percent of its C for a week and 66 percent for two weeks.

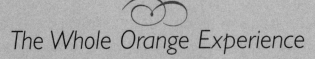

The Whole Orange Experience

Yes, an orange looks like a blazing little sun, and its various parts certainly offer some hot health benefits.

• *The skin.* The benefits start when you peel an orange and get that pungent smell on your hands. The oil in orange skin is 90 to 95 percent limonene, a natural chemical that's been linked to preventing breast and cervical cancers, at least in the laboratory. Limonene ends up in the orange juice you buy, because commercial machines squeeze the oranges so hard. That's a good thing.

• *The pith.* Then there's that white stuff just under the skin. It's packed with pectin, a type of soluble fiber known for lowering cholesterol, and it's higher in vitamin C than the juice is. If you eat a little of the pith along with your orange, that, too, is a good thing.

• *The flesh and the juice.* They're good sources of cryptoxanthin, one of the beta-carotene cousins, which may fight cervical cancer. Canned mandarin oranges are loaded with it, too.

Oranges are also an important source of folate, the B vitamin that's essential for preventing neural tube birth defects and for keeping blood levels of homocysteine under control. Minute increases in homocysteine can trigger a heart attack.

oranges, don't judge by their color, because all oranges are picked when they're fully ripe. Some, especially those from Florida, remain slightly green even at their ripest. Others, such as those from California, turn completely, evenly orange. Instead, look for fruits that are firm, heavy, and evenly shaped.

Here's what to do with your orange-arama.

Grate for flavor. Grate orange peel into vanilla yogurt to make the very best dressing for melon and berry salads. Also grate it into vegetable salads, muffins, and quick breads. You'll capitalize on the limonene in the peel.

Sub for vinegar. Use orange juice instead of vinegar to whip up a heart-healthy salad dressing. Or arrange thinly sliced, peeled navel oranges on greens for a different look.

Go bananas. When you're slicing bananas for fruit salad, stir them into orange juice to keep them from turning brown.

Have a peach melba breakfast. In a blender, combine orange juice, fresh raspberries, and sliced peaches. Fill your travel mug, then GO!

Go stir crazy. When you're sizzling up your next stir-fry, add a can of well-drained mandarin oranges for a zesty counterpoint.

PASTA

Heart Lines

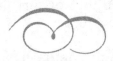

When my friend Karen was growing up, she went to her grandparents' house every Sunday for a special pasta meal. Often, it was just the usual spaghetti and meatballs, but sometimes it was gnocchi (potato dumplings) or manicotti (tubes filled with cheese or meat). Whatever her grandmother made, it was delicious.

These days, Karen doesn't limit pasta to Sundays. To hear her husband tell it, she'd make pasta every night of the week if she could. On Valentine's Day, he even cooks it for her. He must instinctively know that pasta is powerful stuff for the heart!

THE POWER OF LOVE

Pasta pumps up your ticker in two ways. First, it's rich in complex carbohy-

...Just the facts

Spaghetti (1 cup cooked)
Calories: 197
Fat: 1 g
Saturated fat: 0 g
Cholesterol: 0 mg
Sodium: 1 mg
Total carbohydrates: 40 g
Dietary fiber: 2 g
Protein: 7 g
Folic acid: 25% of Daily
    Value
Niacin (vitamin B_3): 9%
Iron: 11%

drates—carbs, for short. When you eat more carbs and less saturated fat, your cholesterol takes a nosedive. With less cholesterol clogging your arteries, you may find that you have less angina pain. And of course, when you toss your pasta with heart-smart olive oil or twirl it with prostate-protective tomatoes, you do even more for your love life. (Bury it in Alfredo sauce, however, and all bets are off!)

Second, most of the pasta that you pick up at the supermarket is enriched with folic acid, a B vitamin. In a Harvard study of more than 80,000 women, the researchers found that participants who had the highest intakes of folic acid and vitamin B_6 were about 45 percent less likely to develop heart disease than those who had the lowest intakes.

Folic acid offers another important benefit for women: Getting the recommended 400 micrograms daily cuts the risk of neural tube birth defects in half. One cup of cooked pasta supplies about 25 percent of your daily requirement.

FOOD NEWS

Does that gorgeous red, green, or striped pasta pack more nutrients than the standard kind? The answer: Maybe. Pasta flavored with tomatoes or red peppers may kick in some extra vitamins A and C, but the kind made with herbs or spinach doesn't usually offer any extras. Do, however, check the Nutrition Facts label on the package to be sure.

DISH UP STAMINA

The complex carbs in pasta aren't just good for your heart; they improve your stamina, too. Athletes often load up on pasta before a competition because it supplies time-released energy. In other words, you won't get a huge burst of energy at the beginning of your performance and then tire out at the end.

Granted, you're probably not going for Olympic gold anytime soon, but this concept can help you if you're taking a hike, walking a charity 5K, or even doing a lot of gardening. You'll eat less than a pro athlete, of course, but the principle is the same.

Plagued by premenstrual syndrome? Sit down to a bowl of pasta. A diet rich in carbohydrates, such as pasta and whole wheat bread, helps increase levels of an amino acid that produces serotonin, a brain chemical that elevates your mood.

SERVING ESSENTIALS

You may be thinking, "But won't pasta make me fat and tax my heart?" No! No! No! I've been dying to set the record straight: Despite what those diet books tell you, calories from pasta are not more likely to pack on the pounds than calories from any other food.

The real problem is that portion sizes of pasta (especially in restaurants) have gotten out of control. For instance, when Karen ordered Linguini Pomodoro (that's just pasta with chopped tomatoes, garlic, basil, and olive oil) at an Italian restaurant, she received a mammoth bowlful—the equivalent of five servings! If you clean that size plate, you will gain weight.

So what's a serving? Not much, according to the USDA—just ½ cup of cooked pasta. Our recommendation is to eat about 1 cup and have it count as 2 of the 6 to 11 servings of grains that the USDA recommends you eat daily. Top it off with about ⅓ cup of sauce, ⅓ cup of veggies, and 1 tablespoon of cheese.

PICK OF THE PASTA

Pasta is available in quite a few different forms. Of course, there are the boxes of regular dried spaghetti, linguine, lasagna, and so on found on supermarket shelves. Then there's the "gourmet" fresh pasta found in the refrigerated case. If you're lucky enough to live near a good Italian market, you may also find homemade pasta, either dried or fresh. In addition, there is whole wheat pasta, and finally, pasta in an array of cheery colors! No matter which shape or color you choose, each of the two main types—regular and whole wheat—offers its own perks.

• *Regular pasta.* Most regular pasta—even the refrigerated kind—is made with flour that has been enriched with extra nutrients, including, as of late, folic acid. To be certain, just look for the words "enriched flour" on the ingredients list. (I hate to break it to you, but the delicious pasta at Italian markets probably isn't enriched, so be sure to ask.)

• *Whole wheat pasta.* This type, on the other hand, naturally contains small amounts of a wide range of vitamins and minerals, but while it boasts three times the fiber of regular pasta, it's not required to include the extra folic

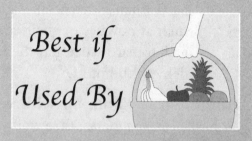

Best if Used By

How long can you keep pasta hanging around?

• Dried pasta maintains its flavor for up to a year when stored in a cool, dry place, such as your cupboard.

• Fresh pasta lasts until the expiration date on the package. Tightly cover opened, unused portions to keep it from drying out. If you don't think you'll use it by the expiration date, you can freeze it for about a month. You don't need to thaw it before using; it'll just take a minute or two longer to cook.

• Frozen pasta can be stored for up to nine months if unopened. Tightly sealed leftover portions will keep for about three months.

acid. Like regular pasta, it comes in dried and fresh varieties.

So which one's best? It's hard to say. We think you should keep both on hand. Then, using either type, follow this step-by-step guide to building a great pasta dinner.

Choose a slimming sauce. Delicate pasta, such as angel hair or thin spaghetti, works best with thin sauces. Thicker pasta (such as fettuccine) goes well with heavier sauces. Shapes such as bowties or shells are perfect for chunky sauces. In general, tomato sauce has the least fat and calories, while Alfredo delivers the most.

Bulk up with veggies. When you add veggies to spaghetti sauce, you can fill up your pasta bowl for fewer calories. Toss broccoli florets into tomato or marinara sauce; add green beans to pesto sauce; dice red bell peppers into garlic and olive oil sauce; or add a medley of colorful chopped veggies, such as carrots, squash, and green bell peppers, to white sauce.

Pour on the protein. It'll help balance all the carbs you're consuming—and keep you full longer. Karen's husband thinks meatballs are a must, but she's of a different mindset, preferring grilled chicken or shrimp.

Add a kiss of cheese. A tablespoon of grated Parmesan or Romano will give your dish a boost in calcium and flavor.

SEEDS

Ease Ticker Trouble

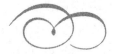

BAKING FRESH YEAST ROLLS WITH MY MOM IS ONE OF MY warmest memories. Before I was old enough to shape the dough, I got to sprinkle the poppy seeds or sesame seeds on top. As it turns out, those seeds were more than just tasty decorations, since all seeds are packed with the unsaturated fat that your body needs for flexible arteries and healthy cell walls, which is great protection against angina.

What's more, seeds are more than just little drops of fat. They're storehouses for all the goodies a plant needs to reproduce itself. They're packed with protein, vitamins, and minerals as well as good fat—just about everything it takes to get growing when the seed meets soil and water. All those heart-thumping and bone-building nutrients can be yours when you start

...Just the facts

Sunflower seeds (1 oz)
Calories: 165
Fat: 14 g
Saturated fat: 1 g
Cholesterol: 0 mg
Sodium: 1 mg
Total carbohydrates: 7 g
Dietary fiber: 3 g
Protein: 5 g
Vitamin E: 70% of Daily
   Value
Calcium: 20%

lightly scattering these nourishing nuggets over your meals and snacks.

TAST-E

Sunflower seeds are nature's powerhouse source of vitamin E. Unless you eat lots of whole wheat bread, green leafy vegetables, and high-calorie vegetable oil, you're probably not getting enough vitamin E from foods, so adding sunflower seeds to a normal diet is a big plus. Just ¼ cup of crunchy little hulled sunflower seeds provides 70 percent of your daily requirement.

Numerous studies suggest that vitamin E may play an important role in preventing heart disease. In one six-year study of 34,000 postmenopausal women, those who got the most vitamin E from foods had the lowest risk of heart disease. In that study, taking a vitamin E supplement appeared to have no effect. Scientists speculate that the benefit may come from the vitamin E itself or from some other element in the whole, natural food that is milled out of most processed foods or isn't added to supplements.

Best if Used By

Store open seed packages in the refrigerator, at least until you get into the habit of using them.

BONE BOOSTER

Sesame seeds give you a surprising little calcium jolt where you least expect it. Just 1 ounce (about ¼ cup) supplies 280 milligrams—more than one-fourth of the Daily Value! Those tiny seeds also pack a walloping dose of magnesium and manganese, now thought to protect against odd bone formations and calcium loss from bones after menopause.

One of the most pleasant ways to eat lots of sesame seeds is in tahini, a paste of ground seeds that's a standard ingredient in hummus. It also delivers the goods.

IMMUNE TUNER

Pumpkin seeds are one of the best plant sources of zinc, a critical mineral in the maze of reactions that build immunity against invaders such as viruses and cancer. Just 1 ounce of pumpkin seeds delivers 3 milligrams of zinc, which is more than you get from 2 ounces of lean beef or 3 ounces of chicken breast.

WAIST WATCHER

Seeds are yummy, but they are pretty calorie dense, which counts in the battle of the bulge. Sunflower and sesame seeds weigh in at about 165 calories per ounce, while pumpkin seeds save you a few calories at 126. Thus, you can't curl up in front of the TV with a can of seeds and just munch away. Instead, use them to garnish or enhance the flavors of your foods. If you're crazy for trail mix, eat it for lunch instead of as a snack.

SENSATIONAL SEEDS

Since fat is a major ingredient in seeds, they can become rancid, so shop and store carefully. Check the "sell-by" or "use-by" date on cans or sealed jars of seeds. If you're bargain hunt-

FOOD NEWS

Sesame seeds are at their tastiest when toasted. Here's how to do it: Place a nonstick skillet over high heat and sprinkle in a tablespoon or two of seeds. As the pan begins to heat up, the kernels will start to pop. Begin shaking the pan like mad, just as you would when making popcorn the old-fashioned way, and shake until the seeds are golden brown and smell too good to resist. Sprinkle them over tossed salads; cooked vegetables; stir-fries; or broiled chicken, fish, or shrimp.

← *Mineral Magnates* →

Seeds pack all the nutrients needed to get a new plant started and offer you great benefits as well, but the details make the difference. Mix and match for best nutrition.

Seed (1 oz)	Copper (% of Daily Value)	Iron (% DV)	Magnesium (% DV)	Manganese (% DV)	Zinc (% DV)
Pumpkin	10	5	19	7	19
Sesame	21	12	25	20	19
Sunflower	26	6	9	30	10

ing at bulk bins, take a good sniff to be sure the odor of loose seeds is fresh. The nose knows!

Here's how to sow seeds into your daily life.

Stir into cereal. Add seeds to hot or cold whole grain cereal to maximize your morning minerals. Keep all three kinds on hand, then alternate from day to day for taste variety and optimal nutrition.

Spin into smoothies. Toss a tablespoon or two of seeds into your next fruit smoothie as it whirls away in your blender. It'll taste terrific, and the fat from the seeds will keep you from getting hungry too soon.

Sprinkle on dessert. Mix luscious summer melon cubes and berries with plain or vanilla yogurt, then top with pumpkin seeds and a dash of ground nutmeg.

DASH Hypertension

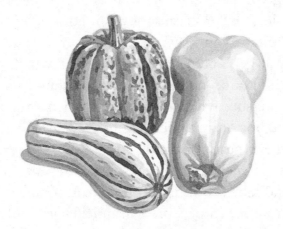

YOU MAY THINK THAT THE ONLY PEOPLE WITH HIGH blood pressure are those who are reckless with the saltshaker. Not so. An astounding 60 million Americans have high blood pressure, and although many keep their shakers in the cupboard, their "pressures" still climb sky-high.

THE QUIET COLLUSION

Salt does boost blood volume, making the heart work harder to pump all that blood and increasing pressure on the walls of blood vessels as it courses through. It turns out, though, that salt is only one factor in the development of high blood pressure. Other dietary and lifestyle factors—such as a high-fat diet, obesity, and a highly stressful life—also contribute because they narrow arteries. Since smaller arteries mean that blood has less room in which to move, the pressure on the vessel walls increases, and the arteries weaken. When this happens, you're a prime candidate for a heart attack, a stroke, and/or kidney failure. Your risk is greatest if you smoke, abuse alcohol, have a family history of high blood pressure, or are male or African American.

The really scary part, though, is that this book may be the only warning you get. High blood pressure, or hypertension, is dubbed the silent killer because it often goes undetected until it's too late. In fact, you may not know your arteries are in distress unless you get a blood pressure reading, which consists of two numbers: The top number (systolic reading) is a measurement of the pressure within the arteries when your heart's pumping. The bottom number (diastolic reading) measures the pressure between beats. Anything above 140/90 on three separate readings means you have high blood pressure, but experts say you should take action if you have readings higher than 120/80, because blood pressure can quickly shift into the high, dangerous range.

A SIMPLE SOLUTION

Reach out and touch someone. Touch lowers levels of the stress hormone cortisol, which constricts blood vessels and bumps up blood pressure. To try this antidote, simply get in close touch with your loved ones today! Holding hands is a great way to start.

PRESSURE-RELEASE VALVE

Many people with high blood pressure take prescription diuretics to help their bodies eliminate sodium, thus reducing blood volume and blood pressure. The problem is, some diuretics tend to flush out potassium and other vital minerals along with sodium. Fortunately, other medications are available. What's more, Harvard researchers have found that a low-fat, plant-based diet such as the DASH (Dietary Approaches to Stop Hypertension) diet can lower blood pressure as well as, if not better than, the most potent prescription drugs—and with none of their side effects, such as constipation or sexual dysfunction. Consult your doctor about your options, and never go off your medications without medical approval.

Nondrug remedies (such as herbal diuretics, which don't flush out potassium and other vital minerals) and lifestyle changes may be enough to keep borderline hypertension from going over the line or at the very least help you lower dosages of prescription meds. Here's where to start.

FOOD NEWS

Avocado is packed with potassium, a mineral that helps keep all the other minerals in balance and is vital for lowering blood pressure, says Jeremy Appleton, N.D., chairman of the National College of Naturopathic Medicine in Portland, Oregon.

Try an amazing diet. Following the DASH diet—that is, eating 8 to 10 servings of fruits and vegetables and 3 servings of dairy foods each day, limiting saturated fat, and consuming less than 2,000 milligrams of salt daily—for a month could shave up to 11 points off your top number and 5 points off the bottom one, and the beneficial effects start kicking in after two weeks.

After two months, your blood pressure could return to normal, especially if, as studies have shown, you reduce your salt intake to less than 1,200 milligrams a day.

Maximize omega-3's.
Omega-3 essential fatty acids, which are found mainly in salmon, tuna, and other cold-water fish, can help lower blood pressure, but you

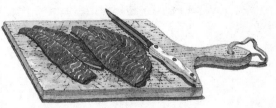

Maximize Your Minerals

Calcium and magnesium help lower blood pressure by reducing the tension on artery walls and relaxing the muscles that control blood vessels, so blood flows more easily. Feast on magnesium-rich navy, pinto, and kidney beans and the calcium king, bok choy, along with low-fat dairy foods, such as milk, cheese, and yogurt, to get what you need.

Even a moderate deficiency of another mineral, potassium, can increase blood pressure. Fruits and vegetables, especially oranges, kiwifruit, bananas, and potatoes, as well as low-fat dairy foods, are packed with potassium.

need about 5 grams a day for the best effect. To reach your quota, Darin Ingels, N.D., a naturopathic physician and director of New England Family Health in Southport, Connecticut, suggests that you check with your doctor about taking fish-oil capsules, along with 400 IU of vitamin E to offset any fishiness. Check your drugstore or health food store for both—or opt for 1 to 3 table-spoons daily of flaxseed oil, also available at health food stores. Both fish and flax may help inhibit inflammatory reactions that can cause arteries to narrow. Since they both thin the blood, however, don't use them if you take aspirin or prescription blood thinners.

Consider CoQ$_{10}$. This antioxidant, available at health food stores and drugstores, makes arteries less vulnerable to con-striction. Stephen T. Sinatra, M.D., a cardiologist and director of medical education at Manchester Memorial Hospital in Hartford, Connecticut, reports that people who took 100 mil-ligrams a day were able to cut their doses of blood pressure medications in half.

Snack on celery. Crunching your way through just four stalks a day could ease down your blood pressure. A component in celery (3-n-butyl phthalide) acts as a diuretic and vasodilator and helps relax the muscles lining the blood vessels.

Dig up dandelions. The greens are an excellent diuretic that won't flush out potassium and are in fact rich in the mineral. Don't like the idea of munching from your lawn? Ask your doctor if you can substitute three or four cups of dandelion tea—which you can find at health food stores—a day, suggests Dr. Ingels, but don't combine it with medication, especially diuretics or potassium supplements.

Curl up with kitty. Just 10 minutes spent with a pet can lower your blood pressure. In fact, if you have borderline hypertension, there's even a holdover effect: If you spend time with Benji or Tiger before work, you may be less vulnerable to blood pressure–raising stress on the job.

Toss your salad with sesame. Loaded with unsaturated fatty acids and calcium, sesame oil may help lower blood pressure and let you reduce your dose of calcium channel blockers. Try downing 2 tablespoons daily for two months, then have your blood pressure rechecked. If your numbers go down, ask your doctor about cutting down your drug dosage, too.

BOK CHOY

Stalking Potassium

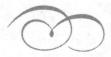

I LOVE TO STIR-FRY—IT'S SUCH A GREAT WAY TO TURN A little bit of meat or poultry into a big pile of food when I mix it with lots and lots of veggies. In fact, it's one of my secret weapons for changing the portions on my husband's plate. Lately, to keep our blood pressure on an even keel, I've started adding bok choy, a vegetable with a secret.

Think of bok choy as Chinese celery. It's about the same size as the hefty celery stalks that show up around Thanksgiving, but the ribs are stark white, and the flat, ruffled leaves are deep hunter green. Very striking. More likely, you'll remember it from Asian dishes you've eaten in restaurants. There it appears as crosswise slices, in the style of romaine lettuce cut for Caesar salad. "Oh, that stuff," you're probably saying.

...Just the facts

Bok choy (1 cup, raw)
Calories: 20
Fat: 0 g
Saturated fat: 0 g
Cholesterol: 0 mg
Sodium: 58 mg
Total carbohydrates: 3 g
Dietary fiber: 3 g
Protein: 3 g
Folate: 17% of Daily Value
Vitamin A: 87%
Vitamin C: 49%
Calcium: 16%

Bok choy is a very mild-mannered Asian member of the cabbage, or cruciferous, family. As a crucifer, bok choy is related not just to cabbage but also to broccoli, cauliflower, kale, kohlrabi, and the new baby in the family, broccolini. Cruciferous vegetables have long been recognized as powerful cancer fighters, but that's not bok choy's big secret.

POTASSIUM POWER

The word is out that eating plenty of fruits and vegetables (8 to 11 servings) each day, along with a couple of dairy foods, can lower blood pressure just as well as medication can. The reason? It's probably because all the nutrients work together in ways we can't yet even imagine, but part of the answer is potassium, which, in large amounts, has been shown to lower blood pressure. Bok choy is packed with potassium—more, in fact, than your breakfast banana or glass of orange juice—but that's not its secret, either.

CALCIUM CONTRIBUTOR

Okay, it's time to let the cat out of the bag: Bok choy's secret is that it's loaded with calcium! Just 1 cup serves up as much of this bone builder as half a glass of milk, an unusually large quantity for a nondairy food. The especially cool part is that unlike the calcium in some other greens (such as spinach), you can absorb bok choy's plentiful calcium as easily as you can the calcium in milk. For that reason, bok choy is especially

Best if Used By

Store bok choy in the vegetable crisper of your refrigerator and use it within a few days. Cruciferous vegetables tend to fade fast, and the flavor changes if they're kept too long. When you're ready to use your bok choy, just separate the ribs, wash them thoroughly, and pat dry.

important for vegetarians who don't "do" dairy.

Perhaps equally important, calcium is crucial for controlling blood pressure. For folks who have a hard time fitting in three dairy foods a day, bok choy can boost calcium totals to respectable levels.

Bok choy is also brimming with vitamin C, so just 1 cup provides half of what you need for the day. And although vitamin C won't cure your cold, it will help heal your wounds, from paper cuts and hangnails to surgical incisions.

STALK THE BEST

Although bok choy was once considered fairly exotic, today many supermarkets carry it in the produce aisle. Look for stalks with sturdy, crisp, white ribs with no cuts or bruises and leaves that are dark green. If they're turning pale green or yellow, they're getting old and losing their vitamins, so move on and look for a better bunch.

Now you're ready for some exotic little adventures. Cut across the ribs and slip some slices of bok choy into everyday fare that's all in good taste. Try these serving suggestions.

Create colorful salads. Replace half the lettuce in your next salad with bok choy. The dark leaves create a lush backdrop for colorful veggies.

Make mountains out of molehills. Bok choy adds bulk, fiber, vitamins, and minerals to stir-fries, with very few calories.

Produce powerful soups. Double the nutrition in canned soups by stirring in a cup or two of bok choy and simmering for 2 to 3 minutes.

CELERY

Crunch Those Numbers

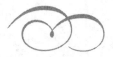

I LOVE TO USE THICK CHUNKS OF CELERY IN MY TUNA salad. The recommended serving of tuna, about 3 ounces, just isn't enough to fill up my pita pocket, so I pack the mix with celery and fold it, along with a tomato slice, into a large red lettuce leaf. Then I stuff the whole thing into a whole wheat pita pocket, and—voilà!—I've gotten in three of my vegetable servings for the day. Better still, researchers have uncovered a naturally occurring chemical in celery, called phthalide, that actually helps lower blood pressure (at least in rats) by dilating blood vessels. Too cool!

CELERY RUMORS 101

Celery has a reputation for being high in sodium, but is this something to worry

...Just the facts

Celery (8-in stalk)
Calories: 6
Fat: 0 g
Saturated fat: 0 g
Cholesterol: 0 mg
Sodium: 35 mg
Total carbohydrates: 2 g
Dietary fiber: Less than 1 g
Protein: Less than 1 g
Folate: 3% of Daily Value
Vitamin A: 1%
Vitamin C: 3%
Calcium: 2%
Iron: 1%
Potassium: 3%

When you're ready to eat your celery:

- Wash the stalks thoroughly and trim off the ends.
- If the bunch has become limp, trim off the root end and the tops, then stand it in a glass of water for an hour or two. It will stiffen right up.

about? Maybe. If you have kidney disease and are on dialysis, the sodium content in a couple of stalks of celery could be an issue. Somehow, though, that concern has been picked up by folks with high blood pressure who've been advised to eat a low-sodium (2,000 milligrams) diet.

Yet a celery stalk serves up only 35 milligrams of sodium, less than a carrot, which has almost 40 milligrams! Add to that the recommendation of the Dietary Approaches to Stop Hypertension (DASH) diet to eat 8 to 11 servings of fruit and vegetables daily to lower blood pressure, and celery takes its rightful place in the healthy foods parade.

CELERY RUMORS 202

Every dieter has heard the "negative calorie" rumor—you know, the one that says you burn more calories by chewing celery than you get from digesting it. And it's almost true! An 8-inch celery stalk nets about 6 (count 'em, 6) calories after chewing. Technically, that's not negative, but it's darn close. You'd have to nosh an entire farm field of celery to get into calorie trouble at that rate.

Thus, you can pretty much eat celery at will and still drop pounds (that will help lower your blood pressure, too). Substitute a celery rib for a couple of Oreos, and you'll save 100 calories. If your usual afternoon snack is a candy bar, you'll save more than 200. It also helps that celery tastes so good, especially the sweet inner stalks. (Okay, it's not chocolate, but what do you want from a simple stem?) Celery is also fat- and cholesterol-free, and since it consists mostly of water, it will even help keep you hydrated.

GET A CHARGE
OUT OF CELERY

Celery is "in season" year-round, and stalking the best is a snap if you just use your eyes and nose. Look for a tight, shiny, well-shaped green bunch with bright

Best if Used By

Store celery in a plastic bag in the vegetable drawer of your fridge and pull off the stalks as you need them. They're good for about a week.

green, fresh-looking leaves. Yellow leaves are a sure sign of old age. The stalks should feel firm and crisp; leave limp or yellow ones behind. Avoid celery that looks abused, with cuts, bruises, or ragged stalks. Then give it the "sniff" test. If it smells bitter, better leave it alone.

Celery's calories may not be negative, but you'll positively enjoy the flavor and texture this veggie gives to everyday foods. Try these ideas.

Chop and cook. Add chopped celery to soups and stews. For best flavor and firm texture, toss it in about 20 minutes before the dish is finished cooking.

Ladle some leaves. Freshen canned soups by adding a few celery leaves.

Shovel it in. Use the wide ends of large stalks as edible spoons for soup. The kids will love it!

CUCUMBERS

Nutrient Hideaways

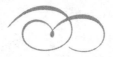

FOR A LONG TIME, MOST OF US THOUGHT CUCUMBERS were, well, blah. They were just one more green ingredient in a salad—nothing special, really. Now we've learned that when you give cucumbers a starring role in a dish, they come alive. Nutritionists have done an about-face with cucumbers, too. While they once regarded them as a nothing vegetable—with few calories but also few nutrients—dietitians now realize that there's more to cucumbers, especially when it comes to high blood pressure.

MORE THAN MEETS THE EYE

Let's start with the basics. An average-size cucumber contributes 30 percent of the vitamin C and roughly 15 percent of the potassium you need for the day.

...Just the facts

Cucumber (1 medium)
Calories: 45
Fat: 0 g
Saturated fat: 0 g
Cholesterol: 0 mg
Sodium: 0 mg
Total carbohydrates: 9 g
Dietary fiber: 3 g
Protein: 3 g
Vitamin C: 30% of Daily
    Value
Calcium: 6%
Iron: 6%
Potassium: 15%

Maybe that sounds paltry, but it's practically free—costing you only 45 calories. What's more, that potassium chips away at your risk of heart disease by helping to lower your blood pressure.

Plus, all along, I've pointed out to anyone who will listen that although cucumbers don't have much in the way of traditional vitamins and minerals, I wouldn't be surprised if scientists uncovered beneficial phytochemicals—plant compounds—in them. I was right on the money. Researchers now know that cucumbers contain phytosterols and terpenes, both believed to diminish the risk of cancer.

Best if Used By

Keep cucumbers in the crisper drawer. If they're waxed and uncut, they'll last for about a week. Otherwise, check them every day or two.

WEIGHT-WATCHER BENEFITS

Not a convert yet? See how this one grabs you: Cucumbers may help you lose weight. Research at Pennsylvania State University in University Park has shown that foods with low energy density—that is, they take up a lot of room in your stomach but provide few calories—can help you shed some pounds. The theory suggests that when you eat these foods, you feel full on fewer calories, so you stop eating.

Cucumbers and romaine lettuce are tied for the position of the vegetable with the lowest energy density. Add them to sandwiches and salads for extra bulk—and pack them in your picnic basket, especially on hot days. Cucumbers are mainly water and may provide you with the extra fluid you need to ward off dehydration.

Good to Go

Before you dig in to a cuke, wash it, even if you're planning to peel it. That way, you won't transfer bacteria from the outside to the delicious inside. Waxed cucumbers should be peeled. With unwaxed cukes, it's your choice, but you'll get more fiber if you eat the skin.

PICKY ABOUT CUCUMBERS

Good news: You can usually find a wide variety of cucumbers at your supermarket all year long. Choose cukes that are very firm and rounded right to the ends. Opt for those that are a rich green. If you're not a big fan of the seeds (and who is, really?), pick up one of the slender European varieties; they're usually seedless, or close to it.

Now, here's what to do with your cucumbers besides adding them to plain old green salad.

Have high tea. Spread thin slices of pumpernickel bread with light cream cheese and top it with cucumber slices. Add a little grated carrot for extra crunch, and you have a great "tea sandwich" to serve at high tea.

Get saucy. Stir chopped peeled cucumber into low-fat plain yogurt seasoned with your favorite herbs (we like to use chives). Serve with grilled chicken or fish.

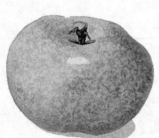

Boost salads. Add diced cucumbers to egg, chicken, or tuna salad, along with sliced celery and radishes, for a big mouthful.

Get dicey. Add diced cucumbers and tomatoes to your favorite pasta salad.

FISH

Reel In Big Benefits

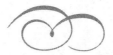

I'M ALWAYS SURPRISED WHEN I TALK TO FOLKS WITH HIGH blood pressure or high cholesterol who admit that they'd like to eat more fish, but they just don't know how to cook it. Nothing could be easier. Fish is so thin and tender that it requires minimal fuss. Nothing could be healthier, either. Fish arrives packed with omega-3 fatty acids—essential fats that our bodies can't make, so we have to get from foods.

UP THE FOOD CHAIN

Strangely, omega-3's actually come from green plants, such as plankton and tree leaves. We get our omega-3's by eating fish that have eaten the plankton. Our forebears got theirs from the meat of animals that fed on tree leaves, such as deer

> ## ...Just the facts
>
> Wild Atlantic salmon (3 oz broiled)
> Calories: 155
> Fat: 7 g
> Saturated fat: 1 g
> Cholesterol: 60 mg
> Sodium: 48 mg
> Total carbohydrates: 0 g
> Dietary fiber: 0 g
> Protein: 22 g
> Vitamin E: 13% of Daily Value
> Iron: 5%
> Zinc: 13%

and antelope, but those days are long gone. Nowadays, our meat comes from the feedlot, where the cattle grow fat eating silage and hay, which contain only traces of omega-3's.

While a few other foods, such as canola oil, flaxseed, walnuts, and some green leafy vegetables, deliver alpha-linolenic acid, which our bodies can use to create omega-3's, by and large, fish is the answer.

Why focus on fish? Numerous studies have shown that people who eat just two 3-ounce portions of fish weekly have lower rates of heart disease, stroke, irregular heartbeat, and high blood pressure. Researchers speculate that omega-3's are the source of fish's power, because these fats are incorporated into cell walls throughout your body and change the way cells work.

When omega-3's become part of blood platelets, for instance, the platelets are less sticky and less likely to clump, so there's less chance that they'll block an artery and cause a heart attack.

ANGLE FOR EXTRAS

Here are some other findings.

• A Danish study found that women with severe menstrual pain tended to have low intakes of fish.

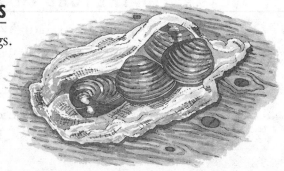

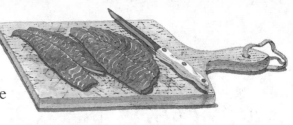

• Researchers have found that supplementing women's diets with omega-3 fatty acids makes their menstrual cycles more regular—no more guessing!

• In a study at Albany Medical College, 33 patients with rheumatoid arthritis who took fish oil had much less joint pain, and some were able to stop taking nonsteroidal anti-inflammatory drugs, such as ibuprofen, for pain relief.

• Finnish research suggests that people with low levels of omega-3's in their brains are more likely to have depression.

← Angling for the Fattiest Fish →

When you're fishing for omega-3 fatty acids, net these beautiful swimmers for a bountiful catch.

Fish (3 oz)	Omega-3 Fatty Acids (g)
Sardines in sardine oil	3.3
Lake trout	1.6
European anchovy	1.4
Bluefish	1.2
Pink salmon	1.0
Striped bass	0.8
Pacific oysters	0.6
Tuna	0.5
Shrimp	0.4
Alaska king crab	0.3
Northern lobster	0.2
Scallops	0.2
Swordfish	0.2

Best if Used By

Now that you've bought the best, keep it tasty and fresh!

• Store fresh fish in its original wrapper in the coldest part of your refrigerator. Use it within two days.

• Keep raw fish away from cooked fish to avoid contamination from the uncooked juices.

BEAR A BRAINCHILD

On the child development front, researchers have learned that when a pregnant woman eats fish, the omega-3's are passed on to her fetus and used for brain and vision development. Later, during breastfeeding, omega-3's are also passed on to the infant. Currently, there is great debate over adding omega-3's to infant formula in the United States, as is being done in Europe.

FRESH CATCH!

Buying delicious fresh fish is easier than you might think. Just look for plump, moist fish that smells fresh and breezy, not fishy. Look for whole fish with bright, clear eyes and clean, tight scales. Choose moist-looking steaks and filets.

Here's how to get your omega-3's in fine style.

Make chunky chowder. Add fresh fish bits to commercial vegetable soup and simmer for at least 5 minutes to be sure the fish is cooked through. You can also use leftover cooked fish pieces.

Reach for anchovies. Along with peppers, onions, and olives, order anchovies on your pizza. Have them on your Caesar salad, too.

Make a double batch. When you're grilling salmon, cook more than you need. Chill the leftovers to mix into pasta salad to take to work the next day.

Pop the top of a sardine can. Have a couple of sardines with some whole grain crackers for lunch or a snack.

ON THE TABLE

Cooking fish is oh, so easy. Here's how to do it safely.

Time the marinade. Since fish is very tender, don't marinate it for more than 10 minutes, or it will become mushy.

Cook lightly. While you shouldn't overcook fish, because that makes it tough, do make sure it's completely cooked. Eating "medium-rare" fish can be risky because it can harbor parasites and bacteria that cause food poisoning. But relax: Thoroughly cooked fish is safe.

Do the math. Baking, broiling, poaching, frying, or stewing fish takes about 10 minutes per inch of thickness. You can tell fish is done when it changes from translucent to opaque.

Be smart about fashion food. The USDA says raw fish dishes, such as sushi and sashimi, can be safe for most people (except for those with diabetes) if they are made with very fresh fish, commercially frozen (at temperatures lower than those of home freezers), and thawed before eating. Commercial freezing kills any parasites that may be present, eliminating any danger to you.

FOOD NEWS

Recent research has revealed that in spite of the health benefits of fish, some contain such high levels of mercury that pregnant women, nursing mothers, and children under age 18 should avoid them. The problem? Mercury can slow brain development in growing children. Here are the recommendations.

• Avoid King mackerel, shark, swordfish, and tilefish.

• Limit white albacore tuna to one serving per week. Chunk light tuna is okay twice a week.

• Many other fish and shellfish are safe to eat twice a week. Some kinds that kids love are shrimp, tilapia, haddock, trout, catfish, flounder, scallops, pollock, cod, perch, halibut, monkfish, and snapper.

MILK

Zap High Blood Pressure

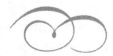

...Just the facts

Fat-free milk (1 cup)
Calories: 85
Fat: 0 g
Saturated fat: 0 g
Cholesterol: 4 mg
Sodium: 126 mg
Total carbohydrates: 12 g
Dietary fiber: 0 g
Protein: 8 g
Vitamin A: 10% of Daily
  Value
Riboflavin (vitamin B$_2$): 20%
Vitamin C: 3%
Vitamin D: 25%
Calcium: 30%

OH, BABY, BABY. YOU STARTED YOUR life drinking milk. In fact, until you were six months old, milk, and milk alone, was the perfect healthy diet. Of course, as you grew older, milk had to make room for other important foods, but it's still critical for maintaining a healthy body—and healthy blood pressure—no matter what your age.

Milk's image has suffered a little because of whole milk's high saturated fat content, but fat-free and 1% milk pack the same nutrition without the fat. Don't like the taste? Neither did I when I was little, so my dad added a little sweetener and vanilla and called it "skookie," and I was good to go!

DIAL DOWN BLOOD PRESSURE

Which do you think works better for lower-ing blood pressure—taking calcium supplements or drinking milk? You're correct if you guessed milk. All sorts of dietary supplements, including calcium and magnesium, have been tested for their ability to lower blood pressure, but what works best is real food.

In a study called Dietary Approaches to Stop Hypertension (DASH), researchers in several centers around the country found that when they switched people with moderately high blood pressure from a typical American high-fat diet to a low-fat diet rich in fruits and vegetables, the participants' blood pressures started to come down. When the participants were given three servings of dairy foods daily, even better things happened. In just two weeks, their readings dropped as much as if they had taken blood pressure medication. Bottoms up!

BUILD UP BONES

When you consider the benefits of milk, you probably think of calcium, which is so important in the fight against osteoporosis. Well, you're right: Milk and products made from milk, such as cheese and yogurt, supply about 300 milligrams of calcium per serving. That's about one-third of the Daily Value for folks under 50 and about one-fourth of what you need if you're older.

What you may not realize is that only milk is fortified with vitamin D, which delivers an osteoporosis-preventing bonus. Without the "sunshine vitamin," you might as well take a bath in milk for all the good it will do your bones. You simply can-not absorb calcium if you're D-ficient.

Most younger adults make enough vitamin D when the sun shines on their skin. Even so, a study at Harvard found that 42 percent of adults under age 65 were deficient in vitamin D. Worse, the study found that 99 percent of older adults who don't spend any time outdoors, or who live in northern areas where the sun's rays are too slanted to get the job done, also didn't have enough. So baby yourself: Drink your milk.

TAKE THE WEIGHT OFF

If you're struggling to control your weight (and who isn't?), milk could be a great ally. Although several studies have pointed in this direction, a recent clinical trial (the gold standard in research) sealed the deal. Under the direction of Michael B. Zemel, Ph.D., professor and head of the department of nutrition at the University of Tennessee in Knoxville, 32 obese adults spent 24 weeks eating 500 calories less per day than they needed to maintain their weight. One group received 400 milligrams of calcium daily from food and lost 6

← Cow Calories →

Cup for cup, fat-free milk has all the vitamins and minerals of whole milk, but fewer calories, less fat, and less cholesterol. See how the cow cartons (8 ounces each) stack up.

Milk	Calories	Fat (g)	Saturated Fat (g)	Cholesterol (mg)
Fat-free	85	0	0	4
1%	102	3	2	10
2%	121	5	3	18
Whole	150	8	5	33

percent of their body weight. A second group, which received 800 milligrams daily from supplements, lost 8.6 percent of their body weight. The third group ate a diet that delivered 1,200 milligrams of calcium per day from dairy foods and were the big losers at 10.9 percent. Also, more of their weight loss was fat rather than muscle, and more of their fat loss came from the dangerous abdominal area. Thus, adding calcium can be a big help, but nothing does weight loss like milk!

Unfortunately, dieters often spurn milk while trying to lose weight, and that's a bad move. Carrying excess pounds is a weight-bearing activity that helps keep calcium in your bones (one of the rare benefits of being overweight). When you lose weight, you start to lose calcium, even if you exercise, so keep that low-calorie milk in your diet plan to minimize bone loss.

BEAT PMS

For women (and their partners!) who cope with premenstrual syndrome, boosting calcium intake to 1,200 milligrams daily can cut symptoms in half. It may take about three months before changes are really noticeable, but it just keeps getting better after that, according to Susan Thys-Jacobs, M.D., of St, Luke's–Roosevelt Hospital Center in New York City. She notes, "I tell all my women patients to get two dairy foods and to take two Tums" to reach 1,200 milligrams. So don't be a cranky baby: Drink your milk!

IN THE MOOD FOR MOO

Need milk? To get the best, check the "sell-by" date to be sure it's fresh, and always buy pasteurized milk. The brief, mild heat treatment kills dangerous bacteria without changing the taste or nutrition. Heat and light are milk's enemies, destroying vitamins with exposure, so keep your milk in the refrigerator.

Here are some easy ways to help you get your daily dose of moo juice.

Create a cocktail. Fight premenstrual syndrome by adding fat-free chocolate syrup to a glass of calcium-rich fat-free milk. Flavor sweetened fat-free milk with vanilla, almond, or peppermint, or maybe make peppermint chocolate milk!

Add extra. For a real calcium jolt, add ⅓ cup of nonfat dry milk to your next smoothie. It has all the nutrition of a full cup of liquid milk.

Double up. Use fat-free evaporated milk to lighten your coffee. Half the water has been removed, so measure for measure, it has twice the nutrition of regular milk.

Replace water. Use fat-free milk instead of water when you microwave your oatmeal or cook creamed soups.

Get comfy. Need some comfort food? Have a glass of milk and a couple of cookies or half a peanut butter sandwich.

POTATOES

Potassium Powerhouses

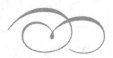

THE RECENT LOW-CARB MANIA MAY have you thinking twice about eating potatoes. If so, listen up: That baked potato you've been passing up packs more potassium than a banana, and potassium is crucial for helping you beat high blood pressure.

PORTION PROMISE

Okay, it's true Americans have been eating way too many French fries. A super-sized serving packs 540 calories, and that's without your sandwich and glass of milk. That's a problem for your body, but a medium potato as part of a meal? It's nutritional dynamite!

In fact, a recently published study led by Ronald Prior, Ph.D., a chemist and

...Just the facts

Potato (1 medium baked, plain with skin)
Calories: 133
Fat: 0 g
Saturated fat: 0 g
Cholesterol: 0 mg
Sodium: 10 mg
Total carbohydrates: 31 g
Dietary fiber: 3 g
Protein: 3 g
Vitamin B_6: 21% of Daily Value
Vitamin C: 26%
Copper: 19%
Iron: 9%
Potassium: 15%

A SIMPLE SOLUTION

Are you on a low-sodium diet to lower your blood pressure? Drop a peeled potato into your soup or stew, then discard it. It will absorb some of the sodium.

nutritionist with the USDA Arkansas Children's Nutrition Center in Little Rock, placed potatoes in the top group of fruits and vegetables for their total antioxidant capacity. It's true! When it comes to having the right stuff to fend off high blood pressure, heart disease, cancer, and other ailments too numerous to mention, potatoes beat out expected favorites such as sweet potatoes, red bell peppers, broccoli, and cantaloupe.

Even if you're struggling with diabetes or insulin resistance, you can still enjoy potatoes. Just eat them in small portions, include the skins, season them with a little heart-healthy fat (such as olive oil), and have them as part of a meal. That will slow their digestion so you don't get a sugar jolt. Why not just avoid them? Because they're good for you in so many ways. So get out your measuring cup and practice serving yourself one portion of delicious health benefits.

MANY-SPLENDORED THINGS

Having mood problems? Potatoes may be your best friend (or maybe second only to chocolate). One medium baked potato delivers 24 grams of pure carbohydrate, known to soothe jangled nerves and elevate mood.

Not enough to chill you out? That potato is also studded with vitamin B_6, which is needed to boost serotonin, the natural brain chemical that makes you feel happy.

Want more? Your potato is bursting with copper, magnesium, and manganese, which boost bone health. And there's even some vitamin C in there to help heal those little shaving cuts. No wonder folks love potatoes!

REENERGIZE WITH "SPUDDIES"

Athletes may start the day with Wheaties, but endurance specialists, such as marathon runners and triathletes, follow their exhaustive workouts with high-carbohydrate foods. Nothing refuels a jock better than potatoes—whether the jock is a Los Angeles Laker in California or a Milltown Midget in your backyard.

Here's why: As athletes train, their muscles learn to suck up carbohydrates from food, turn them into blood sugar, and store the sugar in muscles as glycogen. That's the energy for tomorrow's workout. But all carbs are not created equal. Some are digested and stashed faster than others, and potatoes lead the pack in the race to reenergize.

Think that's just for kids or superstars? Not so. I've been checking out the Senior Olympics, and grownup athletes are just as focused on carbs. So have a guilt-free potato as part of your post-workout meal.

'TATER TALK

Potatoes come in two basic types. Idahos and russets are dry, mealy, and fluffy, so they have to soak up a ton of butter or sour cream to be palatable. Waxy potatoes, such as red-skin, new, or Yukon Gold, have higher water content and need little fat to make them delicious. Guess which ones I prefer.

Fabulous Fill-In!

Want easy? Try peeled, sliced, diced, or mashed potatoes from the supermarket refrigerated case. Canned and frozen potatoes work well, too.

When selecting potatoes, consider buying them loose so you can handpick each one and get the size you prefer. While you're at it, you can also check for cuts, bruises, and mold. If you buy potatoes already bagged, try to get a bag you can see through or, if all else fails, use the sniff test to check for rotten stowaways.

Try these various ways to enjoy your fantastic spuds.

Hook up with fish. Top a baked potato with ¼ cup of canned salmon for a heart-healthy treat that's teeming with flavor. Or stuff your potato with shrimp salad and let the mayo do double duty.

Think Mexican. Dress your potato with salsa for a spicy side dish.

Try Mediterranean. Top a potato with olive spread; you'll do your arteries a favor.

Be a cowboy. Stir powdered ranch dressing seasoning into mashed potatoes for a ton of flavor without the fat, or sprinkle some on a baked potato.

Hurry up. Buy canned cubed or sliced potatoes for quick preparation and add them to soups, stews, and other vegetable dishes.

Recapture the vitamins. When you boil potatoes, use some of the cooking water along with nonfat dry milk to make mashed potatoes. You'll round up some of the vitamins that escaped into the water.

SQUASH

The Color of Health

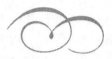

Maybe you've been eating lots of bananas for potassium, and that's a good thing. If you'd like a change of routine, though, have squash occasionally instead (not for breakfast, of course). A mere ½-cup serving, enough to fill half a tennis ball, provides 20 percent more potassium than a banana, and for half the calories!

Potassium is especially important for heavy exercisers and anyone taking diuretic medication, because this mineral regulates heartbeat and keeps blood pressure under control—and that reduces your risk of having a heart attack or stroke.

ORANGE YOU AGLOW!

It turns out that color is key for zeroing in on the healthiest foods from

...Just the facts

Butternut squash (½ cup mashed)
Calories: 49
Fat: 0 g
Saturated fat: 0 g
Cholesterol: 0 mg
Sodium: 5 mg
Total carbohydrates: 13 g
Dietary fiber: 3 g
Protein: 1 g
Vitamin A: 172% of Daily Value
Vitamin C: 20%
Calcium: 5%
Iron: 4%

Think squash is hard to keep? Wrong. Just scrub off the dirt, and you're done. With that hard outer shell, squash is tough enough to survive for months without refrigeration, so you can arrange an assortment in a spectacular autumn centerpiece. They'll last until you serve the squash as a side dish with your Thanksgiving turkey.

Mother Nature's garden. The very ingredients that produce the pretty colors are the same ones that enhance your vision, protect your cells against cancer, and defend your arteries against cholesterol buildup.

The beautiful, deep orange color of winter squash is a sure sign that it's loaded with beta-carotene, a carotenoid that turns into vitamin A in your body. Just a tiny, ½-cup serving of acorn squash delivers enough beta-carotene to meet half your vitamin A needs for a day. The same amount of Hubbard squash delivers a whole day's worth. And get this—a small dollop of butternut squash is over the top, providing enough vitamin A for a day and a half!

THE RAINBOW CONNECTION

Dark green, deep orange, and bright red fruits and vegetables can deliver more than 400 different carotenoids. About 50 of these can create some vitamin A, but beta-carotene is by far the biggest supplier, and it has a lot of jobs to do.

• *Halt cancer.* Beta-carotene helps prevent cancer by draining the energy out of singlet oxygen, an "excited" type of oxygen that can wreck cell membranes, destroy enzymes, and confuse your DNA into making cancer cells instead of normal cells.

• *Trigger immunity.* Beta-carotene also appears to be a powerful stimulant for your immune system, keeping it alert to invading organisms and helping to remove potentially cancerous cells from your body.

• *Screen out sun damage.* Beta-carotene may help protect your skin against sunburn. In one study, women who got lots of beta-carotene and used sunscreen got more sunburn protection than those who used sunscreen alone.

• *Aid eyesight.* A study in Nepal showed that high beta-carotene intake reduced night blindness among pregnant women by 50 percent.

• *Boost bones.* Beta-carotene can enhance vitamin A's efforts to lengthen and strengthen bones.

LEARN TO PLAY SQUASH

One especially nice thing about winter squash is that it shows up just when all those tender summer veggies begin to vanish. In September, you'll find winter squash in an array of colors, shapes, and sizes at supermarkets and roadside stands. Choose squash that are firm, smooth, and evenly shaped, with no cuts or mold.

A SIMPLE SOLUTION

Having a hard time getting your family to eat squash? The secret to success may be in the presentation, so try this approach. Start with four different colors of acorn squash. Cut them crosswise into 1-inch-thick slices, remove the seeds, and—voilà—squash flowers! Spritz them with olive oil, sprinkle with a little brown sugar and cinnamon, and bake at 350°F for 20 minutes. They'll be a surprise hit. Piled on a platter, they make a blooming garden of colors. We bet no one at your table will say, "Yuck!"

Here are some fun and easy ideas for serving up squash in a family-friendly way.

Baby it. Choose a tiny acorn squash, split it lengthwise, and scoop out the seeds, then microwave until fork-tender. (The amount of cooking time depends on the size.) Sprinkle with nutmeg and chopped walnuts for two perfect ½-cup servings.

Make it soup. Use baked squash or the frozen pureed kind to make wonderfully silky soup, or add leftover chunks of baked squash to canned vegetable soup.

Make great gravy. Turn pureed golden squash into heavenly, healthy "gravy" for lean pork, pot roast, or chicken breasts by mixing it with onion flakes and garlic powder.

Make it dinner. Split a small butternut squash and remove the seeds. Fill the cavity with a mixture of ground turkey breast, chopped celery, grated carrots, and cooked brown rice and bake at 350°F until tender.

WHEAT GERM

E-Z Mineral Supply

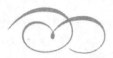

IT WASN'T UNTIL AFTER I WAS ALL GROWN UP THAT I realized my mom had stealthily led our family into the world of healthier food. One of her best-kept secrets was to hide wheat germ in meat loaf and other dishes where no one noticed. Her goal: to thwart the high blood pressure and heart disease that stalked our family. Good move, Mom. As it turns out, wheat germ may be the twinkle in Mother Nature's eye, too.

Wheat germ is that tiny bit of the wheat kernel that gets left behind in making white-flour "balloon" bread and all that other white stuff we're addicted to, such as pasta, most flake cereals, pastries, cakes, and cookies.

But the joke's on us. The germ is

> ### ...Just the facts
>
> Wheat germ (2 Tbsp)
> Calories: 50
> Fat: 1 g
> Saturated fat: 0 g
> Cholesterol: 0 mg
> Sodium: 0 mg
> Total carbohydrates: 6 g
> Dietary fiber: 2 g
> Protein: 4 g
> Folate: 20% of Daily Value
> Vitamin E: 20%
> Magnesium: 10%
> Manganese: 140%

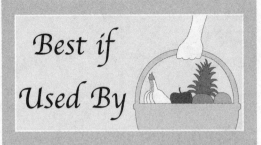

Best if Used By

Store unopened wheat germ in your pantry, away from heat, where it'll keep for about a year. Once the jar is opened, put it in the refrigerator, because the oil becomes rancid easily when exposed to air.

where the goodies are stored, and that just goes to show you why it's not smart to mess with Mother Nature—or my mom!

KEYS TO THE KERNEL

A kernel of wheat has three basic parts.

• *The endosperm*. This is the fluffy white inside of the kernel, the part that is milled to make white flour. It's carbohydrate rich and packs gluten, the protein that makes dough stretchy and elastic enough to capture and hold air while bread bakes.

• *The bran*. The outer coating, or bran, provides the "rough" in roughage. It's the insoluble fibrous part that keeps you regular. Just 2 tablespoons provide 10 percent of the fiber you need for the day, with no calories. What a bargain!

• *The germ*. It contains some unsaturated fat, vitamin E, the B vitamins niacin and thiamin, and the minerals copper, iron, magnesium, manganese, and zinc. Magnesium, in particular, helps reduce the tension on artery walls and relax the muscles that control blood vessels so blood flows freely—the key to lowering blood pressure. Imagine all that in such a tiny package. It's practically a miracle.

If you're fat phobic, you may fear that little bit of oil in wheat germ, but relax. It's essential for carrying the fat-soluble vitamin E so your body can absorb it. Most of us get far too little vitamin E from foods.

Unless you've been living on another planet, you probably

know at least a little about vitamin E. It has been linked to fighting heart disease, stroke, and Alzheimer's disease. The oil is also a good source of phytosterols, a plant version of cholesterol that has been shown to lower cholesterol levels in humans and, at least in test tubes and lab animals, to fight cancer.

FOLATE FINDER

Fortified wheat germ is also an excellent source of folate, a proven protector against neural tube birth defects. Experts at the Centers for Disease Control and Prevention estimate that half of all neural tube defects could be prevented if women just got enough folate before getting pregnant. This B vitamin is also known for managing out-of-control blood homocysteine levels, which can trigger a heart attack.

BONE BUILDER

Wheat germ delivers a truckload of minor minerals that now appear to be critical for bones. No, there's not much calcium in there, and you're right—calcium provides the bulk of bone matter. Nevertheless, bit players such as copper, iron, magnesium, manganese, and zinc play critical roles that make calcium look like a star. Their interaction seems to create a kind of synergy, where working together makes the total greater than the sum of its parts—a sort of one-plus-one-equals-three, if you will.

WHEAT GERM GUIDELINES

The rules for buying wheat germ are simple. You'll probably get it in a vacuum-sealed jar, so look for the "best-used-by" date to make sure it's fresh. If you buy wheat germ in bulk, give the barrel a serious sniff. The heart of the grain should smell fresh. If it has a sour or musty odor, pass on it.

Now what do you do with your wheat germ? Here are some ideas.

Sprinkle it on. After you've tossed your greens until they're glistening with dressing, sprinkle a tablespoon of wheat germ on top. It will stick to the leaves instead of falling to the bottom of the bowl.

Stir it in. Just use your favorite muffin or quick bread recipe, but replace up to ½ cup of the flour with wheat germ. You can add wheat germ to piecrust, too.

Top it off. Sprinkle wheat germ on your favorite hot or cold cereal for a toasty taste and a big measure of minor minerals.

Fold it in. For a speedy dose of vitamins, fold fresh fruit into blueberry yogurt along with a tablespoon of wheat germ.

Trade up. Be loyal to your arteries! It isn't treason to trade white flour for wheat germ when you coat chicken or fish for oven frying.

HIGH CHOLESTEROL

Dump the Gunk

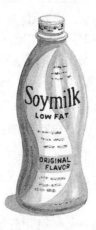

MARIE COULD BE A POSTER GAL FOR THE AMERICAN Heart Association. She savors salads, stays slim with daily runs, and lets off steam with pals at lively book club meetings. Yet she was recently shocked to discover that her total cholesterol level had shot up since her last checkup. Since her mother took potent heart medication for most of her life, Marie worried that she faced the same fate.

It's a common concern. About 98 million Americans—a third of us!—have unhealthy levels of cholesterol, the waxy substance made in the liver that attaches to proteins and travels through the bloodstream as lipoproteins.

Low-density lipoprotein (LDL) is the "bad" cholesterol that can cling to artery walls and set the stage for heart attacks. High-density lipoprotein (HDL) is the "good" cholesterol that sweeps the gunk out of the bloodstream. LDL plus HDL (along with other blood fats, such as triglycerides) equal your "total cholesterol." The idea is to minimize LDL and maximize HDL, but unfortunately, many of us inadvertently do the opposite.

THE HEART OF THE MATTER

A number of out-of-your-hands factors can make LDL levels rise and HDL levels fall—including loss of estrogen at menopause, diabetes, a thyroid disorder, or, as with Marie, a genetic predisposition to hold on to excess cholesterol in the bloodstream. Yet, as one expert put it, "Genetics may load the gun, but lifestyle habits like a fat-laden diet pull the trigger."

Smoking lowers HDL levels by 15 percent, while animal foods from beef to butter are loaded with saturated fat and drive up LDL levels, as do the trans fatty acids in prepared foods such as doughnuts and deep-fried chicken. And starchy, sugary foods don't just raise triglycerides, which are associated with unhealthy total cholesterol levels, they lower HDL, too.

TAKE THE LOW ROAD

A healthy cholesterol profile is one in which total cholesterol is below 200 mg/dl (milligrams per deciliter of blood), LDL is lower than 129 mg/dl, HDL is above 40 mg/dl, and, most important, the ratio of total cholesterol to HDL is below 5. The best way to get there? That depends on your profile.

More than 15 million Americans take cholesterol-lowering drugs called statins (atorvastatin, sold as Lipitor, is the leading prescription medication in the United States). These drugs help block the production of cholesterol in the liver, so they're a tremendous boon to people who have very elevated cholesterol levels. But the side effects can include everything from headaches and muscle weakness to a failing liver.

Consult your doctor to see if you need cholesterol-lowering medication. If you have borderline or mildly elevated cholesterol, though, you may be better off turning to nondrug therapies and making lifestyle changes—or, to get your cholesterol levels as low as possible, doing both in combination with medication. Limiting saturated fat to no more than 10 percent of your total calories, for instance, may help you reduce LDL and your statin dosage. Plus, if you combine a low-fat diet with 45 minutes of aerobic exercise three times a week, you may lower your LDL by a whopping 20 points in just three months. Here are more drug-free ways to go low.

A SIMPLE SOLUTION

Trading cholesterol-raising steak for salmon, which is filled to the gills with cholesterol-lowering omega-3 essential fatty acids (EFAs), just three times a week could slash your cholesterol by nearly half, say some studies. Not big on fish? Take 2 tablespoons of flaxseed oil daily (try drizzling it over your salad) to get an equivalent amount of EFAs, says Melissa Stevens, R.D., nutrition program coordinator for preventive cardiology at the Cleveland Clinic in Ohio. If you're taking aspirin or blood-thinning medication, though, check with your doctor first.

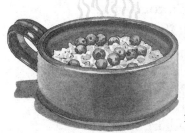

Start with oatmeal. The soluble fiber in oats clears out excess cholesterol better than any other type of fiber. In fact, eating about ⅓ cup of dried oats daily can lower your LDL by more than 5 percent after just one month.

Mix in soy milk. Soy contains isoflavones, estrogen-like compounds that can lower LDL by 10 to 15 percent, says

Looking for a double bang for your nutritional buck? Eat beans. When used in place of meat, beans zap cholesterol with 18 grams of fiber. They also help lower blood pressure with a mineral combo of calcium, magnesium, and potassium.

Michael Miller, M.D., director of the Center for Preventive Cardiology at the University of Maryland Medical Center in Baltimore. You need 25 to 30 grams (about 2 cups) of soy milk daily to reap the benefits.

Manage with margarine. The best way to dress steamed veggies is with 2 tablespoons of a margarine-like spread such as Benecol or Take Control. These spreads contain plant sterols, substances that have been shown to block cholesterol from being absorbed, thus lowering total cholesterol by 10 percent and LDL by nearly 15 percent. Or simply take 200 to 250 milligrams of phytosterols in capsule form three times a day with meals. Most supermarkets carry the spreads; check health food stores for capsules.

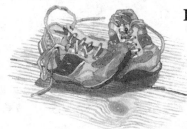

Log more miles. Researchers at Duke University in Durham, North Carolina, have found that people who walk a total of 12 miles a week have bigger HDL molecules that are better at clearing out bad cholesterol than their punier cousins.

Sub for garlic. Allicin, the active component in garlic, quashes cholesterol-producing enzymes. Taking garlic in enteric-coated capsules (which you can find at health food stores) may be more effective than eating it, since the allicin isn't destroyed by stomach acid. Take two capsules daily.

Try a new spin on sugar. For mildly elevated cholesterol, new research indicates that a waxy substance called policosanol, which is derived from sugar cane, may help lower LDL as well as or better than statins and may raise HDL, too. Darin Ingels, N.D., a naturopathic physician and director of New England Family Health in Southport, Connecticut, recommends taking no more than 20 milligrams daily in capsule form (available in health food stores and from the Internet). Talk to your doctor first if you're taking a statin drug or have diabetes.

Sip red wine. According to a study at the University of California, Davis, drinking three to six glasses of red wine a week lowers LDL levels, possibly due to its relatively high concentration of saponins. These plant compounds—believed to bind to and prevent the absorption of cholesterol—are 10 times more abundant in red grapes, especially those in red zinfandel, than in white. You could just eat the grapes, of course, but alcohol seems to release saponins and may also raise levels of estrogen, an HDL booster.

Warm the cockles of your heart. A frothy cup of hot chocolate made with pure cocoa powder (or an ounce of dark chocolate with a high cocoa content) does more than stave off winter's chill: Cocoa is rich in flavonoids, which have been shown to lower LDL and raise HDL.

Two Good!

An apple with its peel is a two-for-the-price-of-one treat, providing both soluble fiber to help lower cholesterol and insoluble fiber to keep your bowels working.

AVOCADOS

Lower Cholesterol Fruitfully

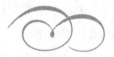

LITTLE CAN COMPARE TO THE TASTE OF A CRISPY TORtilla chip dunked in a dish of creamy guacamole. Mmm! Unfortunately, in the past decade, as we counted fat grams ad nauseam, guacamole got a bad rap. Avocados had the distinction of being one of the few fruits that are high in fat—up to 15 grams in a medium fruit. But now, surprise! Nutritionists have discovered that 80 percent of the fat in avocados is the kind that lowers cholesterol. What's more, avocados outpace every other fruit in certain plant compounds that scientists believe may help prevent cancer and heart disease.

A DIFFERENT ANGLE

When you look at the vitamin and mineral content of avocados, it doesn't seem impressive. Sure, they have a bit of

...Just the facts

California avocado (⅕ medium; about ¼ cup)

Calories: 55

Fat: 5 g

Saturated fat: 1 g

Cholesterol: 0 mg

Sodium: 1 mg

Total carbohydrates: 3 g

Dietary fiber: 3 g

Protein: 1 g

Folate: 6% of Daily Value

folate, potassium, and vitamins B_6, C, and E, but the amounts are scrawny compared with those found in other fruits.

However, researchers at the University of California, Los Angeles, recently dug deeper and found that avocados (at least the ones grown in California) boast 76 milligrams of beta-sitosterol per 3½ ounces. This plant compound can inhibit the absorption of cholesterol from your intestines so you'll have less in your bloodstream, reducing your risk of heart disease. What's more, animal studies have shown that beta-sitosterol inhibits the growth of cancerous tumors.

Ounce for ounce, avocados pack more than four times the beta-sitosterol of commonly eaten fruits such as oranges (17 milligrams), apples (11 milligrams), and strawberries (10 milligrams). They also contain at least twice the amount found in other good sources, such as corn, olives, and soybeans.

That's not all. Avocados are loaded with glutathione, a plant compound that neutralizes free radicals, which cause cell

Good to Go

When you're ready to use your avocado, you'll have to tackle seeding and peeling it. Relax. It looks a lot harder than it is. For safety's sake, we prefer to use this technique recommended by the California Avocado Commission.

• Cut the avocado lengthwise around the seed.

• Rotate the halves to separate them.

• Remove the seed by sliding the tip of a spoon gently underneath it and lifting it out.

• Peel the fruit by placing the cut side down and removing the skin with a knife. Or you can scoop out the insides with a spoon.

• Use the avocado immediately or sprinkle it with lemon juice or white vinegar to prevent discoloration.

damage. Studies suggest that glutathione helps prevent cancers of the mouth and pharynx, as well as heart disease. Avocados offer about 28 milligrams of glutathione in 3½ ounces, while many other fruits, such as watermelon (7 milligrams), pears (5 milligrams), and bananas (4 milligrams), contribute considerably less.

FABULOUS FAT

Yep, it's fabulous. Here's why: A diet rich in unsaturated fat, the main type in avocados, helps lower your level of low-density lipoprotein (LDL) cholesterol—the bad kind—while maintaining your level of high-density lipoprotein (HDL) cholesterol—the good kind. Dozens of studies have linked unsaturated fat to a reduced risk of ticker trouble, although most of them examined the amount of olive oil consumed rather than the amount of avocados.

To pinpoint the benefits of avocados specifically, researchers

← The Skinny Fat →

You can drop a few pounds simply by replacing your usual topping on bagels, baked potatoes, sandwiches, and toast with lower-calorie fare. Check out how 1 ounce (about ¼ cup) of avocado stacks up against an ounce (2 tablespoons) of typical condiments.

Topping	Calories	Healthy Fat (g)	Saturated Fat (g)
Avocado spread	55	5	1
Butter	215	8	15
Cream cheese	105	3	7
Mayonnaise	215	17	4

in Australia asked a group of women ages 37 to 58 to follow a high-carbohydrate, low-fat diet for three weeks and a diet rich in unsaturated fat from avocados for another three weeks. Depending on how much the women weighed, they ate ½ to 1½ avocados daily.

The impressive results: When the participants were on the avocado diet, their total cholesterol levels dropped by 8 percent on average, compared with just 4 percent when they followed the high-carb, low-fat plan. It gets better. While the high-carb, low-fat plan lowered the women's levels of good cholesterol by 14 percent, the avocado diet didn't lower it at all!

Best if Used By

If you buy an unripe avocado, put it in a paper bag and keep it at room temperature to ripen in two to five days. If you need it sooner, add an apple to the bag to speed the process.

THE WEIGHT-LOSS FAT

We know what you're thinking: "This sounds good, but if I start eating avocados and olive oil, my jeans won't fit." That's where you're wrong. If you substitute these foods for less healthy low-fat ones (such as fat-free cookies), you won't gain a pound. In fact, following a high-fat diet may even help you lose weight.

Here's the proof: An 18-month study at Brigham and Women's Hospital in Boston compared a diet rich in unsaturated fat with a low-fat diet. Those on the high-fat plan were allowed about 45 grams of fat a day, mostly from foods such as avocados, nuts, and olive oil. The group on the low-fat diet received only 25 grams of fat a day. After six months, both groups dropped the same amount of weight (about 13 pounds), but a year later, the low-fat group had gained back about 7 pounds, while the high-fat folks had put on just 2 pounds.

"The participants on the high-fat plan seemed to like the diet better, so they were far more likely to stick to it," says study leader Kathy McManus, R.D. It's your choice: steamed vegetables, fat-free salad dressings, and dry bagels—or veggies grilled in olive oil, plus avocados and nuts. Which sounds better to you?

PICK YOUR FAVORITE

There are more than 100 varieties of avocados, but—thankfully—just two main types: California and Florida. You'll be able to find California avocados year-round, while the Sunshine State's avocados are usually available from June through March.

Because they have distinctly different flavors, buy both types to determine which you prefer. In general, California avocados taste more buttery than their southern cousins do, probably because they have twice the fat and about one-third more calories. Everything else about the avocados—including their nutrient content—is identical.

No matter which type you try, determine how ripe the fruit is before you buy. Look for a slightly soft avocado if you want to use it right away. To test it, squeeze it gently in the palm of your hand. Look for a firm avocado if you're not planning to enjoy it until later in the week.

You can incorporate your beautiful green avocado into dozens of dishes besides guacamole. Here are a few.

Smooth out salsa. To quiet salsa's heat and boost nutrients and flavor, just stir chopped avocado into any commercial or homemade tomato salsa.

Spread on bread. For a sandwich, skip the mayo and use mashed avocado as your spread. Top with turkey, provolone cheese, and tomato slices.

Reinvent pasta. Tired of tomato sauce? Cook a pound of fettuccine (plain fettuccine is fine, but try the red-pepper variety, too), then immediately toss with 2 tablespoons of olive oil, ¼ cup of white wine vinegar, ½ cup of chopped fresh cilantro, ½ cup of diced red bell pepper, ½ cup of diced green or yellow bell pepper, 1 cup of diced sun-dried tomatoes, and, of course, 1 diced avocado. Serves 6.

BEANS

Cholesterol Tamers

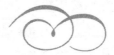

WHEN MY FRIEND KAREN WAS A KID, HER FAMILY OFTEN made minestrone soup. While everyone else heartily dug in, Karen carefully navigated around the soup bowl, pushing the kidney beans aside. Today, her family still makes a mean minestrone, but now she eats the beans. Why? Because study after study has shown her that these luscious legumes are loaded with fiber and other nutrients that keep cholesterol in check and the rest of her body running in top shape.

THE FIBER FOLLIES

Just ½ cup of cooked beans kicks in 3 to 6 grams of fiber, both soluble (the cholesterol controller) and insoluble (a colon cancer fighter). All that fiber is great for your body in so many ways.

...Just the facts

Dried red kidney beans
　　(½ cup cooked)
Calories: 110
Fat: 0 g
Saturated fat: 0 g
Cholesterol: 0 mg
Sodium: 4 mg
Total carbohydrates: 20 g
Dietary fiber: 4 g
Protein: 8 g
Folate: 16% of Daily Value
Calcium: 5%
Iron: 14%

• A study at the University of Kentucky in Lexington found that eating 1 cup of canned beans in tomato sauce daily for three weeks lowered cholesterol in middle-aged men by about 10 percent. Of course, lower cholesterol means less risk of heart disease.

• People with type 2 diabetes may also benefit from the soluble fiber in beans, because it slows the passage of carbohydrates from foods into the bloodstream. As a result, less insulin is needed to control blood sugar levels. By eating a diet rich in beans and other legumes, such as lentils, people with diabetes may be able to get away with using less medication to control their blood sugar levels. Just be sure to check with your doctor before altering your dosage.

• The poky release of carbohydrates into your bloodstream offers another perk: long-lasting energy. "Beans will sustain you longer than a food such as a potato, which quickly releases its carbohydrates," says Kim Galeaz, R.D., of Galeaz Food and Nutrition Communications in Indianapolis.

• If that weren't enough, beans also fight the battle of the bulge. Studies at Pennsylvania State University in University Park suggest that foods low in calories but high in volume and fiber (such as beans) help control your appetite simply by taking up a lot of room in your tummy.

BEYOND FIBER

Beans are also loaded with the B vitamin folate, which reduces blood levels of homocysteine, an amino acid implicated in heart disease. (Yes, folate is the same vitamin that wards off birth defects.) Second, a recent study of 111 women suggests that bean eaters have more flexible arteries than legume loathers. Researchers at Cedars-Sinai Medical Center in Los Angeles planned to do follow-ups, but in the meantime, they recommend eating at least ½ cup of beans a day.

Anybody with asthma knows the scary feeling that constricted airways cause, but now British scientists have found that people who have asthma are half as likely to develop constricted airways if they regularly eat foods rich in magnesium. One of the best? Black-eyed peas, which are actually a type of bean.

BEAN COUNTERS

Many good cooks prefer using dried beans, but if you're a bean novice, start with canned. There's no doubt about it—they're bushels more convenient than dried. Here are some tips to get you off to a successful start using canned beans.

• *Try several brands.* Flavors vary slightly from brand to brand, so experiment to see which you prefer.

← The Bean Bake-Off →

Size up the nutritional differences among your favorite beans.

Bean (½ cup cooked)	Calories	Fat (g)	Fiber (g)	Folate (% of Daily Value)	Calcium (% DV)
Black	114	0.5	4	32	2
Garbanzo (chickpeas)	135	2	3	35	3
Great Northern	105	0.5	5	22	6
Lima	115	0.5	6	34	2
Navy	130	0.5	5	32	6
Pinto	118	0.5	6	36	4
Red kidney	110	0	4	16	5

• *Check for salt content.* Look for brands that contain 350 milligrams or less of sodium per serving.

• *Rinse.* Tests by the nutrition advocacy group Center for Science in the Public Interest in Washington, D.C., have shown that you can eliminate one-quarter to one-third of the sodium in canned beans simply by rinsing them in cold water for about a minute.

Now you're ready to try these bountiful, beautiful bean dishes.

Streamline nachos. At a restaurant, the calories and fat in nachos add up quickly. At home, just dig into this low-fat recipe: Top baked tortilla chips with black beans, reduced-fat Cheddar cheese, lettuce, chopped tomatoes, chopped sweet or hot peppers, and low-fat sour cream.

Improve on hummus. Sure, you can buy this spread, which is an ideal topping for crackers or a great alternative to mayo on bread, but it tastes so good when it's homemade. Try this: In a large bowl, mash one 15½-ounce can of chickpeas (garbanzo beans) or 1½ cups of cooked dried chickpeas. Mix in 2 tablespoons of lemon juice, 1 tablespoon of olive oil, 1 teaspoon of minced garlic, 1 teaspoon of dried oregano, and salt and ground black pepper to taste.

Create instant entrées. Open a can of beans, drain, rinse, and add to salads or soups (such as tomato or vegetable). You can also use them to make a pot of chili or heat them up and mix with cooked brown rice.

CANOLA OIL

The Heartiest Oil

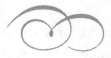

EATING HEALTHIER OFTEN REQUIRES A SACRIFICE—ditching Danish pastries for granola, replacing Alfredo sauce with tomato sauce, or trading French fries for a baked potato. But switching your cooking oil from vegetable to canola isn't a hardship. In fact, the odds are that no one will know but you—and your family's cholesterol levels!

If you don't try canola oil for your ticker, do it for all its other health benefits. Its alpha-linolenic acid may help reduce the risk of stroke, protect against cancer, ease rheumatoid arthritis, and boost your immune system.

LEADER OF THE PACK

You probably think that olive oil is the only healthy fat, and why shouldn't you?

> ## ...Just the facts
>
> Canola oil (1 Tbsp)
> Calories: 120
> Fat: 14 g
> Saturated fat: 1 g
> Cholesterol: 0 mg
> Sodium: 0 mg
> Total carbohydrates: 0 g
> Dietary fiber: 0 g
> Protein: 0 g
> Vitamin E: 31% of Daily
>   Value

It's the one that grabs all the headlines. While olive oil certainly qualifies as healthy, it contains twice as much saturated fat—and only half as much vitamin E—as canola oil.

What's more, canola oil is the only cooking oil rich in heart-healthy alpha-linolenic acid. This substance protects against heart disease by lowering levels of low-density lipoprotein (LDL) cholesterol (the bad kind) and triglycerides (another troublesome component of cholesterol), as well as by reducing the stickiness of blood cells. And, yes, canola oil packs a lot of the healthy monounsaturated fat that has made olive oil famous.

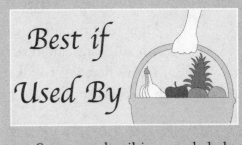

Best if Used By

Store canola oil in a cool, dark place or in the refrigerator. It should keep for up to a year.

THE FRENCH CONNECTION

Because canola oil battles heart disease from a variety of angles, it makes a big impact. Scientists studied 600 men and women in Lyons, France, who had recently had heart attacks. They put half of the participants on a Mediterranean-style diet that derived most of its fat from canola oil, while the other half of the group followed an American diet.

Although both groups ate about the same amount of fat, those on the canola oil diet were 68 percent less likely to have subsequent heart attacks in the following four years than those on the American plan. The results were so dramatic that the researchers stopped the study early so that all the participants could enjoy canola oil's benefits!

IN A HEALTHIER VEIN

After hearing about the promise shown by canola oil in the French study, researchers at the University of Maryland at Baltimore decided to take a closer look. They gave 10 men with normal cholesterol levels meals that contained 50 grams of fat. One day, the men received bread and canola oil (not much of a meal); on another day, they got bread and olive oil; and on a third day, salmon (now we're talking!).

Before and after each meal, the researchers measured blood flow in the men's arteries. The canola oil and the salmon didn't

← The Big Fat Difference →

Tablespoon for tablespoon, all oils have the exact same number of calories (120) and grams of fat (14). But they're far from nutritionally equal. Depending on the type of oil, the 14 grams of fat are split in different ways among saturated (bad), polyunsaturated (good), and monounsaturated (very good). Check out the percentage of each in your favorite oil.

Oil	Saturated Fat (g)	Polyunsaturated Fat (g)	Monounsaturated Fat (g)
Canola	7	32	61
Corn	13	58	29
Olive	15	10	75
Peanut	19	33	48
Safflower	10	76	14
Sunflower	12	72	16
Vegetable	14	64	22

cause any significant changes—which was good—but the olive oil actually decreased blood vessel function.

What did the researchers make of this? "We were surprised," says Robert Vogel, M.D., chief of cardiology at the university. "We expected to see a benefit with all the oils." Dr. Vogel is now conducting the study with a large number of participants. In the meantime, he suggests that you consider cooking with canola oil more often. Check with your doctor first if you're taking the blood thinner Coumadin (warfarin), because canola oil contains quite a bit of vitamin K, which actually encourages blood clotting.

CANOLA CONNOISSEUR

You'll spot several brands of canola oil at your supermarket. Consider buying the type that says "first press" or "expeller press" on the label, even though it's a little pricey.

Canola oil producers extract about 35 percent of the plant's oil by rolling or flaking the seeds. To get the remaining oil, some manufacturers soak the seeds in a chemical solvent, and traces of it probably end up in your oil. No one knows for sure whether it will cause you any harm, but to be on the safe side, look for a bottle from the first press—before the solvent was added.

Unlike olive oil, canola oil doesn't have a strong taste, so it's ideal for dishes that require fat without overwhelming flavor. Here are some ways to use it.

Bake better brownies. You can substitute canola oil for the butter or margarine in your homemade cookie, cake, and brownie recipes and in treats made from boxed mixes. If the recipe requires less than ¼ cup of butter or margarine, use the same amount of canola oil. If it calls for ¼ cup or more, use about 20 percent less oil. For instance, substitute 3½ tablespoons of canola oil for ¼ cup (4 tablespoons) of butter or margarine or 7 tablespoons of oil for ½ cup of shortening. If the recipe calls for vegetable oil, make it with the same amount of canola oil.

Go stir crazy. Heat 2 tablespoons of canola oil in a nonstick wok or skillet, add onions and garlic (as much as you like!), and stir-fry your favorite veggies along with chicken, pork, or lean beef.

Stave off sticking. Use canola oil spray to prevent food from sticking to your pans, baking sheets, or grill rack.

Be the best dressed. Substitute canola oil for vegetable oil in your homemade dressing recipes. It blends well with many herbs and doesn't separate in a dressing.

CHIVES

Make Cholesterol Dive

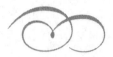

A COUPLE OF YEARS AGO, I STARTED GROWING MY OWN chives. It's so easy: You just throw the seeds in the ground and up they come, edible right from the start. Better still, they come back year after year without prompting. These powerful little onions (or are they garlic?) add incredible flavor to meals while they help lower cholesterol and add other health benefits. That's because chives have pretty darn good genes. Depending on the type you choose, they're related to either onions or garlic. Whatever your choice, they contain compounds that head off heart disease, curb cancer, and more.

THE MAGIC INGREDIENT

The most-studied compound in chives is called allium. Research suggests that allium has antibacterial and antifungal

> ## ...Just the facts
>
> Chives (1 Tbsp)
> Calories: 1
> Fat: 0 g
> Saturated fat: 0 g
> Cholesterol: 0 mg
> Sodium: 0 mg
> Total carbohydrates: 0 g
> Dietary fiber: 0 g
> Protein: 0 g
> Vitamin C: 3% of Daily
>   Value

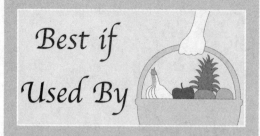

Best if Used By

Store fresh chives in your fridge, where they'll keep for up to a week. If you can't find fresh chives in the produce section, head to the freezer case, where you may be able to snag a bag of frozen ones. When all else fails, swing by the spice rack and pick up a jar of freeze-dried chives.

properties that may help stave off infections. What's more, it guards against cancer of the stomach and colon and lowers cholesterol.

Want to cut back on fat in your diet, as I have? Your taste buds will probably cry foul when you deprive them of some tasty fats. Mine sure did—but only until it dawned on me to add fresh herbs to my recipes.

Think about it: One tablespoon of butter has about 100 calories; 1 tablespoon of chives has just 1 calorie. If you were to replace a tablespoon of butter with a tablespoon of chives every day, you'd lose about a pound a month and not miss a thing. What's more, losing weight helps lower your cholesterol!

SNIP SOME CHIVES

Fresh chives are available year-round in the produce section of your supermarket. When buying them, you first need to decide whether you want onion or garlic chives. Onion chives, the most common type, taste like a mild onion. Garlic chives have the air of the "stinking rose," but they're not quite as strong. Choosing a good bunch of either kind isn't a challenge. Just look for those that have uniformly green leaves and avoid any that show signs of yellowing or wilting.

Ready to add some spice to your life? Try these uses for chives.

Make salad come alive. Line a plate with romaine lettuce leaves and top them with red grapes, chopped pecans, a little blue cheese, a splash of olive oil vinaigrette, and fresh garlic chives.

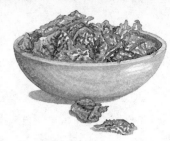

Perk up dip. Mix 1 tablespoon of onion chives with 1 cup of low-fat sour cream or low-fat plain yogurt. Serve with baked chips at your next party.

Magnify flavor. For an extra kick, top cooked shrimp with a sprinkling of garlic or onion chives.

Energize breakfast. Throw some onion chives into your next omelet or mix them into some low-fat cream cheese for a great bagel topping.

CHOCOLATE

Chipping In with Health Benefits

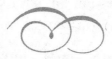

NUTRITION EXPERTS KNOW THERE'S A SPECIAL, LOVING relationship between chocolate and cholesterol, and they're willing to kiss and tell—or at least model great behavior. Sneak a peek.

...Just the facts

Dove Promises Dark
    Chocolate (1 miniature)
Calories: 31
Fat: 2 g
Saturated fat: 1 g
Cholesterol: 0 mg
Sodium: 5 mg
Total carbohydrates: 4 g
Dietary fiber: 0 g
Protein: 0 g

When a roomful of registered dietitians, nutrition researchers, and health writers sit down for dinner, the scene is pretty much as you'd expect. Everybody wants salad dressing on the side. Nobody touches the saltshaker. They all fill their plates with more broccoli than most people eat in a week.

After the main course has been eaten, though, something surprising happens: They start whispering about dessert, how they hope it's chocolate. Chocolate! Not fruit, not angel food cake, not sugar-free

Jell-O. Chocolate! Men and women (but mostly women) who know by heart the calorie, fat, and nutrient content of virtually every food still want chocolate.

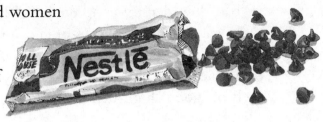

The point: If nutritionists aren't phobic about chocolate, maybe you don't have to feel guilty either. Quite the opposite, in fact. New research suggests that chocolate is good for you. It's not wishful thinking—really!

BARS CHOLESTEROL

No doubt you've heard about fruits such as strawberries being superior sources of antioxidants, compounds that battle heart disease and cancer. Five strawberries offer about 2,400 antioxidant units.

Well, chocolate offers more! Dark chocolate packs 5,700 antioxidant units in 1½ ounces (about the size of a standard candy bar), and milk chocolate weighs in at nearly 3,000.

"Ounce for ounce, dark chocolate has 10 times the antioxidants in strawberries," says Penny Kris-Etherton, R.D., Ph.D., distinguished professor of nutrition at Pennsylvania State University in University Park. "But when you look at serving sizes, it's more like twice as many."

What do these antioxidants have to offer? For one thing, they may help us live longer. At Harvard, a study of nearly 8,000 men found that those who ate chocolate and other candy—regardless of how much they indulged—lived a year longer than those who passed up these treats.

Dr. Kris-Etherton's research suggests that the type of saturated fat in cocoa butter—called stearic acid—doesn't raise "bad" low-density lipoprotein (LDL) cholesterol. In one study, she gave men 1⅓ ounces of cocoa powder (added to milk or pudding) and 2 tablespoons of chocolate chips. As expected, their levels of LDL remained steady, but surprisingly, their levels of "good" high-density lipoprotein (HDL) cholesterol increased.

"We used to think all saturated fat was bad for your heart," she says, "but now we know that there are some types of saturated fat, like the kind found in chocolate, that have neutral or beneficial effects."

Test-tube research has shown that chocolate may prevent bad cholesterol from undergoing a process that makes it more damaging to your heart. Animal studies suggest that an antioxidant in cocoa powder may halt the growth of skin tumors. Scientists have also long known—although they didn't need a study to prove it—that chocolate contains a chemical that improves mood!

HEALTHY MORSELS

Given all the good news about chocolate, how often should you pass the candy dish? No one knows for sure, but the Harvard study indicated that moderate candy eaters—those who reached for one to three candy bars a month—fared the best, reducing their risk of dying by 36 percent over those who didn't eat chocolate.

"It also has a lot to do with the portions," points out Judith Stern, R.D., Ph.D., nutrition researcher at the University of California, Davis. "You can have a full-size chocolate bar a couple of times a month or a mini one every day." Her choice? You guessed it—the mini.

Researchers figure that you're also better off reaching for

either solid chocolate candies or those with nuts rather than those with creamy fillings, which contribute extra calories but very few antioxidants. Also be careful of chocolate in desserts such as cake, cookies, and ice cream. Although you get the health benefits of the chocolate, they come with a lot of calories and other ingredients that could spell trouble for your heart. The bottom line: Settle for a kiss.

What's more, if you have trouble digesting milk, stirring in a few teaspoons of cocoa may help, according to a study at the University of Rhode Island in Kingston. The cocoa may stimulate an enzyme that breaks down lactose, the compound in milk that may be responsible for your bloating and gas.

COCOA LOCO

Shopping for chocolate is almost always fun! In general, look for chocolate that's made with cocoa butter rather than palm kernel oil. Cocoa butter won't raise your cholesterol, says Margo Denke, M.D., professor of internal medicine at the University of Texas Southwestern Medical Center in Dallas and one of the first researchers to break the news that chocolate has redeeming health qualities. Let your taste buds decide the rest.

Dr. Denke would rather opt for a single piece of wonderful chocolate than an entire bar of something that tastes just so-so. You can apply her suggestion to chocolate chips, too. The more flavorful they are, the fewer you'll need to feel satisfied.

Since you're already a pro at using chocolate in desserts, we thought you'd appreciate these healthier options.

Have an eye opener. Stir a tablespoon of unsweetened cocoa into your morning coffee. Dust with cinnamon for a perfect south-of-the-border treat.

Dip into dessert. For an easy dessert, microwave chocolate chips on medium, stirring once or twice until melted, then dunk the tips of strawberries, banana slices, pineapple rings, or prunes.

Go a little nutty. Core and slice an apple. Give the slices a thin coating of peanut butter, then sprinkle with a few mini chocolate chips. It makes a great snack.

Make kid stuff. Love those sugar-laden kids' cereals? We won't tell, but you have to try this instead. Pour yourself a bowl of low-sugar, high-fiber cereal and add a tablespoon of mini chocolate chips and a tablespoon of mini marshmallows along with low-fat milk.

Add yum to yogurt. Trade ice cream for low-fat frozen yogurt, top with berries, and drizzle with a little chocolate syrup.

FENNEL

Fend Off Heart Disease

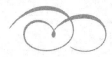

SEVERAL YEARS AGO, WHILE VACATIONING IN THE SONOMA Valley in northern California, I stumbled upon some fennel growing wild. I collected the seeds and planted them in my own backyard in Maryland. They grew into tall, top-heavy plants that reseed every year, so I always have fresh fennel to add to pork dishes. Eventually, I gave some of the seeds to my daughter Bobbi, and now I have grandchild fennel!

Little did I know at the time that those fennel seeds could help my entire family tamp down cholesterol. I just kept on having fun with fennel. Each fall, after I harvest my seeds, I cut the plants off at the ground, gather them into a bunch, and stand them in a large pot that Bobbi made in ceramics class. At nearly 6 feet tall, the

...Just the facts

Fennel seeds (1 Tbsp)
Calories: 20
Fat: 1 g
Saturated fat: 0 g
Cholesterol: 0 mg
Sodium: 5 mg
Total carbohydrates: 3 g
Dietary fiber: 2 g
Protein: 1 g
Calcium: 7% of Daily Value
Iron: 6%
Magnesium: 6%
Manganese: 19%

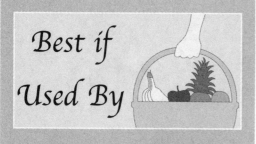
arrangement is quite impressive, and it makes the house smell so good! To enhance the natural room-freshening effect, I add last year's bundle to the woodpile and burn it bit by bit in the fireplace over the winter. Sure smells like home!

FRAGRANT CARROT

Fennel seeds have been around practically forever. The ancient Egyptians called the fennel plant fragrant hay, but it's actually part of the carrot clan. Close relatives include anise (you'll find it in Italian sausage), caraway (in rye bread), coriander (the seed from which you grow cilantro), cumin (essential for Mexican and Indian dishes), parsley (the worldwide garnish), and dill (the best in red-skin potato salad). When they all get together, what a flavorful family!

Although fennel seeds are ancient, scientists with their test tubes and lab mice have just started discovering natural ingredients in the seeds that may help keep you alive and well long enough to enjoy all that delicious flavor.

One recent discovery is anethole, which has been shown to block inflammation and prevent the development of cancer. Fennel seeds also provide modest amounts of flavonols, including quercetin (a more powerful antioxidant than vitamin E), suggesting that these seeds may add to the protective army of fruits and vegetables, such as apples, onions, and tea, that ward off heart disease. And, of course, flavoring with fennel instead of saturated fat such as butter or cream is heart smart and waist conscious, too!

If you need a breath mint, chew on a few fennel seeds. They'll make you kissing-sweet! Hint: They're often served for free at the end of a meal in Indian restaurants.

FINE FEATHERED FRIEND

Fennel bulb is the edible base of one type of fennel plant. It looks like fat celery with green feathers. Like celery, it's very low in calories (about 27 per cup), but it packs more fiber (about 3 grams) and a little vitamin A (about 2 percent of the Daily Value), which is important for protecting all your mucous membranes against invading bacteria and viruses. Fennel bulb makes a top-notch diet food because it tastes a lot like licorice, is bulky and filling, and, best of all, is nearly calorie-free! Fending off the pounds is a super way to control your cholesterol.

FANTASTIC FENNEL

Fennel bulb is available in large supermarkets, mostly in winter. The finest fennel bulb looks nice and clean, is firm and has straight stalks, and sports fresh-looking, green, feathery leaves.

You'll find fennel seeds in the spice aisle. They should be fresh looking and deeply colored rather than dried out and pale.

Here are a few neat ways to add a different taste to everyday dishes.

Make tasty tuna. Instead of celery, dice a fennel bulb into your chicken or tuna salad.

Simmer a side dish. Thinly slice a fennel bulb, mix with chopped onion and garlic, and simmer in chicken broth for about 15 minutes. Drain and serve with a squeeze of fresh lemon juice. It's great with chicken or lean pork!

Order with onions. Toss fennel bulb shavings with red onion shavings and green leaf lettuce. Dress with oil and balsamic vinegar and garnish with freshly grated Parmesan cheese.

Make feathery salad. Snip fennel leaves into salad.

Bake savory bread. Throw some fennel seeds into bread dough just before shaping and baking.

MARGARINE

The Super Sub

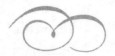

WHEN MY FRIEND KAREN WAS GROWING UP, HER PARents always kept margarine in the house—even though she preferred the taste of butter. Her mom would remind her that margarine was better for her heart than butter and that if she preferred, she could always eat her bread dry.

Years later, Harvard researchers shocked the country by saying that margarine could actually increase your risk of heart disease. Why? Unfortunately, when margarine manufacturers made liquid vegetable oils creamy, they created trans fats, a type that the brainiacs at Harvard have shown is worse for you than the saturated fat in butter!

Now, some manufacturers are offering

...Just the facts

Benecol Light Spread (1 Tbsp)
Calories: 45
Fat: 5 g
Saturated fat: less than 1 g
Cholesterol: 0 mg
Sodium: 110 mg
Total carbohydrates: 0 g
Dietary fiber: 0 g
Protein: 0 g
Vitamin A: 10% of Daily Value
Vitamin E: 20%

You can cook the same way with trans fat–free margarine (except Take Control) as you can with the regular stuff. Baking results, however, may vary depending on the brand and the recipe you're using, so you'll have to experiment. Take Control's manufacturer recommends that you not use that particular product for baking.

margarines that don't contain any trans fats, and a couple of these products are actually made with a compound to lower your cholesterol. Cool, huh?

NEW KIDS ON THE BLOCK

Let's start with the trans fat–free margarines that lower cholesterol—Benecol and Take Control. They boast a cholesterol-like plant fat that blocks the absorption of cholesterol in the small intestine. As a result, the amount of low-density lipoprotein (LDL) cholesterol in the blood drops. How much? The American Heart Association (AHA) says that eating 2 tablespoons of Benecol or 3 tablespoons of Take Control daily lowers LDL cholesterol levels by 7 to 10 percent—and more if used in conjunction with a heart-healthy diet.

Amazingly, these margarines don't seem to lower levels of high-density lipoprotein (HDL) cholesterol, but the AHA warns that you should discuss trying these margarines with your doctor so the two of you can monitor the impact and make adjustments to your medication if necessary.

What's more, Benecol and Take Control are really just for people with high cholesterol. The AHA recently emphasized: "Children and adults who have not been diagnosed as having

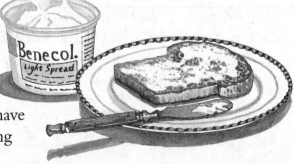

← *Spread Yourself Thin* →

The following spreads are all trans fat–free (and that's fabulous), but their calories and fat content per tablespoon vary tremendously. I suggest sticking with the lower-calorie and lower-fat versions, especially if you're watching your weight. Take a look.

Spread	Type	Calories	Fat (g)	Saturated Fat (g)	Cholesterol	Sodium (mg)	Vitamin E (% of Daily Value)
Benecol	Tub	90	9	1	0	110	20
Benecol Light	Tub	45	5	0.5	0	110	20
Brummel & Brown	Tub	45	5	1	0	90	0
Promise	Stick	90	10	2.5	0	90	15
Promise (Cholesterol Balance)	Tub	80	8	2	0	70	15
Promise Light (Cholesterol Balance)	Tub	45	5	1	0	85	15
Smart Balance	Tub	80	9	2.5	0	90	10
Smart Balance Light	Tub	45	5	1.5	0	90	10
Smart Beat	Tub	20	2	0	0	105	10
Take Control	Tub	80	6	1	Less than 5	110	6
Take Control Light	Tub	40	4.5	0.5	Less than 5	110	10

elevated levels of LDL cholesterol should not consume the product as a 'preventive' measure. While cholesterol-lowering margarines may be used as part of a treatment plan, they do not prevent the underlying cause of elevated LDL."

Somewhere between the new cholesterol-reducing margarines and the old trans fat margarines, you'll find new margarines that are trans fat–free but don't contain cholesterol-lowering plant compounds. These "in-betweens" would be better for kids and adults without high cholesterol.

OLD NEMESIS

Some butter substitutes, especially the stick kinds, are a major source of trans fats in the diet, supplying 1 to 3 grams per tablespoon. A Harvard study of 85,000 nurses found that those who took in the most trans fats (about 5 grams daily) had a 50 percent greater risk of heart disease than those who ate the least, even though their overall fat intakes were the same.

"About 15,000 women die prematurely every year because of heart disease resulting from a high trans fat intake," explains study author Walter Willett, M.D., chairman of the nutrition department at the Harvard School of Public Health.

STICK OR TUB?

If you're in a hurry, the margarine aisle in your supermarket can be a nightmare. If you bear with us for a minute, though, we'll get you through it in a flash. When selecting margarine, choose a brand such as Promise for Cholesterol Balance or Smart Beat, both of which are free of trans fats. Consider liquid margarine labeled trans fat–free. Or, if you have high cholesterol, talk to your doctor about using Benecol or Take Control. These are specifically designed to lower levels of bad cholesterol.

NUTS

Nonpareil Nuggets

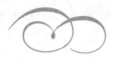

OFFER MY FAMILY A CHOICE OF ANYTHING—MUFFINS, breakfast cereal, salad—plain or nut-studded, and you'll get an instant answer: "We're nuts about nuts!" From applesauce to zabaglione, those crunchy little nuggets make every dish taste better. True, they've been in a dark period because of their high fat content, but through the marvels of modern science, we're beginning to see the light. Nuts are tiny power packets of heart-healthy fat, laced with trace minerals that are critical to health but are often missing from diets built on highly processed (read: white) foods.

BIG FAT BREAKTHROUGH

In 1992, researchers at Loma Linda University in California published a study showing that people who ate a handful of nuts five or more times a week cut their heart attack risk in half compared with folks who never ate nuts.

Since then, one study after another has revealed the same protective effect, whether the nuts studied were walnuts, almonds, macadamias, mixed nuts, or peanuts. (Okay, peanuts are legumes, not nuts, but their fat, calorie, and nutrient profile is a very close match.)

How can all this fat be good for you? While it's true that eating lots of saturated fat from fatty meats, high-fat dairy foods, and baked goods can slam your arteries shut on a moment's notice, the kind of fat in nuts actually opens them up and makes them more pliable.

Walnuts in particular offer something more. The kind of fat in walnuts, alpha-linolenic acid, turns into the same kind of fat you'd get from eating fish. It makes your blood less sticky and less likely to clot, so it reduces your chance of having a heart attack or stroke.

Other varieties of nuts pack big doses of monounsaturated fat, shown to lower "bad" low-density lipoprotein (LDL) cholesterol and triglycerides and to protect "good" high-density lipoprotein (HDL) cholesterol. And with nuts, this isn't just theory. Nut diets have been tested over and over again, and they always work.

TWEAKING DASH

Health professionals have been so excited about this nutty good news that they've incorporated nuts in the Dietary

Approaches to Stop Hypertension (DASH) diet. This incredibly powerful plan combines 8 to 11 servings of fruits and vegetables and 3 servings of dairy foods daily, plus a handful of nuts four or five times a week, along with some lean protein and a few whole grains every day. The result: In just two weeks, people with moderately high blood pressure saw improvements as great as if they had been on blood pressure medication!

MINERAL MEGASTARS

Beyond nuts' special fat, they're also packed with minerals, such as potassium (to help control blood pressure), copper (needed for healthy hemoglobin), and magnesium and phosphorus (great for bones). Plus, they're loaded with vitamins, such as thiamin, or vitamin B_1, which helps turn carbohydrates into energy, and vitamin B_6. which helps make serotonin, insulin, and antibodies that fight infection. In short, nuts are bursting with good stuff!

WEIGH IN ON FAT

Nuts are high in fat and calories, though. If you curl up in front of the TV every night with a can of nuts, you'll quickly pack on the pounds, and that's very bad for your heart and everything attached to it.

We're talking about eating a handful. One ounce. The light side of ¼ cup. The good news is that working nuts into a healthy eating plan that gets 35 percent of its calories from fat can help you lose weight.

In a study at Brigham and Women's Hospital in Boston,

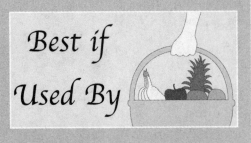
people on this higher-fat diet were compared with a group on a diet containing only 20 percent fat. Although both groups lost the same amount of weight at the outset (an average of about 12 pounds), the nutty dieters kept the weight off for 18 months, while the low-fat dieters regained about half their weight. What's more, twice as many of the low-fat dieters fell off the wagon and dropped out of the study than did those who were enjoying the deliciously nutty plan.

NUTS TO YOU!

You can buy nuts fresh in the shell at most supermarkets, usually from early fall through late winter. The advantage of buying nuts in the shell is that they are unprocessed and unsalted, and they take longer to eat. However, unsalted fresh nuts are also available, already shelled and bagged, in the produce department. You can find smaller packages in the baking aisle.

We recommend these unsalted types. It's also a good idea to keep several varieties on hand so you get a different taste and a different nutrient variety each day. When selecting nuts in the shell, choose those that feel heavy for their size and appear clean, fresh, and free of mold.

Focus on using small servings of nuts in these delicious ways.

Top off your morning. Try a tablespoon or two of nuts

← *Nutrition in a Nutshell* →

Nuts are all packed with protein, heart-healthy fat, vitamins, and the trace minerals often missing from American diets. Each one has its own unique nutrient profile. Pick your favorite from the list below and check its standout qualities. For best nutrition, mix and match. Nutritional values are based on a 1-ounce serving. (The number of nuts in an ounce is listed next to each type.)

Almonds (24 whole)
  Vitamin E: 40
  Magnesium: 20
  Phosphorus: 15
  Calcium: 8

Cashews (18 whole)
  Copper: 30
  Magnesium: 20
  Phosphorus: 15
  Iron: 10
  Zinc: 10
  Selenium: 6

Macadamias (11 whole)
  Monounsaturated fat: 17 g
  Thiamin (vitamin B_1): 15

Peanuts (30 whole)
  Protein: 7 g
  Folate: 10

Pecans (20 halves)
  Monounsaturated fat: 13 g
  Zinc: 10

Pistachios (47 whole)
  Potassium: 290 mg
  Vitamin B_6: 25
  Phosphorus: 15
  Thiamin (vitamin B_1): 15
  Vitamin A: 4

Walnuts (14 halves)
  Polyunsaturated fat: 14 g
  Copper: 25
  Vitamin B_6: 8

NOTE: Values are percent of Recommended Dietary Allowance, unless otherwise noted.

on your hot or cold cereal in the morning. You'll be crazy about your breakfast, and that little bit of fat will help keep you satisfied until lunch.

Hit the machine. When you're starving, grab a bag of peanuts from the vending machine. For 170 calories, you'll be good to go until dinner.

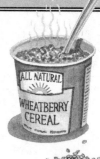

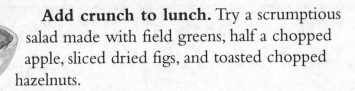

Add crunch to lunch. Try a scrumptious salad made with field greens, half a chopped apple, sliced dried figs, and toasted chopped hazelnuts.

Hide 'em away. Tuck nuts in your desk drawer. Use mini paper bathroom cups to measure out a serving.

Make ants on a log. Stuff celery with reduced-fat ricotta cheese and top with chopped walnuts.

Gussy-up yogurt. Stir in sliced almonds or chopped walnuts—you'll love it!

PARSLEY

Garner Health Gains

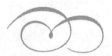

THE NEXT TIME SOMEONE GARNISHES YOUR PLATE WITH parsley, don't just ask, "What's this green stuff?" and then push it aside. Instead, pop it into your mouth! Parsley squeezes so much good nutrition into such a small package that you shouldn't simply compost it.

It starts with your heart. Researchers are reviewing certain plant compounds in parsley called terpenoids, and preliminary results suggest that they can reduce "bad" low-density lipoprotein (LDL) cholesterol and also fight cancer.

A SPRIG OF GOODNESS

A little bit of parsley offers quite a lot of vitamins A, C, and K. Vitamins A and C act as antioxidants, which destroy cell-damaging substances before they can trigger heart disease and cancer. Vitamin K,

> ### ...Just the facts
>
> Fresh parsley (2 Tbsp chopped)
> Calories: 3
> Fat: 0 g
> Saturated fat: 0 g
> Cholesterol: 0 mg
> Sodium: 4 mg
> Total carbohydrates: 0 g
> Dietary fiber: 0 g
> Protein: 0 g
> Vitamin A: 8% of Daily Value
> Vitamin C: 17%

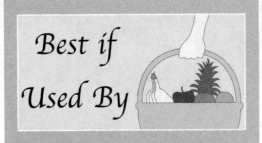
meanwhile, may help strengthen your bones. A recent study at Harvard found that women who had the least vitamin K in their diets were about 70 percent more likely to have hip fractures than those who had the most. Offering protection from debilitating injuries isn't too bad for a garnish, huh?

Then there's parsley's purely cosmetic benefit. This herb can de-funk your breath. The ancient Romans often ate parsley with bread for breakfast, probably to fight morning breath. Try it! It really is an herbal breath mint—and restaurants give it away for free!

FRESH AS A DAISY

Picking fresh parsley is a breeze. Just decide whether you want the curly variety (the kind most often used as a garnish) or the Italian flat-leaf type (better used for cooking). No matter which you choose, look for a bunch with bright green leaves and no signs of wilting or yellowing.

Here are some suggestions to help you use every last parsley sprig.

Buddy with basil. Substitute chopped fresh parsley for half the basil in your pesto recipe.

Pair with potatoes. Add chopped fresh parsley to baked, roasted, or mashed potatoes.

PEANUT BUTTER

Fountain of Youth

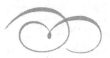

ONE THING THAT MAKES YOU FEEL LIKE A KID AGAIN IS A
peanut butter sandwich. Now, after years
of bad press for being high in fat, peanut
butter is back on the healthy foods list.
Peanut-friendly researchers have clearly
demonstrated that peanut butter's fat is
mostly monounsaturated—the good
kind—and that's probably why studies
show that eating peanuts and peanut butter can lower "bad" low-density lipoprotein (LDL) cholesterol and triglycerides
without lowering "good" high-density
lipoprotein (HDL) cholesterol. That's a
profile that's healthy for your heart.

Ounce for ounce, peanuts contain the
same amount of monounsaturated fat as
tree nuts, such as walnuts, pecans, and
almonds, which have also been shown to

...Just the facts

Creamy peanut butter (2
   Tbsp)
Calories: 190
Fat: 16 g
Saturated fat: 3 g
Monounsaturated fat: 8 g
Cholesterol: 0 mg
Sodium: 150 mg
Total carbohydrates: 6 g
Dietary fiber: 2 g
Protein: 8 g
Niacin (vitamin B$_3$): 21% of
   Daily Value
Vitamin E: 16%
Magnesium: 13%

protect against heart disease. Serving for serving, peanuts contain almost as much protein as beans. Nature's whimsy has created so many delicious ways to nurture a healthy heart!

EAT FAT, LOSE FAT

Of course, if you eat a ton of peanut butter, you'll gain weight, and that's bad for your heart, but if you eat peanut butter in moderation, you should have no problem. Remember, 2 tablespoons (a mound the size of a golf ball) is a serving, and it delivers 190 calories. That's substantial, but it works to keep you satisfied longer than low-fat fare. In fact, in a weight-loss study at Brigham and Women's Hospital in Boston, a group who ate peanut butter and other healthy fats lost weight as well and kept it off better than guys and gals on a very low fat diet.

BREAKING NEWS

The latest nutrition news is that peanuts are packed with sterols, the plant version of cholesterol. Sure, that sounds like a potential problem, but it's not. Plant sterols are absorbed so slowly that they actually get in the way of the cholesterol from foods and prevent it from being absorbed.

At least in the laboratory, those sterols have also been shown to stop the growth of colon, prostate, and breast cancer cells and to cause cancer cells to die. The bad news is that Americans average only 80 milligrams of phytosterols daily. Asians and vegetarians (who rarely get those cancers) get about 400 milligrams daily. Two tablespoons of peanut oil or peanut butter or ¼ cup of roasted peanuts delivers about 50 milligrams of phytosterols.

THE TASTE THAT'S RIGHT FOR YOU

When it comes to peanut butter, buy what you like. Now, you may ask, "What about salt, sugar, and trans fats?" On average, a 2-tablespoon serving of unsalted peanut butter delivers about 5 milligrams of sodium, while the salted kind provides about 155 milligrams (about 6 percent of the recommended daily limit), an amount that doesn't make a huge difference. Some brands also contain a little sugar, but usually not very much (less than 1 teaspoon per serving).

Recently, the biggest flap was over trans fats, the Frankenstein fats created when hydrogen is forced into liquid oil to make it solid. Trans fats can push up your LDL cholesterol while dragging your HDL down, the worst possible scenario for your heart.

Indeed, some hydrogenated oils are added to peanut butter to keep the peanut oil from separating, but these amounts are so small that they rate a zero on the FDA's new labeling scale. Also reassuring is the fact that all the research showing how well peanut butter can lower your cholesterol was done with the hydrogenated kind—so breathe easy.

SPREAD IT AROUND

Now try these simple ways to regain your lost youth.

Berry it. Forget the jelly. Make a grownup sandwich with whole wheat bread, chunky peanut butter, and some fresh blueberries, raspberries, or sliced strawberries. Yum!

Crack it. Forget those neon orange peanut butter crackers from your wasted youth. To get a new lease on life, try some 100 percent stone-ground whole wheat Ak-Mak crackers spread with your favorite peanut butter.

Snack it. Smooth your daily allotment of creamy goobers on celery stalks, carrot sticks, apple slices, or banana circles.

POMEGRANATES

Ancient Healers

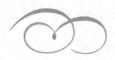

One of autumn's highlights is the arrival of pomegranates, those "jewels of autumn" that remind me of when I was young and shared the sparkling seeds with my friends. Back then, a pomegranate was a special treat—a "fun" food. Now it turns out that it's also a health food. In fact, a pomegranate a day may just keep the cardiologist at bay. The oncologist, too.

LAB LESSONS

Researchers in Israel have been exploring the antioxidant power of pomegranates, with surprising results. The germ of their curiosity came from Middle Eastern folk medicine, in which pomegranates have been used for centuries to tame disease and infections.

In the lab, researchers fermented the

...Just the facts

Pomegranate (1 fruit or ½ cup juice)
Calories: 105
Fat: 0 g
Saturated fat: 0 g
Cholesterol: 0 mg
Sodium: 4 mg
Total carbohydrates: 26 g
Dietary fiber: 1 g
Protein: 1 g
Vitamin C: 16% of Daily Value
Manganese: 44%
Potassium: 11%

juice into wine and cold pressed the oil from the seeds. Then they extracted compounds called flavonoids from both of these liquids and tested their power against that of other known protective foods.

What they learned was that pomegranate flavonoids were equal to green tea and even better than red wine when it came to preventing oxidation of low-density lipoprotein (LDL) cholesterol, the chemical change that allows plaque to clog and harden your arteries. They also found straight pomegranate juice to be more potent than red wine, which means you don't have to get tipsy to get healthy. Another probable benefit of pomegranate flavonoids is the slowing of cell aging.

Going a step further, researchers found that pomegranate juice prevented plaque buildup in mice. And in a group of healthy men, drinking sparkling, sweet-tart pomegranate juice daily for two weeks increased production of an enzyme that can protect against cancerous changes in cells.

It turns out that pomegranates are packed with ellagic acid,

Good to Go

A pomegranate is a sort of leathery red pouch that's about the size of an apple and filled with sparkling, jewel-like seeds. The seeds are packed in a spongy white membrane that acts like bubble wrap. You really can't eat the outer coating (the bubble wrap), so here's how to ditch the debris and get to the good stuff.

• Cut off the crown.

• With a sharp knife, score the leathery rind lightly from top to bottom in several places, being careful not to cut deeply enough to rupture the seeds.

• Put the whole fruit in a bowl of water and soak for 5 minutes.

• Hold the fruit underwater and break the sections apart, separating the seeds from the membranes. The seeds will sink to the bottom of the bowl, and the rind and membranes will float to the top.

• Skim off the rind and membranes and discard them.

• Drain the seeds in a colander, then pat dry. Voilà!

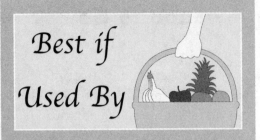

Best if Used By

Even when fully ripe, pomegranates will keep well at room temperature for up to a month, so you could use a few in your Thanksgiving centerpiece and still be able to eat them later. To keep them longer (up to two months), store them in the fridge.

a polyphenolic compound that prevents cancers from getting started. It has been shown to inhibit cancer startup in the lungs, liver, skin, and esophagus of mice.

FALL FOR POMEGRANATES

Pomegranates are available only from September to December, with peak supplies in October and November. During these months, the fruits will arrive at your supermarket ripe and ready to eat. When selecting pomegranates, pick those that have thin, tough, unbroken skin and are heavy for their size—a sign of juiciness.

Here's what to do with your sparkling seeds.

Juice up. Put 1½ to 2 cups of seeds at a time into a blender or food processor and whirl them around until liquefied. Pour the juice into a container through a wire strainer lined with cheesecloth. If you don't drink all of it right away, the juice will keep in the refrigerator for about five days or in the freezer for six months. You can use the juice to make lemonade, to color sliced pears and apples for salads, or as stock for soups and stews. Nifty!

Roll on. Pack a pomegranate in your lunch bag. At your desk, roll the fruit around with the palm of your hand to pop the seed sacs, then just cut off the top and squeeze out the juice. Cool!

Color it beautiful. Just sprinkle the fresh or frozen seeds anywhere you need a brilliant red garnish—on salads, fruit desserts, and even cakes and puddings. Toss seeds into rice or wheatberry salads, stir them into applesauce, or use them as a topping for waffles, pancakes, or frozen yogurt. Pretty!

Chill out. Yes, pomegranates are available only in the fall, but once you find out how good they are, you'll want to eat them year-round. Just scatter the seeds in a single layer on a baking sheet and freeze until firm. Then pack them in freezer containers and store them for up to six months. (Okay, that won't get you through a full year, but half a year is better than nothing.)

Take it easy. Simplest of all, eat them by the handful. They'll be your sweet-tart.

SOY

Lower LDL

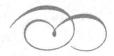

ARE YOU STILL DUBIOUS ABOUT THE TASTE OF SOY FOODS? Childlike, do you simply say "Yuck!" and turn away? Maybe it's time to try again.

One of the big benefits of the low-carb frenzy is that now you can buy pasta made from soy flour. Then there are spicy, Italian sausage–like links made from tofu that add zest to your daily fare. Or how about just eating a bowl of edamame, the boiled green soybeans that are popular as appetizers in sushi restaurants? And finally, you could try a chocolate silk pie made with tofu that will knock your socks off! "Sounds good," you might think, "but why should I bother?" Zing will go the strings of your heart—and there may be other benefits as well.

...Just the facts

Tofu (3 oz)
Calories: 64
Fat: 4 g
Saturated fat: 1 g
Cholesterol: 0 mg
Sodium: 6 mg
Total carbohydrates: 2 g
Dietary fiber: 1 g
Protein: 7 g
Calcium: 4–30% of Daily
    Value
Iron: 25%
Magnesium: 21%
Phosphorus: 8%

PITTER-PATTER

You probably know from watching the news that nutrition researchers like to hedge their bets—they're not certain about much of anything (annoying, isn't it?). But one thing they'd put money on is that two or three servings of soy foods daily lower your cholesterol, reducing your risk of heart disease by about 15 to 30 percent.

The amount of risk reduction depends largely on how high your cholesterol level is, but those numbers were good enough for the FDA to allow food manufacturers to claim heart health benefits on the label of any soy product that contains at least 6.25 grams of soy protein per serving. Also, the American Heart Association recently added soy to its list of ticker-friendly foods. Researchers think that soy keeps your heart healthy in several ways.

• It acts as an antioxidant, gobbling up compounds called free radicals that can cause cell damage that leads to heart disease.

• It decreases blood clotting and inflammation.

• It promotes the expansion of blood vessels when they're under stress, so blood can continue its normal flow.

Many nutrition experts, such as Barry Goldin, Ph.D., professor of family medicine at Tufts University in Boston, recommend that you eat a serving of soy foods in place of something that isn't so healthy for your heart, such as fatty ground beef or whole milk.

FLASH FLUSHER

You've probably heard that soy foods may help ease menopausal discomforts such as hot flashes and vaginal dryness. Research has shown that soy does help cool the midnight fire, but in many studies, a placebo (fake pill) worked almost as well. Scientists are still trying to unravel the mysteries of hot flashes, and they concede that some women may get a lot of relief from soy, while others may see no benefit. Research reported at the Fifth International Symposium on the Role of Soy in Preventing Chronic Disease suggested that women who have the most frequent hot flashes are likely to get the most relief, dropping from eight a day to four or five a day.

BONE BUILDER

Soy may help out with another pesky side effect of menopause: thinning bones. A new three-year study showed that a diet rich in soy lowers the rate at which you lose the bone mineral density that keeps your skeleton strong. Several (but not all) studies have found that soy protein rich in isoflavones reduced bone loss in both perimenopausal and postmenopausal women. Researchers still have to do more work to confirm the connection between soy and your bones, but at this point, it looks promising.

CANCER CURE?

Now here's some news you've been waiting for: Scientists are fairly certain that soy lowers the risk of some types of cancer—especially prostate cancer. That's great news for guys.

Given soy's preventive effects on both heart disease and prostate cancer, "for men, eating soy foods should be a no-brainer," says Bill Helferich, Ph.D., associate professor of food science and human nutrition at the University of Illinois in Urbana.

For women—especially those who have breast cancer or have a strong family history of the disease—soy becomes a lit-

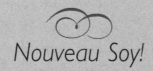

Nouveau Soy!

Have you looked around your supermarket lately? The selection of soy products has exploded in recent years. From staples such as soy milk, tofu, tempeh, and miso to products that use soy as an ingredient (such as soy burgers, cereals, energy bars, low-carb bread, cheese, and yogurt), there's a whole shopping cart of choices.

What's more, major food manufacturers are racing to bring dozens of additional lip-smackin' soy foods to your local market as new processing techniques make them far superior in taste to the gritty brown soy milk or smelly cheese you choked down just a few years ago.

Not all soy products are created nutritionally equal, however. Some of the new products are not-so-healthy foods with a little added dollop of soy. You want to select only the foods that have reasonable amounts of calories, fat (especially the saturated kind), and sodium.

For instance, one new soy cereal packs 200 calories and 440 milligrams of sodium per serving—more than many other cereals, even the kiddie kind.

tle more complicated. Bear with us as we try to explain.

Some types of breast cancer rely on the hormone estrogen to grow. Women make estrogen throughout their lives, although the amount significantly drops after menopause. Soy foods contain plant estrogens called isoflavones. Before menopause, getting about 60 milligrams daily of isoflavones (the amount in a serving or two of soy foods) seems to decrease the body's own estrogen production by about 20 to 40 percent. Since less estrogen means less chance of developing breast cancer, the under-50 crowd probably gains a lot of cancer protection from eating soy foods.

The Serving Sizer

Use this handy guide to determine how much of your favorite soy product equals one serving.

Edamame: ½ cup
Miso: 2 tablespoons
Soy burger: 1 pattie
Soy milk: 1 cup
Soy nuts: ¼ cup
Tempeh: ½ cup
Tofu: ½ cup

As you approach menopause, however, and your body's production of estrogen plummets, the benefits of eating soy start to become iffy. Isoflavones have the potential to stimulate breast tissue, causing changes that may speed growth of cancerous cells.

What's fueling a heated debate is how likely this scenario is to happen. Some experts think that it's a remote possibility; others have staked their careers on its occurrence. Current studies should offer some insight into which theory is right.

Wondering what to do? Try this conservative approach.

• If you have breast cancer or are trying to prevent a recurrence, some researchers advise that you stay away from soy.

• If you have a strong family history of the disease and are postmenopausal, you probably should limit yourself to no more than one serving a day.

• Otherwise, two or three servings daily seem to be fine. More close-to-natural foods (such as tofu and edamame) appear to be better choices than highly processed isoflavone supplements, at least until researchers are able to identify the active ingredients.

SEARCHING FOR SOY MILK?

You'll usually find a brand or two in the refrigerated dairy section near the cow's milk. You'll also find several varieties in aseptic containers in the cereal or baking aisle. No matter where the soy milk's located, the selection guidelines are the same. Make sure it contains no more than 3 grams of fat per cup (about the same as 1% cow's milk). Choose a brand that's fortified with at least 30 percent of the Daily Value for calcium and vitamin D. Otherwise, if you replace cow's milk with soy milk, you won't get as much calcium as you normally would. Store leftover soy milk from aseptic containers in the refrigerator after opening. It will keep for about five days.

TRY OUT TOFU

There are three main types of tofu: firm, soft, and silken. Choose firm tofu for stir-fries or whenever you want it to maintain its shape. Use soft tofu in dishes that require it to be blended and silken tofu in dishes that call for it to be pureed or blended.

Once you know which kind of tofu you need, compare the calcium content among several brands. Most tofu provides from 4 to 30 percent of the Daily Value for calcium. Look for the brand that offers the most of this bone-building mineral.

Keep tofu in the fridge and use it by the expiration date. If you have leftovers, rinse and cover them with fresh water before refrigerating. If you change the water every day, they'll keep for about a week.

BITE INTO A SOY BURGER

Notice that we didn't say "veggie burgers." Some veggie burgers are made from just grains and, well, veggies. They contain no soy at all. Even soy burgers can vary tremendously in the amount of isoflavones they provide.

When selecting soy burgers, check the ingredients list for the words "soy protein isolate" and "soy protein concentrate." Soy burgers made with the isolate have all the isoflavones; those prepared with the concentrate offer just 5 percent, says soy researcher James Anderson, M.D., of the University of Kentucky in Lexington. Keep the burgers in the freezer until you're ready to cook them.

SERVING UP SOY

Once you get your goods, here's how to make the whole family love them.

Call it cow. You can use soy milk in just about any recipe that calls for cow's milk—even cream sauces, puddings, and pancakes. Shop around for a brand you like. My favorite is Silk.

Whip up dip. In a blender, combine your favorite dip mix (such as ranch) with a package of soft or silken tofu. Then open up the low-fat nacho chips and party!

Get fried. Consider using firm tofu instead of beef, chicken, or pork the next time you fire up the wok for a stir-fry.

Go nuts. Instead of noshing on chips and pretzels, curb your craving for crunch with soy nuts. Compared with regular nuts, they have about half the calories and one-third the fat per serving. You can buy them plain or seasoned. Or cook up some crunchy green soybean pods. Even children think that they're yummy—and you know how picky kids can be.

Better your burger. Even though we're tempted, we're not going to lie to you: Even the tastiest soy burger falls short of a mouthwatering real McCoy, but you can come pretty close if you doctor up the burger.

Here are five ways to spruce up a soy pattie.

1. Marinate it in teriyaki sauce before cooking.

2. Add a thin slice of smoked Cheddar cheese and let it melt.

3. Toast the bun (and make sure you pick out a really delicious one).

4. Top it with thin slices of avocado.

5. Spread it with your favorite honey mustard.

Part Three

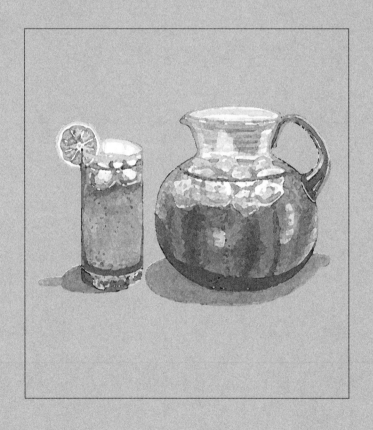

Eat to Calm the Turmoil

As far back as I can remember, peppermint tea has been my family's treatment of choice for soothing upset stomachs. For years, I thought it worked more on my head than in my tummy. After all, who wouldn't feel better when someone makes you a cup of tea, carries it to the couch for you, fluffs your pillow, and coos, "Poor baby!"

Actually, though, the cure wasn't all in my head. It turns out that peppermint is bursting with menthol's natural oils, which can quell tummy spasms, help digestion, and even kill bacteria.

Unfortunately, the truth is that no matter what condition your stomach is in, chances are good that sooner or later, you're going to have a tummy ache. They come in as many shapes and sizes as tummies do, and some need medical attention. Since many digestive woes are temporary, though, and you can treat or prevent them by tweaking what and how you eat, I'll talk about each of the most common digestive problems and how you can find relief. And because what you eat plays a big part in finding that relief, you'll learn about 24 healing foods that will give you a hand. Read on—and never fear tummy troubles again!

Get a Move On

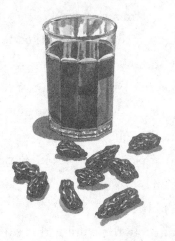

CONSTIPATION MAY SEEM LIKE A MINOR INCONVENIENCE if it's just an occasional thing, but children and adults who are plagued by it may experience major problems with school, work, social life, and how they feel about themselves. If you're really stuck, work with your doctor and/or dietitian to come up with an appropriate diet. That, along with improvements in bathroom habits, can eventually turn things around.

COME UNGLUED

Nearly everyone who has to deal with constipation can reverse it—and more important, prevent it—with some

Two Good!

Double the healing power of dinner by mixing corn and lima beans. Together, they outrank all other vegetables when it comes to forking over fiber.

very basic changes. Here's how to get started.

Pile on the produce. The best diet for beating constipation is the same one that doctors recommend for preventing heart disease, cancer, and dozens of other serious health problems: a lot of plant foods and very little, if any, junk food.

In other words, eat as though processed foods had never been invented. "You want a diet that's high in fiber and complex carbohydrates," says Rob Dramov, N.D., a naturopathic physician in Tigard, Oregon. That means lots of fruits and vegetables, whole grains, and legumes every day, as well as high-fiber cereals such as oatmeal and oat bran.

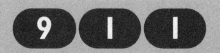

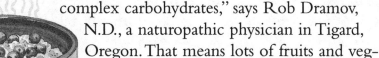

If there's been any change in your usual bathroom habits, get professional advice. There are literally hundreds of things that can cause constipation. It can be a side effect of medications, and lack of exercise, drinking too little water, or not eating enough fiber can also cause it. Sometimes, though, there's a bowel obstruction, and that requires prompt medical attention.

Give fiber a helping hand. It's best to get fiber into your system by eating high-fiber foods, but there's nothing wrong with taking a fiber supplement to help you along. Unlike high-powered laxatives, these supplements are safe enough to use every day. For example, products that contain psyllium, such as Metamucil, can be very helpful. "Try different kinds of supplements until you find the one that works best for you," says Michael P. Spencer, M.D., a colon and rectal surgeon and assistant professor of surgery at the University of Minnesota, Twin Cities.

Dine and unwind. It's the best way to encourage your

A SIMPLE SOLUTION

Constipated? Have a glass of prune juice with a squeeze of fresh lemon juice. Prune juice packs sorbitol, a natural laxative that will get you going quick as a wink. Really stuck? Use your prune juice to wash down a bran muffin.

digestive tract to kick into gear. If you're the type who likes to eat and run, you're diverting blood to other parts of your body and leaving your intestine short-changed. "The old adage, 'rest and digest' is just as true today as it ever was," says Dr. Dramov.

Just say "yes" to Mother Nature. If you're reluctant to use a public restroom no matter how urgent the need, you're setting yourself up for trouble. Resisting the urge to have a bowel movement—whether at home or anywhere else—can make it difficult to go later on. You'll be a lot more regular if you go as soon as possible when you feel the need.

Drown your sorrows. Drink lots of water. It's one of the best ways to treat and prevent constipation. If you don't drink enough, stools will get harder and smaller and be more difficult to pass. As a general rule, plan on drinking at least eight full glasses of water daily, and more if you smoke or drink alcohol, both of which can deplete your body of fluids.

Fabulous Fill-In!

Baby spinach stems are tender enough to eat, so you get twice as much fiber as you would from large spinach leaves with the heavy stems removed.

Make a date, and keep it. Most people find it easiest to have bowel movements in the morning, usually after breakfast or a cup of coffee. Take advantage of this time. Even if you're not sure you can go, plan on spending 5 to

10 minutes in the bathroom. This will help "train" your bowels to move at that time.

Manage with massage. To encourage movement in sluggish bowels, try a simple belly-button rub. Use your favorite massage oil and lightly massage your stomach with the tips of your fingers, starting at your belly button and moving in small clockwise circles. Gradually expand the circles until you're massaging your entire abdomen. If you do this for 10 to 15 minutes every morning, you may find that your daily routine will be a bit more regular.

Move it to move it. Any kind of physical movement—walking, lifting weights, riding a bicycle—helps the intestine work more efficiently. In fact, it's not uncommon for people who have been constipated for years to get completely better once they start exercising for 20 to 30 minutes daily.

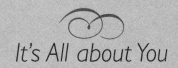

It's All about You

Everyone experiences constipation in different ways. For someone who's accustomed to having a bowel movement every day, a reduction to three or four a week could be a sign of constipation. For others, having three bowel movements a week is normal, but having fewer than that is a problem.

FIGS

Figure on Fiber

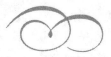

IF I SAID "FIG," YOU'D PROBABLY SAY "NEWTON"—AND that's about as close as most folks get to real figs. But as much as 6,000 years ago, long before there was sugar as we know it, there were figs to sweeten daily fare and keep bowels from getting stuck. Even my grandmother had a fig tree in her backyard! The good news for us modern types is that figs are making a comeback—and not just in natural foods stores. Even larger stores now offer fresh figs in season and dried figs year-round.

ANCIENT JEWELS

Never tried a fig? You don't know what you're missing. Aside from the most amazing flavor, figs supply a boatload of nutrients, benefiting your body in different ways.

...Just the facts

Figs (dried, about 4)
Calories: 120
Fat: 0 g
Saturated fat: 0 g
Cholesterol: 0 mg
Sodium: 5 mg
Total carbohydrates: 28 g
Dietary fiber: 5 g
Protein: 1 g
Calcium: 6% of Daily Value
Iron: 8%

• *Fiber.* Each serving of dried figs (three Calimyrna or four or five Mission figs) provides about 5 grams of fiber. About three-quarters of that, the insoluble form, staves off constipation and may drop your risk of colon cancer.

The other kind of fiber in figs is the soluble type that works to reduce cholesterol levels. A recent study also found that it may help you lose weight. When overweight women were given a soluble fiber supplement, they began eating fewer calories and reported feeling fuller.

• *Potassium.* A serving of figs provides more potassium than a banana does. This mineral lowers your blood pressure, thus reducing your risk of heart disease and stroke.

• *Phenols.* Perhaps the most exciting nutrients found in figs are polyphenols. These compounds may be able to curb cancer, head off heart trouble, and more. Just one serving of dried figs packs 444 milligrams of these disease fighters—twice as much as the average American gets from vegetables in an entire day!

Add to that the fact that figs contain coumarin and benzaldehyde, two other potent cancer fighters, and you'd be silly not to dig into figs at least a couple of times a week.

GET THE BEST

During summer and early fall, you'll be able to buy fresh figs—

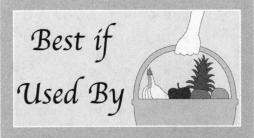

Best if Used By

The one drawback of fresh figs is that they have the shortest shelf life on the planet. Once they're harvested, they last no longer than a week. By the time you pick them up at the store, they may have only two good days left, so handle them with care. To prevent bruising, place them in a container lined with paper towels, then refrigerate them immediately.

and you should, because their taste is unbelievable. Look for figs that are plump and unblemished and soft to the touch but not mushy. Sniff them, too, because a sour smell is a tipoff to spoilage.

When you're ready to add figs to your menu, try these techniques.

Feel your oats. Stir chopped fresh or dried figs into your morning oatmeal for a natural hint of sweetness. If you haven't refrigerated your figs, do so for an hour to make them easier to cut.

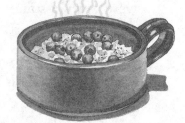

Roll in dough. Toss chopped figs in a little flour and add them to bread or muffin batter just as you would dried apricots or berries. What's the flour for? It prevents the figs from settling to the bottom of the baked goods.

Go gourmet. Top a bed of greens with chopped walnuts and sliced figs and season with a vinaigrette dressing.

Mix 'n match. Put figs along with bananas and your other favorite fruits on skewers for kebabs. Serve as a side dish with grilled chicken or pork.

Get jammed up. Try fig spread instead of jelly or jam on your morning toast for a little extra fiber.

LENTILS

Quick Fix for Constipation

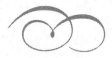

IF YOU'RE OFTEN CONSTIPATED, ADD ½ CUP OF COOKED lentils to your daily diet. They kick in 5 grams of fiber—roughly one-fifth of what you need for the day.

"Well," you may be thinking, "that's fine, but I don't always have the time to plan ahead and presoak dried beans and the like." That's why lentils are your savior: You don't have to remember to do anything in advance. Just take them out of the package and in 5 to 30 minutes, depending on the variety, you have dinner on the table. And you don't have to sacrifice a bit of nutrition for these speedy suppers.

GET YOUR FILL

Lentils are chock-full of fiber, and that means benefits beyond better bowels.

...Just the facts

Lentils (½ cup cooked)
Calories: 115
Fat: 0 g
Saturated fat: 0 g
Cholesterol: 0 mg
Sodium: 2 mg
Total carbohydrates: 20 g
Dietary fiber: 5 g
Protein: 9 g
Folate: 45% of Daily Value
Niacin (vitamin B$_3$): 5%
Copper: 12%
Iron: 18%
Magnesium: 9%
Zinc: 8%

Studies suggest that fiber lowers cholesterol and reduces cancer risk. In fact, a new study suggests that people who eat the most fiber-rich foods have about half the risk of developing mouth and throat cancers compared with those who consume the least.

Also, when it comes to folate, lentils are a powerhouse, supplying 45 percent of your daily requirement in just a ½-cup cooked serving. That's more than many fortified cereals provide! Here's why folate is your lifelong friend.

• *For moms-to-be.* During their childbearing years, women need plenty of folate before they even know they're pregnant, since this B vitamin and its synthetic form, folic acid, are crucial for warding off neural tube birth defects, such as spina bifida. So I, along with nearly every government health organization, strongly urge all women who are capable of becoming pregnant to make sure they get 400 micrograms of folate from foods and 400 micrograms of folic acid from fortified foods or supplements daily. Lentils provide 179 micrograms in ½ cup.

• *For 50-plus.* Even if babies are no longer a concern, you need folate for your heart. Although researchers are still working to solidify the link, it appears that folate lowers levels of homocysteine, an amino acid that could trigger a heart attack when it rises too high. How much is enough? Researchers suspect that it's 400 to 800 micrograms daily.

Best if Used By

When you get your dried lentils home, put them in a tightly sealed container and store in a cool, dry place (not the fridge). They'll keep for up to a year.

LOVIN' LENTILS

You can always find dried lentils in your supermarket, and if you have a good market nearby, you may find more than one variety. Available options include regular lentils, also known as brewers' lentils, a good all-purpose choice; Red Chief lentils, best in purees, dips, and other dishes where soft lentils work well; Pardina or Spanish Brown lentils, which tend to have a lighter flavor; and large green lentils, which are excellent for salads. Look for boxes containing lentils of uniform size.

Good to Go

Unlike beans, you shouldn't presoak lentils. Simply sort, rinse, and then boil most varieties in unsalted water for 15 to 30 minutes; Red Chiefs require only 5 to 10 minutes. Follow the package directions for exact cooking times.

Here are a few ideas to get you started on adding these little packets of goodness to your meals.

Stir into salad. Add cooked lentils to a salad made with spinach or watercress.

Stuff into potatoes. Bake two medium potatoes, scoop out the insides, and mash with ¼ cup of low-fat milk, 2 tablespoons of low-fat plain yogurt, and ½ cup of cooked lentils.

Pile on pizza. Mix a little meat topping (such as sausage) with cooked lentils and top your pizza. Don't forget to load up on veggies, too.

Take a shortcut. For those days when you really have no time, buy a few cans of lentil soup.

NECTARINES

Fiber without the Fuzz

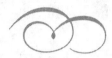

LUSCIOUS NECTARINES ARE IN A CLASS BY THEMSELVES, although they are closely related to peaches (but sweeter). In fact, just one recessive gene, the "fuzz" gene, separates these two fruits on the tree of life. That can be a bonus for folks who get all itchy from eating peach fuzz and end up peeling their peaches. By choosing nectarines, they can eat skin and all, nudging themselves closer to the recommended 25 to 30 grams of fiber a day that will keep them moving regularly. (Most Americans get only halfway to their daily fiber goal.)

ORANGE PLUS

Like peaches, cantaloupe, carrots, and other orange-colored fruits and veggies, nectarines are packed with beta-carotene and cryptoxanthin, two carotenoids that

...Just the facts

Nectarine (1 medium)
Calories: 67
Fat: Less than 1 g
Saturated fat: 0 g
Cholesterol: 0 mg
Sodium: 0 mg
Total carbohydrates: 16 g
Dietary fiber: 2 g
Protein: 1 g
Vitamin A: 13% of Daily
    Value
Vitamin C: 8%
Calcium: 1%
Iron: 1%

can turn into vitamin A in your body. Fully formed vitamin A comes only from liver, fish-liver oils, margarine, butter, milk, and eggs, and while small portions of those foods deliver needed nutrients, overdoing them can be a health hazard.

Indulge in luscious nectarines on a hot summer day. While the juice is dripping off your chin, your body will make enough vitamin A from the fruit to bolster your skin and mucous membranes so they can defend against invading viruses and bacteria and to boost your immune system to destroy invaders that breach the ramparts.

Numerous studies make it clear that people who eat the most foods rich in beta-carotene have better protection against cancer, but it's not clear exactly why. One possibility is that beta-carotene boosts communication between cells. Basically, cells need to talk to each other across the spaces that separate them in order to coordinate their defenses. Two laboratory studies have shown that carotenoids improve this communication, a little like the string between two tin cans.

GO FOR THE EYE DEAL

Nectarines also carry small amounts of another carotenoid, lutein, which has been shown to

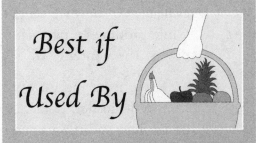

Best if Used By

Once you get your nectarines home, here's how to keep them juicy.

• Put them in a paper bag on your kitchen counter for one to three days. Keep the bag out of the sun. They'll get sweeter and softer day by day, and you'll know they're ripe when they smell heavenly and yield to gentle pressure.

• When they're ripe, put them in the refrigerator so you'll have a nice supply at the peak of flavor.

defend against age-related macular degeneration, the leading cause of blindness in older adults. Even though the amount of lutein in a nectarine is small, researchers have discovered that your body absorbs carotenoids twice as well from fruits as from green leafy vegetables, such as kale or spinach, so nectarines' visual impact may be greater than it first appears. Their vitamin A activity also fends off night blindness, and some studies suggest that beta-carotene battles cataracts, making nectarines the top fruit for your eyes.

HOW SWEET IT IS

Most nectarines come from California's San Joaquin Valley, which produces 175 varieties. Nectarines from California are available all summer long, from mid-May through September. Chile produces a nectarine crop that's on supermarket shelves during the winter.

Each nectarine variety has its own flavor and color, ranging from red-blushed golden yellow to almost entirely red. They'll be firm and a little underripe when you buy them.

Here's how to use nectarines to make your life sweeter.

Bring on the heat. Finely chop a nectarine and toss the pieces into fiery salsa for a sweet-hot sensation.

Go for the frost. Use sliced nectarines to top frozen yogurt. Drizzle with chocolate syrup for a perfect dessert.

Spin until silky. Add chopped nectarines to smoothies.

Create a topper. Finely chop ripe nectarines, mix with some cinnamon, and pour over pancakes or waffles instead of syrup.

PRUNES

Pretty Is as Pretty Does

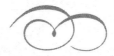

No DOUBT ABOUT IT: PRUNES ARE THE UGLY DUCKLINGS of the dried fruit family. To boost the image of prunes, the FDA recently agreed that their name could be changed to "dried plums." But as Shakespeare once asked, what's in a name? It's what's inside that counts—and in that sense, prunes are plum beautiful!

Prunes are famous (or maybe infamous) for their laxative effect. Researchers still aren't exactly sure why prunes can relieve constipation, but they suspect that it's their unusual combination of insoluble fiber and the sugar sorbitol, each of which bulks up the stool.

While most fruits offer very little sorbitol, prunes are composed of about 15 percent of the sugar. Eating about five prunes or drinking a cup of prune juice

...Just the facts

Prunes (about 5)
Calories: 109
Fat: 0 g
Saturated fat: 0 g
Cholesterol: 0 mg
Sodium: 5 mg
Total carbohydrates: 26 g
Dietary fiber: 2 g
Protein: 1 g
Vitamin A: 17% of Daily
    Value
Iron: 4%

can help curb constipation, although the fruit probably works a little better than the juice because it contains more fiber. Prune juice has one advantage over the fruit, though: Just 1 cup kicks in about 17 percent of the energy-boosting iron you need for the day. Five prunes (oops, dried plums) offer only about 4 percent.

If you'd rather drink prune juice than eat the dried fruit, look for brands without added sugar, to avoid packing on the pounds. One cup of unsweetened prune juice already has 70 more calories than the same amount of orange juice.

RAISINS ON STEROIDS

Ounce for ounce, prunes pack more than twice as many antioxidants as raisins do, according to a study at Tufts University in Boston (and raisins are no lightweights!). Antioxidants are valuable compounds because they help fight cancer and heart disease.

Additional research at the University of California, Davis, suggested that one particular antioxidant in prunes, called neochlorogenic acid, protects the body by riding herd on low-density lipoprotein (LDL) cholesterol—the bad kind—preventing it from undergoing a process that eventually leads to clogged arteries. In one trial, for example, men with slightly high cholesterol who ate about a dozen prunes a day significantly lowered their LDL cholesterol levels.

A PRUNE BY ANY OTHER NAME...

Regardless of whether they're called prunes or dried plums, what you should look for remains the same. Choose packages that are tightly sealed. Properly protected, the prunes will be moist and clean. If your diet falls a little short on iron, B vitamins, and vitamin E, consider picking up Mariani Prunes Plus, which offer 20 percent of the Daily Value for each of these nutrients. Living on a tight budget? Buy unpitted prunes and use a small knife to pit them yourself.

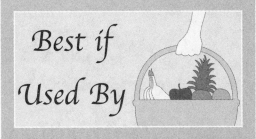

Best if Used By

Once you open the package, tightly reseal it and stash it in the refrigerator or transfer the prunes to an airtight container and store in a cool, dry place. They'll last up to six months.

Check out all the ways that you can perk up foods with prunes.

Go a little nuts. Add chopped pitted prunes to peanut butter for an extra fiber boost.

Pear with onions. Sauté pitted prunes with pears and red onion and serve this intriguing combination with pork.

Get your just desserts. Soak pitted prunes overnight in orange juice, then spoon them over sorbet or low-fat frozen yogurt for a healthy dessert.

Swap for fat. To lower the fat content of baked goods, whip them up with store-bought prune puree. Simply use half the amount of butter or oil called for in the recipe and replace half of the amount removed with prune puree.

RASPBERRIES

Glittering with Good Health

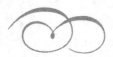

THINK OF RASPBERRIES AS NUTRITIONAL GEMS—RUBIES, really. Just 1 cup packs about 6 grams of fiber—20 to 25 percent of what you need for the entire day! That's more than most other fruits provide. Better yet, raspberries have both soluble and insoluble fiber. The insoluble version wards off constipation, while the soluble type lowers cholesterol, especially the bad kind.

True, the berries are pricey, but you'll be willing to pay up when you realize the bargain you're getting. Raspberries are sparkling with compounds that scientists believe may battle cancer, head off heart disease, and even ease allergies.

MAKE WAR ON CANCER

Raspberries—specifically, the seeds—are chock-full of a compound called ellagic acid. It shows up in small amounts in

...Just the facts

Raspberries (1 cup)
Calories: 60
Fat: Less than 1 g
Saturated fat: 0 g
Cholesterol: 0 mg
Sodium: 0 mg
Total carbohydrates: 14 g
Dietary fiber: 6 g
Protein: 1 g
Vitamin C: 50% of Daily
    Value

most fruits and vegetables, but raspberries boast levels that are five to six times greater than those found in other fruits, such as plums and apples.

Ellagic acid does something really cool: It binds cancer-causing chemicals in your body, renders them inactive, and destroys them. Most of the studies involving ellagic acid have been done in test tubes or on laboratory animals, but the results have been very promising. In these studies, researchers found that ellagic acid stopped cancer cell division within 48 hours and caused breast, prostate, skin, esophageal, pancreatic, and colon cancer cells to die within 72 hours.

To see whether ellagic acid will have the same dramatic effects on people, researchers at the American Health Foundation in New York City are conducting two major studies. One clinical trial is examining whether eating raspberries can reduce the number of colon polyps in people who are at risk for developing colon cancer, and another is determining whether raspberries can stave off cervical cancer in women at increased risk for the disease. The results aren't expected for several years, but in the meantime, lead researcher Daniel Nixon, M.D., says he and his family are eating raspberries as often as they can.

Good to Go

Just before you're ready to use fresh raspberries, arrange them in a shallow pan and carefully wash them, then blot with paper towels. If you're using frozen berries, defrost them by putting them in the fridge for a day or by running cold water over them.

FOOD NEWS

Just 1 cup of fresh raspberries provides half your day's quota of vitamin C—the key to wound healing and a spunky immune system.

Best if Used By

Here's how to keep your berries tasty.

• Refrigerate them as soon as possible. Ideally, you should use them within three days of the time you bought them.

• If you're lucky enough to have a bounty, freeze them. Simply wash the berries, carefully spread them on baking sheets, and freeze them overnight. Transfer them to a plastic container and refreeze. (Freezing them on baking sheets first keeps them from clumping.)

ADD TO THE ARSENAL

As if that weren't plenty, raspberries are rich in quercetin. Like ellagic acid, this antioxidant seems to protect against cancer. Additionally, it may help:

• Prevent "bad" low-density lipoprotein (LDL) cholesterol from causing blood vessel damage, which contributes to heart disease.

• Block the production of histamine, the substance that causes the runny nose, itchy eyes, and sneezing during allergy attacks.

DAZZLING GOOD TASTE

If you can find fresh raspberries at a roadside stand, always buy two pints: one to use in cooking and baking and one to eat just plain! And keep an eye out for black raspberries. They're hard to find, but they contain 10 to 20 times more disease-fighting anthocyanins than red raspberries do. Choose berries that are in dry, unstained containers, because moisture speeds decay.

Can't find fresh berries, or they're too pricey for your wallet? You can pick up frozen berries at your supermarket, but feel the bag or box for ice crystals—a sign that the berries have been thawed and refrozen. In this condition, they won't be as tasty or last as long.

While you're at it, search your store for products such as

sorbet, jam (with the seeds, for more ellagic acid), and vinaigrette made with raspberries.

Once you have your stash, try these berry-good ideas.

Sparkle your salad. Toss a handful of fresh raspberries into a salad made with baby lettuces, crumbled Asiago or feta cheese, shredded carrots, and balsamic vinaigrette. It looks almost too pretty to eat!

Charm your chicken. Marinate chicken breasts in low-fat raspberry vinaigrette, then toss them on the grill.

Take a break. Unwind from a long day with a bowl of raspberries topped with a tablespoon or two of light whipped topping and drizzled with a little chocolate sauce.

Dazzle your crackers. Of course, you can top your bread with raspberry jam or jelly, but if you're worried about the extra sugar, mash very ripe raspberries as a spread for crackers, toast, and bagels.

A SIMPLE SOLUTION

Some older folks find that as they slow up a bit, their intestinal tracts seem to get lazy right along with the rest of their bodies. This quick trick can help: Sprinkle ½ cup or more of raspberries on bran cereal every morning. Practiced daily, this strategy should make everything come out right.

WHEATBERRIES

Nutty Nutrition Nuggets

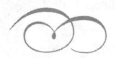

SINCE THE DAWN OF THE FOOD GUIDE PYRAMID, GRAINS have been at its base. Now, the focus is shifting toward whole grains as research continues to reveal their superior power over processed white products. Why? First of all, they're packed with insoluble fiber, known to ward off digestive difficulties, such as constipation and diverticulosis, and the hemorrhoids that can result. Wheatberries are as whole as you can get.

IT'S THE REAL THING

If you're often constipated, add a serving of wheatberries and a couple of extra glasses of water to your diet. Just ½ cup of cooked wheatberries delivers one-fourth of your day's fiber, and you need the water because insoluble fiber soaks up lots of

...Just the facts

Wheatberries (½ cup cooked)
Calories: 158
Fat: 1 g
Saturated fat: 0 g
Cholesterol: 0 mg
Sodium: 1 mg
Total carbohydrates: 33 g
Dietary fiber: 6 g
Protein: 7 g
Copper: 10% of Daily Value
Iron: 10%
Magnesium: 15%
Manganese: 97%
Zinc: 9%

fluid in your digestive tract.

Wheatberries are also packed with a vast array of vitamins, minerals, and phytochemicals that appear to work synergistically to stave off major lifestyle diseases. Here are a few of these natural ingredients.

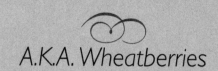

A.K.A. Wheatberries

Can't find wheatberries? Ask for hard, red winter wheat. Wheatberries, it turns out, are just little whole wheat kernels that turn into chewy, nutty-tasting, plump little dark brown nuggets.

• *Phenolic acids, lignans, and phytic acid.* These antioxidants mop up free radicals, the dangerous particles that form when body cells burn oxygen for energy. (Caution: Living is dangerous to your health!)

• *Vitamin E.* Wheatberries are a concentrated source of this vitamin, especially the tocotrienol form (one of the many subparts of vitamin E) that researchers think packs the most antioxidant benefits.

SCIENCE SAYS

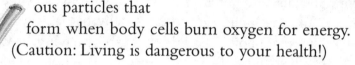

Weight seems out of control in the United States, with one-third of all adults considered overweight or obese, but wheatberries and other whole grains can help those of us who need to shed a few pounds. Wheatberries are very filling, and they contain a little healthy fat to keep you from getting hungry again too soon. Some research even suggests that whole grain foods help you stay satisfied longer. A recent study of more than 74,000 women showed those

FOOD NEWS

Wheatberries contain twice as much fiber as brown rice, wild rice, or oatmeal.

Cooking wheatberries is as easy as pie.

• Put a cupful in a strainer and rinse with cold water to remove any dust or dirt.

• Take this time to separate the wheat from the chaff and any other minor debris.

• Put the wheatberries in a big pot, add 4 cups of water, and put a lid on the pot. Cook over high heat until the water comes to a boil. Reduce the heat to low and simmer for about an hour while you do something else.

• When you think they're done, take out a few, let them cool, and give them the bite test. Continue to simmer until they reach a consistency you like.

• Pour off the excess water.

• Use the berries right away or store them in the fridge for later.

who increased the amount of whole grains they ate had a 49 percent lower risk of gaining weight than those who clung to their white food habits.

Large scientific studies of many populations say whole grains offer great protection for your heart. The Iowa Women's Study, for instance, found that healthy postmenopausal women who ate just one serving of whole grains daily had a 30 percent lower risk of having heart attacks than women who ate them once a week or less.

Two other studies, one of 43,000 men and the other of 65,000 women ages 40 to 65, showed that those who ate the most cereal fiber (such as wheatberries) were least likely to develop type 2 diabetes, the kind that most adults get.

GO FOR IT

Wheatberries aren't very mainstream yet, so they're not available in most local supermarkets. Unless your store has a health food section, you'll probably have to go to a natural foods store to buy your hard, red winter wheat.

You'll probably find wheatberries in a see-through package, and that's good because you'll be able to examine them for bugs. Bugs don't go for white-flour products…they know where the good stuff is!

If wheatberries are new to you, here are some ideas on how to use them. (Prepare the berries ahead of time and keep your cooked supply in the fridge.) We're betting you'll love them both hot and cold.

Hot for breakfast. If Wheaties are the breakfast of champions, then wheatberries could lead to Olympic gold! Warm them up in the microwave with a little honey, dried fruit, nuts, and milk.

Best if Used By

Keep your wheatberries fresh and flavorful!
• If you're not going to cook them right away, put them in an airtight container and store them in your pantry for use within a couple of weeks.
• For longer storage, keep them in the refrigerator to prevent their oils from becoming rancid. They'll keep for up to a year.

Cold for lunch. Mix chilled cooked wheatberries with chopped raw veggies, such as celery, radishes, cucumbers, and carrots, and your favorite salad dressing.

Hot in soup. Stir a big spoonful into canned bean, pea, or lentil soup for protein that's as complete as meat's.

Cold for parties. Combine cooked wheatberries with chopped ripe olives and toasted pine nuts for a fancy treat.

Hot for dinner. Replace pasta, rice, or potatoes with warm wheatberries dressed with olive oil, balsamic vinegar, and Italian herbs, such as basil, oregano, and thyme.

DIARRHEA

Subdue the Storm

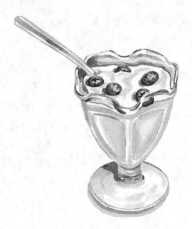

We all get diarrhea from time to time. Usually the bouts are short, lasting a day or two, but occasionally they may be wretchedly prolonged, lasting up to a week and leaving you sore, crampy, and exhausted. Either way, you don't have to just sit there and take it. There are things you can do to ease your troubled gut.

FOOD NEWS

Yogurt manufacturer Stonyfield packs more kinds of tummy-taming live, active cultures into their yogurt than any other brand.

GUT TO GO

Loose stools occur when the large intestine isn't able to absorb the usual amount of fluid from wastes on their journey out of the body. All sorts of things can make this happen. Mild infections are the main cause, but eating too much junk food and even emotional stress can make stools looser than they should be.

Unfortunately, loose stools aren't the only symptom of diarrhea. The underlying problem irritates the intestine and causes painful abdominal cramps, along with sudden "emergencies" that send you running to the bathroom.

GET BACK ON YOUR FEED

Although diarrhea is among the most common intestinal ailments, don't make the mistake of treating it lightly. True, it's usually a result of garden-variety infections that make you miserable for a few days and clear up on their own, but there are plenty of exceptions that require a doctor's attention. That said, it's pretty easy to get through a short bout of diarrhea. Here's what the experts advise.

Stay as sweet as you are. Avoid sugary treats and simple carbohydrates such as honey. Bacteria that invade your digestive tract like sugar just as much as you do. The more you give them to eat, the more likely they'll be to stick around, says Rob Dramov, N.D., a naturopathic physician in Tigard, Oregon.

Focus on fiber. There's a good reason that doctors advise people with diarrhea to eat plenty of fresh fruits and vegetables, along with whole grain cereals and breads. These foods are loaded with fiber, which absorbs water in the intestine and

A SIMPLE SOLUTION

Bet on barley. Bland though it may be, barley can slow intestinal motion and curb diarrhea. To make it tasty, prepare pearl barley according to package directions and add 1 cup of beef broth. The mixture will replace lost fluids and electrolytes in addition to calming your intestines.

Diarrhea is sometimes triggered by heavy-duty infections that require prompt treatment with antibiotics. It can also be a symptom of a serious intestinal disorder, such as inflammatory bowel disease, or even a warning sign of cancer. That's why you should always call your doctor when diarrhea doesn't go away within two days. Don't wait even that long if you have a fever, are nauseated or vomiting, or notice that your stools are black and tarry looking.

makes stools firmer and less watery. Most doctors recommend that you get 25 to 30 grams of fiber a day.

Find your water level. Most people don't drink as much water as their bodies need. If you're also losing fluid from diarrhea, it's easy to see how your water balance can dip dangerously. Dehydration is the reason that doctors take diarrhea seriously. Your body simply can't function without adequate fluid, especially because dehydration invariably results in low levels of essential minerals called electrolytes, which control everything from muscle movements to normal nerve functions.

When you're coping with diarrhea, be sure to drink about half your body weight, in ounces, of water daily. It's also helpful to drink soup, broth, sports drinks, or fruit or vegetable juice.

Unleash the bacterial horde. Diarrhea often occurs when harmful bacteria set up camp in your digestive tract. Actually, your intestine is normally chock-full of bacteria, the good along with the bad, but the bad bugs are usually kept in check by the microscopic good guys. Anything that changes the usual balance—taking antibiotics, for example—can allow harmful germs to proliferate.

A quick way to restore the normal balance is to have one

or two daily servings of live-culture yogurt. It's packed with *Lactobacillus acidophilus*, a type of beneficial organism that makes it harder for diarrhea-causing germs to thrive.

Wash up. We're surrounded by bacteria all the time, and usually our immune systems keep them in check. There are times in life, though—when stress levels are high, for example—when your natural immunity can't keep up with bacterial marauders. An easy way to prevent problems is simply to wash your hands with soap and water several times a day. Studies have shown that many of the common infections that cause diarrhea could be prevented just by keeping your hands clean, says Dr. Dramov.

Take notes. If you get diarrhea fairly frequently, it's possible that something in your diet is behind it. Some people, for example, are sensitive to fatty foods, while others react to artificial sweeteners. It's worth taking the time to keep track of everything you eat long enough to figure out what may be upsetting your intestine.

Drink rice. Boil ½ cup of brown rice in a quart of water for 15 to 20 minutes, stirring constantly, then strain. Drink the liquid throughout the day to soothe your digestive tract and replace lost fluids.

Healing **VITAMINS**

Even if you don't usually supplement your diet with multinutrients, you should certainly take them when you have diarrhea. A once-a-day supplement is all you need. It's a fast way to replace the essential nutrients that diarrhea takes out of your body.

ARTICHOKES

Feed Your Friendly Bacteria

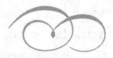

FOR BETTER BOWEL FUNCTION, YOU NEED A CONSTANT parade of fiber-rich fruits and vegetables in your diet. Artichokes really wave the fiber flag, delivering about one-third of a day's supply in just one medium fat-free globe. It turns out that they're probiotics, too. In other words, they deliver just the right kind of carbohydrates to feed the good bacteria in your gut. When they're well fed, these bacteria have the energy to multiply into a huge army that's strong enough to fight off a hostile bacterial invasion and the diarrhea that often comes with it.

Artichokes will help with weight control, too, if you dip them in lemon juice instead of drowning them in butter. Not only are they low in calories (just 60 each), but they also take a long time to eat,

...Just the facts

Artichoke (1 medium, boiled)
Calories: 60
Fat: 0 g
Saturated fat: 0 g
Cholesterol: 0 mg
Sodium: 114 mg
Total carbohydrates: 13 g
Dietary fiber: 6 g
Protein: 4 g
Vitamin A: 4% of Daily Value
Vitamin C: 13%
Calcium: 5%
Iron: 9%

so your body gets a chance to register that you're full before you pack away too many calories.

TAKE HEART

You'll adore what artichokes do for your heart. First, they appear to help keep your blood flowing freely because they're packed with luteolin, one of the naturally occurring plant substances in the flavonoid family that acts as an antioxidant in your body. At least in laboratory petri dishes, concentrated luteolin taken from artichokes prevents the oxidation of "bad" low-density lipoprotein (LDL) cholesterol, the process that makes cholesterol gummy and lazy and very eager to find a resting place on your artery walls, making arteries narrower and ripe for clogging.

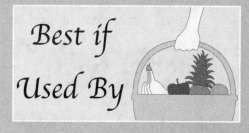

Best if Used By

Sprinkle your artichokes with a little water, place them in an airtight plastic bag, and chill them in the fridge. They'll keep for about a week

Second, one medium artichoke provides about 15 percent of your daily folate requirement. This B vitamin helps control blood levels of homocysteine, which, when out of control, can trigger a heart attack.

Third, artichokes are full of cynarin, which has been shown to lower cholesterol production. The idea here is that if you make less cholesterol, there's less for your body to deal with.

LOVE THE SKIN YOU'RE IN

Cynarin may have benefits for your skin, too. In an Italian study, researchers found that cynarin (this time extracted from the herb echinacea) helped protect collagen, the connective tissue that holds your cells together, against sun damage. More research is needed, of course, and you may have to use it more as a sunscreen than as an appetizer, but the possibilities are intriguing.

Meanwhile, Cleveland researchers have been pursuing the cancer prevention benefits of another artichoke ingredient, silymarin. At least in the lab, silymarin seems to forestall cancer development at several stages.

SIZING UP 'CHOKES

A few fresh artichokes are available year-round, but you'll find tons of them in your supermarket from March through May. Fall and winter globes may have a whitish or blistered look due to a little frostbite, but don't worry—they'll turn green when you cook them. In fact, these are often the tastiest 'chokes.

Artichokes come in three sizes. Babies weigh just 2 to 3 ounces each and are great for appetizers, casseroles, or sautés. Medium 'chokes, which weigh in

Good to Go

Puzzled by how to begin? Start by slicing off the stem so that the artichoke can sit firmly on its bottom, then cut off one-quarter to one-third of the top. Cook by one of these three methods. You'll be dining in style in no time.

• *Boil.* Stand trimmed artichokes in a deep saucepan with 3 inches of boiling water. Add lemon juice or seasonings, if desired. Cover and boil gently for 25 to 40 minutes, depending on size, or until a petal near the center pulls out easily. Stand the artichokes upside down to drain.

• *Steam.* Place trimmed artichokes on a rack above boiling water. Cover and steam for 25 to 40 minutes, or until done.

• *Microwave.* Place trimmed artichokes in a deep microwavable cup or bowl. Add water, cover, and microwave on high until done. For one artichoke, use 1/2 cup of water and microwave for 5 to 8 minutes; for two, use 1 cup of water and cook for 7 to 11 minutes.

at 8 to 10 ounces each, are perfect for dipping, stuffing, or as a light entrée. Large artichokes weigh about 1 pound each, big enough for a shared appetizer for two or more people.

Here are some easy ways to use a cooked artichoke.

Strip it. Pull off the petals one at a time and dip each into something healthy, such as salsa. Holding on to the tip, put the petal in your mouth and gently bite down, then pull the petal out of your mouth, scraping off the tender flesh with your teeth. Throw away the skeleton, then take another petal. It's the most fun appetizer.

Fill it. With a spoon, scrape the fuzzy center out of the artichoke. Fill the 'choke with something cold, such as chicken or tuna salad, or something hot, such as warm crabmeat.

Cut it. Again, de-fuzz the artichoke center, then remove some of the outer leaves for decoration. Thinly slice the artichoke and toss the slices into salad.

Can it. In a rush? Fill the center of a canned artichoke heart with a jumbo ripe olive. Use it as a garnish for your dinner plate or salad.

BANANAS

Helping Hands

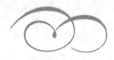

...Just the facts

Banana (1 medium)
Calories: 109
Fat: 0 g
Saturated fat: 0 g
Cholesterol: 0 mg
Sodium: 1 mg
Total carbohydrates: 28 g
Dietary fiber: 3 g
Protein: 1 g
Vitamin A: 2% of Daily Value
Vitamin B$_6$: 34%
Vitamin C: 12%
Calcium: 1%
Iron: 2%
Potassium: 12%

BANANAS ARE MOTHER NATURE'S most perfect fast-food snack. They require no preparation (not even washing!) or refrigeration. They come prepackaged in a biodegradable wrapper and require no utensils for perfect enjoyment. Babies love them. In fact, bananas are often a first food because they're so digestible. Folks with tummy troubles rely on their digestibility, too, especially during times of intestinal distress such as diarrhea, because they are so soothing. Athletes thrive on the quick, sustained carbohydrate energy they supply. Gym rats toss them into their bags for the perfect preworkout boost. Women coping with premenstrual syndrome can get a healthy serotonin surge by indulging in them. What could be better?

PUT THE FINGER ON HEART DISEASE

Besides being yummy and easy on your tummy, bananas help build a shield against heart disease. To start with, they're packed with potassium, which helps fend off high blood pressure, a big risk factor for heart disease and stroke—but you probably already knew that. (Getting more potassium may also help prevent kidney stones, especially if you eat a high-sodium diet.)

What may surprise you is that bananas are a powerful package of pyridoxine (better known as vitamin B_6), delivering one-third of your daily requirement in each medium-size finger. In a study of 80,000 healthy professional women, those whose diets included the most vitamin B_6 and folate (another B vitamin) were least likely to have heart attacks. In another study of almost 500 people at high risk for heart disease, increasing their intake of B_6, folate, and vitamin B_{12} helped control their blood homocysteine levels, another risk factor for heart attack. So whatever your risk level, have a banana.

Best if Used By

Store bananas at room temperature until they ripen to the stage that you prefer, then refrigerate them. They'll be good for three or four days. Worried about the skins turning black in the fridge? Don't be. The skins may turn dark, but the insides stay luscious longer when they're cold.

KNOCK OUT CANCER

Reports about the beneficial effects of fiber in preventing bowel, colon, and colorectal cancers change from yes to no and back again day after day. The issues are complex, and fiber itself has many parts. In one Hawaiian study, researchers looked at an array of fiber fractions, such as soluble and insoluble fiber, crude fiber, dietary fiber, and nonstarch polysaccharides. No wonder we're all confused!

In that study, only vegetable fiber worked, but one thing the researchers learned along the way was that fiber aside, eating certain plant foods, such as bananas, broccoli, carrots, and corn, had an inverse relationship to colorectal cancer risk. That means that the more of those foods the study participants ate, the less likely they were to get that cancer. In another study, bananas were ranked with oranges, peaches, and asparagus for ability to hamper the creation of new cancer cells—so while you're working on your five a day, say "Make mine banana."

POINTING OUT THE BEST

Bananas are available year-round. Choosing the right ones is largely a matter of taste, although short, thick bananas seem to be the sweetest. Avoid bananas with cuts or bruises. Aside from that, the degree of ripeness you prefer is what counts.

Once you've found your perfect hand of bananas, enjoy them as a sweet treat or use them to add natural sweetness to other dishes. Here are a few ideas.

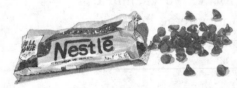

Kiss 'em with chocolate. Insert wooden sticks into peeled, overripe bananas. Dip the bananas in chocolate and freeze them for a tasty snack.

Give 'em a yogurt spin. In a blender, whirl ripe bananas with yogurt or milk and vanilla for a cool milkshake.

Sauté 'em with sugar. Sauté banana slices, toss with brown sugar, and serve over your favorite broiled fish.

HORSERADISH

A Toxin Terminator

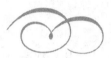

HAVE YOU BEEN TAKING HORSERADISH FOR GRANTED? Well, let's have a little more respect here. Just a dab of this powerful root vegetable provides a surprising amount of good nutrition. Some of its most important compounds, isothiocyanates, have nutrition researchers doing cartwheels. Studies suggest that they help fight *Listeria, E. coli,* and other harmful bacteria that cause food poisoning and, along with it, vomiting and diarrhea. There's no telling when these bacteria may end up in your food, especially sandwiches. So why not top your sandwich with some horseradish? It'll taste great, and you can rest a little easier.

That's not the only promising news about these compounds. Research has found that, at least in test tubes, isothiocyanates seem to deactivate chemicals

...Just the facts

Prepared horseradish (2 Tbsp)
Calories: 14
Fat: 0 g
Saturated fat: 0 g
Cholesterol: 0 mg
Sodium: 94 mg
Total carbohydrates: 3 g
Dietary fiber: 6 g
Protein: 1 g
Folate: 4% of Daily Value
Vitamin C: 12%

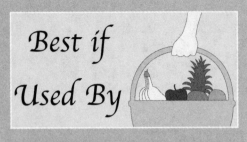

Best if Used By

If you buy fresh horseradish, store the roots in a plastic bag in the refrigerator, where they'll keep for up to a week.

before they trigger cancer. Scientists think that they may be especially helpful in staving off cancers of the mouth, pharynx, lung, stomach, colon, and rectum.

HEAL THE CRUELEST CUTS

Fresh or prepared, just 2 tablespoons of horseradish provide 12 percent of the vitamin C you need daily. Who would have guessed it? Over the long haul, vitamin C seems to fend off heart disease and cancer. In the short run, it speeds up wound healing, so you recover from razor cuts or even a root canal a little faster. Perk up your sauces and dips with a little horseradish. You'll get a kick out of it.

If a head cold has you down and you can't breathe, slather a teaspoon of prepared horseradish on a cracker, then eat it slowly. The horseradish vapors will reach into the back of your nose and liquefy the stuffy stuff. Even the most clogged-up nose will respond to three crackers' worth!

ROOTING AROUND FOR THE BEST

When you're in the market for horseradish, you have three choices: the prepared version, fresh root, or horseradish sauce.

Most people choose prepared horseradish. It comes in a jar and is usually mixed with vinegar. (If the horseradish is red, it's been mixed with vinegar and beet juice.)

Rather take the fresh route? Be warned: Fresh horseradish is much more pungent than the prepared type. If you opt for fresh, select firm roots.

Here's how horseradish can take root in your kitchen.

Add magic to mustard. Stir some horseradish into your favorite brand of mustard to breathe new life into your roast beef, turkey, or ham sandwich! Sure, you could buy prepared horseradish mustard, but it costs more and may have too much or too little horseradish for your taste.

Good to Go

Just before you're ready to grate the fleshy white roots of fresh horseradish, clean them by removing their outer skin.

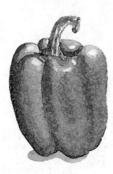

Add zest to dip. Stir 3 tablespoons of horseradish into 1 cup of low-fat sour cream, plain yogurt, or French dressing. It makes a tangy dip for red bell pepper strips, broccoli florets, and baby carrots.

TURKEY

Gobble Up the Nutrition

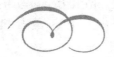

...Just the facts

White meat turkey (3 oz roasted, no skin)
Calories: 119
Fat: 1 g
Saturated fat: 0 g
Cholesterol: 73 mg
Sodium: 48 mg
Total carbohydrates: 0 g
Dietary fiber: 0 g
Protein: 26 g
Niacin (vitamin B_3): 30% of Daily Value
Vitamin B_6: 24%
Vitamin B_{12}: 6%
Iron: 7%
Phosphorus: 18%
Zinc: 12%

MY FRIEND KAREN HAS "THANKS-giving dinner" with her mom at least a half-dozen times a year—even in July. Mom's got the right idea! Turkey is so healthy, why should you enjoy it only on holidays? Turkey is a feast in itself, with generous contributions of a half-dozen important nutrients. Topping the list is niacin, needed to produce energy in all the cells of your body. If you don't get enough, you may become mentally disoriented or have diarrhea.

BENEFICIAL BANQUET

Here's the lowdown on the remaining five.

• *Vitamin B_6.* This vitamin helps convert an amino acid into serotonin, an important brain chemical that affects your mood. It also helps manufacture other crucial substances, such as insulin and infection-fighting antibodies.

• *Vitamin B₁₂.* Working in conjunction with folate and its synthetic counterpart, folic acid, B_{12} helps make red blood cells. They may also team up to fight heart disease.

• *Iron.* You know the deal on this one: If you don't meet your iron requirements, you may feel tired and lethargic. Eventually, you could develop iron-deficiency anemia, which would make your symptoms much worse.

• *Phosphorus.* Next to calcium, this is the most abundant mineral in your bones and teeth. It also helps generate energy in your body's cells and helps regulate metabolism in your organs.

• *Zinc.* Several studies have shown that this mineral is essential for a strong immune system.

THE BIG FAT DILEMMA

If you're really watching your fat intake—say you're on the American Heart Association's Step 2 Diet, you're having gallbladder problems, or you're fighting off diarrhea—you should stick to white meat turkey without the skin, which has only 1 gram of fat per 3-ounce serving. Otherwise, you can enjoy both white and dark meat.

Dark meat isn't as fatty as you think, costing you just 30 extra calories and 3 additional grams of fat for a skinless, 3½-ounce serving. On the plus side, dark meat turkey offers about twice as much zinc, iron, copper, calcium, and vitamin E as

Since its inception more than 20 years ago, the Butterball Turkey Talk Line has been answering questions from panicked home chefs. Here's its advice on the best way to thaw a turkey.

Thawing at room temperature isn't recommended, as it could promote bacterial growth. To thaw a turkey in the refrigerator, just place it breast side up in its unopened wrapper on a tray or large platter in the fridge. For every 4 pounds of turkey, allow at least one day of thawing time. If you're short on time, put the wrapped turkey breast side down in cold water to cover, changing the water every 30 minutes to keep the surface cold. The estimated minimum thawing time is 30 minutes per pound for a whole turkey.

white meat does, so you get a lot of bang for your calorie buck. Whether you can get away with eating the skin really depends on your personal calorie allotment. For 3 ounces of dark meat with skin, the fat content can jump up to 8 grams per serving, depending on the part of the turkey that you choose, and add another 40 calories to your portion. If your figure can handle it, though, don't fear the fat. More than half of it is the unsaturated, heart-healthy kind. What's more, the 2.6 grams of saturated fat in that 3-ounce portion is just 13 percent of your day's allotment.

PICKING UP THE PIECES

Fortunately, you no longer have to buy a whole turkey or even a turkey breast to enjoy this delicious, nutritious meat. Many manufacturers sell sliced turkey cutlets or ground turkey that's healthy and easy to incorporate into your meals.

Choose ground turkey that's made from skinless white meat. Avoid types that contain dark meat and skin; its fat content rivals that of ground beef.

When selecting a fresh or frozen turkey, choose one in a tightly sealed package. On frozen turkeys, you shouldn't spot any freezer burn or ice crystals, although the turkey should be very hard.

You know the most obvious way to serve a whole turkey, but what can you make with the leftovers, turkey cutlets, or ground turkey? I'm glad you asked. Try these suggestions.

Head south of the border. One of Karen's friends makes quesadillas with leftover Thanksgiving turkey. She simply tucks small turkey pieces, vegetables, and cranberry relish into flour tortillas, then heats the whole she-bang in the oven.

Create great soup. Skinless dark meat is a great addition to practically any noodle or vegetable soup.

Trade in chicken. Did you already have chicken three times this week? You can use turkey cutlets in many of the same recipes that call for chicken breasts.

Streamline burgers. Substitute ground white meat turkey for half of the ground beef you use for hamburgers.

YOGURT

Live, Active Protection

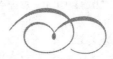

YOGURT IS YUMMY, WHICH IS REALLY WHY WE LIKE IT SO much. Thick and creamy, it's packed with calcium, that wonderful mineral that protects your bones and fights off osteoporosis—but even its bounty of calcium may not be the healthiest thing about yogurt. Instead, it's more likely to be its bugs. Not insects, but microscopic forms of friendly bacteria. In fact, studies suggest that they help destroy the bad guys that give us diarrhea, yeast infections, and—sit down for this—possibly cancer.

MICROBIAL MADNESS

Here's what research has found.

• A new study reported that among 200 hospitalized patients receiving antibiotics, those who also ate yogurt had both fewer

...Just the facts

Low-fat plain yogurt (1 cup)
Calories: 155
Fat: 4 g
Saturated fat: 2 g
Cholesterol: 15 mg
Sodium: 172 mg
Total carbohydrates: 17 g
Dietary fiber: 0 g
Protein: 13 g
Riboflavin (vitamin B_2): 30% of Daily Value
Calcium: 45%
Phosphorus: 35%
Zinc: 15%

bouts and fewer days of diarrhea.

• Another study found that eating 8 ounces of yogurt containing the bacterial culture *Lactobacillus acidophilus* reduced the risk of yeast infections threefold.

• A clinical trial showed that dieters who got 1,200 milligrams of calcium from dairy foods lost more weight, more body fat, and more dangerous abdominal fat than those on low-calcium plans.

• Animal research suggests that *L. acidophilus* may decrease the risk of breast, colon, and liver tumors triggered by carcinogens. "Although we have to conduct clinical human trials, the relationship between active cultures in yogurt and the reduced risk of breast and colon cancers looks very promising," says yogurt researcher Ian Rowland, Ph.D., of the University of Ulster in Ireland.

ANTICANCER COMMANDOS

Beyond bacteria, other compounds in yogurt may have anticancer benefits. "Certain lipids, acids, and peptides in yogurt may play a role in fighting cancer," says M. E. Sanders, Ph.D., of Dairy and Food Culture Technologies in Colorado. In fact, yogurt may rev up the entire immune system.

A recent review of studies at Tufts University in Boston suggested that people with compromised immune systems, especially older folks, may increase their resistance to certain diseases by eating yogurt. Researchers point out, however, that more studies are needed to make the connection for sure.

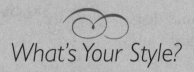

What's Your Style?

Yogurt with fruit on the bottom. Yogurt with fruit on the top. Yogurt topped with crushed nuts! Yogurt with a spoon included!! The yogurt section of your supermarket keeps growing larger and more confusing.

What kind of yogurt should you buy? We'll make it easy. Hands down, your best bet is plain yogurt, either low-fat or fat-free, with live, active cultures. Why? Plain yogurt usually kicks in more calcium than the flavored fare. Plus, the fruit and sweeteners that manufacturers add may, over time, inhibit the healthy bacteria.

If you like your yogurt flavored, customize it with all kinds of healthy goodies. Try fresh berries, chopped pineapple or peaches, raisins, cereal, chopped nuts, or even a few mini chocolate chips.

Is frozen yogurt as fabulous for you as regular yogurt? Sorry, but no, says Manfred Kroger, Ph.D., professor of food science at Pennsylvania State University in University Park. The sweeteners and fruit added to frozen yogurt inhibit some of the beneficial yogurt cultures.

THE CULTURE CLUB

When choosing yogurt, check the label to be sure it contains active cultures, such as *L. acidophilus* or *L. bifidus*. These additional cultures may provide much of yogurt's stomach-soothing benefits. Look for the latest expiration date, because the amount of beneficial cultures declines with age. Skip any yogurt that claims to be "heat-treated" or "pasteurized after culturing," because the cultures may been destroyed by processing.

MINERAL DEPOSITS

The minerals in yogurt deserve some special attention, too. A 1-cup serving of low-fat plain yogurt offers 100 milligrams more potassium than a banana. Getting plenty of potassium may help keep your blood pressure in check, reducing the risk of heart disease and stroke.

Then, of course, there's calcium. One cup of low-fat plain yogurt delivers about 150 milligrams more calcium than a glass of milk. That's good news for your bones!

If you're wedded to flavored yogurt, all the rules for plain yogurt apply, plus these two: opt for fruit-on-the-bottom yogurt, which usually contains more beneficial cultures than yogurt with fruit mixed throughout the container, and compare the calorie and calcium contents among brands, since they vary widely. Select a brand that packs at least 30 percent of the Daily Value for calcium in a 6-ounce serving.

Once you've made your selection, see all the healthy ways that you can use your yogurt.

Streamline your mayo. Substitute plain yogurt for one-third of the mayo that you typically use in tuna, chicken, or potato salad. You can also use it instead of all the sour cream called for in dip recipes.

Turn dinner into dessert. Have leftover white or brown rice from Chinese takeout? The next day, mix it with vanilla yogurt, ground cinnamon, nutmeg, and raisins for instant rice pudding.

Make wonderful waffles. Instead of syrup, top your waffles with yogurt and berries.

Skip the campfire. When your sweet tooth starts acting up, satisfy it with S'Mores Yogurt: Just combine 1 cup of low-fat plain yogurt, 2 teaspoons of mini marshmallows, 2 teaspoons of mini chocolate chips, and 1 crushed graham cracker.

IRRITABLE BOWEL SYNDROME

Solve Your Personal Puzzle

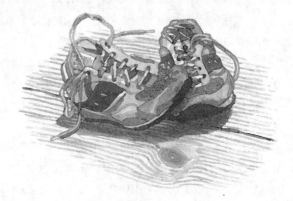

Even though irritable bowel syndrome, or IBS, is among the most common conditions treated by doctors, they still don't know what causes it. For some reason, people with IBS have intestines that are, well…irritable. They seem to have abnormal electrical activity that causes frequent, uncomfortable muscle contractions, or spasms.

Everyone with IBS has a slightly different pattern of problems. Some people have mainly cramps, some have episodes of diarrhea and/or constipation, and others have gas and bloating. The symptoms may occur daily for years, or they may disappear for a while, then come roaring back without any warning.

Whatever your symptoms, though, there are ways to find relief. Here's what we mean.

CALM YOUR IBS

Irritable bowel syndrome is a frustrating condition because there aren't any one-size-fits-all treatments. It isn't dangerous in the long run, but the symptoms can make it impossible for people to live normal lives, not only because of the discomfort but also because of insecurity about being too far from a bathroom.

If your symptoms are so severe that they interfere with your day-to-day life, you should see a doctor right away. For one thing, there are a number of other conditions that cause similar symptoms. For another, the doctor may be able to prescribe medication to reduce the intensity and frequency of intestinal contractions.

If your physician tells you that you do have IBS, lifestyle changes may be just as important as medical care. Here's what doctors advise.

Two Good!

Apples and pears are twin remedies for IBS because they're loaded with fiber, which helps tame intestinal spasms and encourages regular bowel movements. They're also easy to snack on as you go about your day. Other foods that offer a lot of fiber bang for your buck include oat bran and ground flaxseed. Try sprinkling a tablespoon of either on salads, cereal, or yogurt.

Make friends with high-fiber foods. You should have five daily servings of fruit and vegetables. While that's good advice for everyone, it's especially important if you have IBS, since the fiber in these foods is very effective at reducing symptoms.

"Five servings a day is a good start," says Michael A. Visconti, N.D., a naturopathic physician in Orlando, Florida. But more is even better. The more fiber you eat, the less painful—and frequent—your symptoms are likely to be.

Eat smaller meals. Many people with IBS find that it helps to split their day's calories among five or six small meals rather than following the traditional break-fast-lunch-dinner schedule. Eating less food at one time puts less strain on the large intestine.

Chew, chew, chew. When you have IBS, your goal should be to make life as easy as possible for your digestive system. If you eat slowly and chew food thoroughly, your intestine has less work to do, which can reduce or even eliminate some of the discomfort.

Go fish! Some foods can help quell the intestinal inflammation that contributes to IBS symptoms. For example, salmon and other cold-water fish, as well as ground flaxseed, contain omega-3 essential fatty acids, which help your body suppress inflammation.

Work it out. You may not be up to it when your symptoms are in high gear, but 15 to 20 minutes of exercise every day is an important IBS-stopping strategy. Physical activity helps in two ways: It reduces levels of emotional stress, and it helps your bowel work more regularly. "People who exercise have a significant reduction of symptoms," says Dr. Visconti.

Develop a yen for yogurt. Live-culture yogurt contains beneficial *Lactobacillus acidophilus* organisms, which appear to reduce IBS symptoms. Plan on having at least a few servings of live-culture yogurt a week.

De-stress. For many people with IBS, the best way to ease discomfort is to change the ways in which they respond to stress, says Dr. Visconti. "You have to learn to manage stress without sending it to your digestive tract," he explains.

Turn off the tube. If you watch TV during meals, you could be setting yourself up for an IBS attack. Disquieting news programs and annoying commercials tend to ratchet up stress levels, which invariably makes symptoms worse, says Dr. Visconti. You'll also tend to eat too quickly because you're not paying attention to your food. His advice: Turn off the TV and enjoy your meals in peace and quiet.

FOOD NEWS

Raw fruits and vegetables are notorious gas promoters in people with IBS, but you can still get your fiber (which will also ease constipation) and nutrients by roasting or grilling fresh produce, says Gary Gitnick, M.D., chief of the division of digestive diseases at the University of California, Los Angeles, School of Medicine. Try roasted red peppers tossed with grilled eggplant and pineapple and splashed with ginger dressing. Mmm!

APPLES

Roughage from Eden

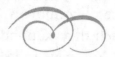

I GREW UP WITH A GOLDEN DELICIOUS APPLE TREE IN MY backyard, so I understand the apple's reputation for temptation. I also think Eve may have seduced Adam with an apple to be sure his bowels didn't get in an uproar. Why? Apples are bursting with fiber. In fact, one medium apple with skin delivers 20 percent of your daily fiber quota. The best news of all is that apples offer the insoluble kind of fiber that keeps bowels in good working order, as well as pectin, a type of soluble fiber that can help calm diarrhea.

What's more, pectin, in combination with the fruit sugars in apples, slows nutrient absorption, which helps people with diabetes keep their blood sugar under control. Soluble fiber also works to lower blood cholesterol—by as much as 16 per-

...Just the facts

Apple (1 medium)
Calories: 81
Fat: 0 g
Saturated fat: 0 g
Cholesterol: 0 mg
Sodium: 0 mg
Total carbohydrates: 21 g
Dietary fiber: 4 g
Protein: 3 g
Vitamin A: 1% of Daily Value
Vitamin C: 9%
Calcium: 1%
Iron: 1%

cent in one study! So don't fight temptation. Have an apple!

AN APPLE FOR THE TEACHERS

If Adam and Eve had lived in Finland, they might have been part of a study showing that men and women who munched an apple every day had a lower risk of ischemic stroke (the kind caused by a tiny blood clot blocking an artery in the brain) than those who were halfhearted in their pursuit of the Isaac Newton special. Exactly why the apples were so powerful isn't clear. (Stay tuned. Scientists are hunting for yet another secret ingredient. Just have another apple while you're waiting!)

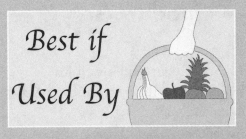

Best if Used By

Apples are already fully ripe when you buy them, so take them home and put them right in the fridge, where they'll keep for up to six weeks. At room temperature, they'll get mushy—fast.

POWERFUL TEMPTATION

The first couple was probably short on knives and peelers, so they undoubtedly ate their apples with the skin on—and that's good. Apple skins are brimming with quercetin, a much-studied plant chemical that accounts for other health benefits. Quercetin fights heart disease by preventing cholesterol from transforming itself into the muck that plasters itself to your artery walls, narrowing them and setting you up for a heart attack.

Quercetin fights cancer, too, possibly by deactivating carcinogens or causing them to just give up and die. One apple with skin

Scrub your apples well just before eating them to remove pesticides and wax.

delivers as much quercetin as ½ cup of tea or ⅔ cup of raw onion, so indulge yourself.

SHAKING THE TREE

More than 2,500 varieties of apples are grown in the United States (good job, Johnny Appleseed!), but just 8 make up 80 percent of what we buy and eat. Apples are at their juicy best when picked fresh in the fall, but modern, controlled-atmosphere storage techniques keep us supplied with crisp, crunchy apples all year long.

When choosing apples, select firm to hard ones. If a gentle squeeze produces a dent, the apple is too soft. Pick out the smaller ones, because little apples are usually better than big ones. And look for pretty ones; apples should have nice color for their type, tight skins, and no bruises or cuts.

Here's how to get your apple a day.

Chunk it into Waldorf salad. Mix apples, light mayo, walnuts, raisins, and celery for a side dish. Add cooked chicken bits for a main dish. Serving a crowd? Combine red, green, and yellow apples for a color fest!

Bake it. Core a large Rome Beauty. Fill the center with yellow raisins, cinnamon, brown sugar, and chopped pecans. Microwave until tender, about 5 minutes.

Wedge it. Cut an apple into thin slices and spread them with peanut butter for a super snack.

Stash it. Tuck it in your gym bag for a preworkout energy boost.

CHILES

Red-Hot Help for Your Gut

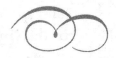

HERE'S A HOT TIP. WHILE SOME PEOPLE WITH IBS HAVE painful flare-ups when they eat spicy foods, others find that a little culinary heat makes them feel better. "The right kinds of spices seem to help," says Michael A. Visconti, N.D., a naturopathic physician in Orlando, Florida.

TURN UP THE HEAT

The ribs and seeds of chiles are packed with capsaicin, a heat-producing chemical with bountiful benefits. While your body is feeling the heat, your brain is chilling out with a flood of endorphins—high-flying, mood-lifting natural painkillers that create a sense of well-being (a sort of "eater's high"). One Thai dish called Drunken Noodles contains

...Just the facts

Red chile (1 pod)
Calories: 18
Fat: 0 g
Saturated fat: 0 g
Cholesterol: 0 mg
Sodium: 0 mg
Total carbohydrates: 4 g
Dietary fiber: 1 g
Protein: 1 g
Vitamin A: 97% of Daily
    Value
Vitamin C: 121%
Calcium: 1%
Iron: 3%

Looking for mild chiles? Banana peppers, cherry peppers, and jalapeños show up, sliced or whole, in jars at your supermarket. You almost can't go wrong with them. Then there's always paprika, crushed red pepper, and ground red pepper in the spice section. These should be a deep red color and a little lumpy (because they've hung on to their fresh, natural flavoring oils), rather than dusty and dry.

not a drop of alcohol but packs enough heat from chiles to make diners downright woozy!

Capsaicin fires up a nerve ending by activating its personal receptor, which turns right around and desensitizes nerves to pain. Eventually, that helps you become tolerant when you eat chiles and they bring on the heat. For the same reason, capsaicin is now being incorporated into a topical cream that helps fight the pain of osteoarthritis and diabetic neuropathy.

Capsaicin also turns out to be an antioxidant that helps lower "bad" low-density lipoprotein (LDL) cholesterol and reduce the stickiness of blood platelets so they don't clot and cause a heart attack or stroke. Each chile also comes packed with plenty of additional heart-smart ingredients. One fresh chile provides 121 percent of the vitamin C and 97 percent of the vitamin A you need daily, creating a powerful antioxidant team that fights the kind of cell damage that sets you up for heart disease, cancer, and premature aging.

What's more, capsaicin is heat stable, so if you don't want to bother with fresh chiles, dried or ground peppers will do.

Now here's some funny news: For years, part of ulcer treatment was to avoid hot, spicy foods, but today, chiles are being explored as a treatment for ulcers because of their bacteria-fighting ability.

CHILE CHOICES

Chiles are available fresh, dried, frozen, canned, and ground. When selecting fresh chiles, choose pods that are firm and bright looking and avoid those with any signs of bruising or decay.

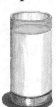

Here are a few quick ways to spice up your life with chiles. (If the fire gets too hot, have milk, yogurt, or frozen yogurt available to douse the flames.)

Perk up pizza. Sprinkle crushed red pepper and a small amount of aniseed on your pizza to mimic the taste of Italian sausage—without the fat. Add pepperoncini to your salad.

Say Olé! Spice up a can of vegetarian chili with a dash of ground red pepper, chopped onions, and a little cilantro.

Try Thai. Mix chilled, thinly sliced filet mignon with garlic, ginger, soy sauce, and fish

Learning to eat chiles is a lot like learning to drink alcohol. When you first taste alcoholic beverages, you're taken aback by the fiery breathlessness they cause, but with experience, you taste different flavors in red and white wines, beer, and bourbon. It's the same with chiles.

Each type boasts a unique flavor, and many offer mild fruit flavors with tinges of coffee, licorice, dried plum, or raisin. And each type is armed with its own amount of firepower. The biggest chiles are fairly mild—it's those tiny ones that will take your head off!

Has a cold got you all stuffed up? Cook up a pot of chicken soup (canned will do), then add fresh garlic and plenty of ground red pepper. Inhale the fumes while you eat the soup. You'll be breathing freely in no time, but keep the tissues handy. Your nose will run freely, too!

sauce. Toss with sliced red onions and jalapeños and some lime juice and serve on Butterhead lettuce.

Put a cherry on top. Add some Hungarian cherry peppers (they're sweet and mild—usually!) to your next pickle and olive tray.

Enjoy Asian. Toss a couple of small dried red chiles into your next stir-fry. They'll fire up the flavor even if you don't eat them.

GREEN BEANS

Jack-of-All-Nutrients

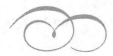

MY FRIEND KAREN HAS ALWAYS HAD A THING ABOUT green beans. As a little girl, she was the official bean snapper at her grandmother's house. (Together, they whipped up a mean green bean and ham soup.) In high school, she often cooked green beans Lyonnaise-style, following a recipe from her French teacher. Now, she steams and seasons them for a quick side dish or orders chicken and green beans from her local Chinese restaurant. All the green bean goodness now gives her family a head start on better bowel function.

The thing about green beans is that they're mild tasting as vegetables go, making them an all-American favorite. Also, while they don't have one standout nutrient, they pack a sprinkling of lots of goodies. Take a look at what they have to offer.

> ## ...Just the facts
>
> Green beans (½ cup cooked)
> Calories: 22
> Fat: 0 g
> Saturated fat: 0 g
> Cholesterol: 0 mg
> Sodium: 2 mg
> Total carbohydrates: 5 g
> Dietary fiber: 2 g
> Protein: 1 g
> Folate: 5% of Daily Value
> Vitamin A: 7%
> Vitamin C: 10%

Once you get your beans home, refrigerate them. They'll keep for about three days.

MANY-SPLENDORED BEANS

Green beans contribute fiber, potassium, folate, and vitamins A and C, which keep your entire body humming along so your bowels don't bother you and all your other moving parts get a tuneup. Here's how they do it.

• Fiber helps keep your bowels tiptop while reduc-ing your cholesterol.

• Potassium lowers blood pressure.

• Folate decreases your level of an amino acid that researchers suspect con-tributes to ticker trouble.

• Vitamins A and C also contribute, gobbling up free radicals, those bad guys that may trig-ger both heart disease and cancer.

• Scientists have also identified two additional cancer-fighting compounds in green beans—coumarin and quercetin. Researchers aren't sure yet exactly how much green beans contain or specifically how the compounds work, but they know that they do work!

The bottom line: With green beans, you're in good hands.

SNAPPING UP GREEN BEANS

Fresh green beans are available in the produce department of

Good to Go

When you're ready to use your green beans, rinse, then scrub off any dirt with a veggie brush and remove the stem ends before cooking.

your supermarket all year long. Choosing great fresh beans is, well, a snap. Be sure the pods are bright green, firm, and smooth. If they feel bumpy, it's probably because the beans were picked past their prime and the seeds have grown very large. Leave these at the store.

Now here are some delicious ways to eat your green beans.

Say cheese. Cook the beans, toss them with olive oil, and top with a little goat cheese.

Cool it. Make a cold green bean salad for a summer picnic. Just marinate cooked beans in vinaigrette (such as Ken's Basil and Balsamic Vinaigrette), then add a little minced garlic and chopped fresh tomatoes.

Go savory. Sauté green beans with sliced mushrooms and minced garlic.

Bulk up Chinese. Add plenty of green beans to stir-fries. In restaurants, order extra beans on the side.

Fabulous Fill-In!

If you can't find fresh green beans, there are always plenty of frozen and canned beans to meet your needs. They're good choices, too. Despite common myths, studies show that they have about the same amount of nutrients as fresh. (In case you're curious, this is true for all the veggies that were tested.) Just be careful about the sodium content of canned veggies if you're following a low-salt diet.

PEARS

Unparalleled Fiber

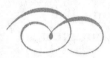

IN LATE AUGUST, JUST WHEN YOU'RE BEGINNING TO HOPE for a cool autumn breeze, check out local roadside stands, as well as your favorite supermarket, for the season's first succulent, tree-ripened pears. Eat them out of hand until you just can't stand it any more, then use them in salads, sandwiches, and anything else that comes to mind. You can't go wrong, because pears pack a mighty health punch—and you'd be crazy to pass up this delicious treat! Not only will your taste buds thank you, but your iffy bowels will be high-fiving you, too!

FIBER TWO-FER

Hands down, the healthiest thing about pears is their high fiber content. A medium-size Bartlett pear boasts about 4 grams, and a study is under way to deter-

---

...Just the facts

Bartlett pear (1 medium)
Calories: 100
Fat: 1 g
Saturated fat: 0 g
Cholesterol: 0 mg
Sodium: 0 mg
Total carbohydrates: 25 g
Dietary fiber: 4 g
Protein: 1 g
Vitamin C: 10% of Daily
    Value

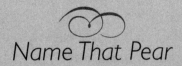

Name That Pear

Pears were all the rage in France from the 12th to the 19th century, and breeders continually developed new varieties. Eventually, 3,000 separate types came into existence. Fortunately for those of us who have a hard time making up our minds, only a handful of pear varieties are grown commercially. Here are five of the most plentiful types.

• *Anjou.* The most popular pear, the Anjou is egg shaped and remains green when ripe.

• *Yellow Bartlett.* A sweet and most aromatic pear, the yellow Bartlett is usually green at the supermarket and turns yellow while ripening in your kitchen.

• *Red Bartlett.* This variety tastes and smells just as good as its yellow cousin. It is dark red at the supermarket and ripens to bright red in your home.

• *Bosc.* With firm, dense flesh and super flavor, this variety is ideal for cooking and baking. You can easily spot a Bosc by its earthy brown color.

• *Seckel.* This maroon-and-olive-green petite pear (about half the size of an Anjou) is the sweetest of all.

mine whether thicker-skinned varieties, such as Bosc pears, offer even more of this important nutrient.

Better yet, pears pack a 50-50 blend of the two main types of fiber: soluble and insoluble. Lignin, the insoluble fiber in pears, helps bulk up stools and makes them pass through the intestines faster, possibly reducing the risk of colon cancer. It also binds up the male hormone testosterone and thus may lower the chance of prostate cancer.

The soluble fiber in pears, called pectin, may help lower

cholesterol levels, a critical way to reduce your risk of heart disease. Here's how it works.

• Soluble fiber helps bind together bile acids, enabling pectin to draw cholesterol out of your blood.

• It also helps block the fat and cholesterol in your foods from getting to the interior wall of the intestines, where it would be absorbed.

Researchers at Purdue University in West Lafayette, Indiana, found that eating about 9 grams of pectin daily reduced cholesterol by 10 percent. Pears have at least 2 grams of pectin in each fruit!

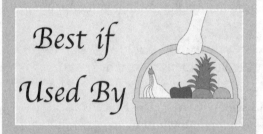

Best if Used By

Here's what to do when you get home with your pears.

• If they're ripe, refrigerate them immediately. Left at room temperature, they may turn brown inside. They'll last about a week in the refrigerator.

• Place unripe pears in a brown paper bag along with a damp cotton ball (the moisture will help prevent shriveling) and store at 60° to 70°F. Check them every day to see if they've ripened. If not, replace the cotton ball.

PEAR WITH A-PEEL

Some people peel a pear before they eat it, but you shouldn't let them! According to a recent study at the University of California, Davis, almost all of the phyto-chemicals (healthy plant compounds) that pears have to offer lie in the skin. Red Bartletts pack about one-third more of these beneficial compounds—particularly anticancer flavones and antho-cyanins—than green varieties do.

While pears in general don't contribute as many of these compounds as some other fruits do (scientists consider the amounts to be moderate), you'll want to hang on to every bit. So no peeling!

PERFECTLY PEARED

Once you choose your variety, determine how ripe you'd like your pears to be. Do you want to eat them today or save them for a few days? Most supermarket pears are about one to three days from being ripe. To tell the degree of ripeness, you could rely on color, since some pears do change color when they're ripe. Other varieties remain the same hue, so you could use the thumb test by gently pressing down near the base of the stem with your thumb. If it yields slightly, it's ripe and ready to eat. If not, you'll have to ripen it at home.

Try these unusual ways to enjoy this exceptional fruit.

Edge out bread. Forget croutons; toss pear slices into your salad instead. If you're making the salad ahead of time, drizzle the pears with lemon juice to prevent browning.

Slice for toast. For a hint of sweetness (and extra fiber), top a piece of toasted whole wheat bread with peanut butter and pear slices.

Nudge potatoes aside. Bake pear halves with ham or pork during the last 15 minutes of cooking, basting them with the juices from the meat, then serve them as a side dish. It's a lot easier than making mashed potatoes!

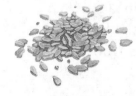

Sweeten your snack. Slice a pear, then dip one end in honey and coat it with chopped nuts or sunflower seeds.

A SIMPLE SOLUTION

The next time your internal plumbing gets clogged, slice up a pear and mix it with a couple of prunes and a teaspoon of bran for a before-bed snack. Your plumbing will be fixed by morning—guaranteed!

QUINOA

A Mini Grain with Maxi Goodness

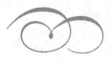

SMELL IS THE SHORTEST DISTANCE BETWEEN TWO MEMORIES, and the earthy bouquet of quinoa (pronounced *keen-wah*) takes me right back to the best part of my childhood. When I was a little girl, I spent a lot of time with horses, and I've never gotten over the wonderful smells that wafted out of their grain bins. Now that I'm a big girl, I rely on quinoa to keep my bowels running smoothly.

THE SAME BUT DIFFERENT

Quinoa isn't the same grain that I fed my horses, but it does have a similar clean, fresh fragrance. And when it comes to whole grains for humans, quinoa is as good as it gets, providing all the benefits of other whole grains, such as whole wheat or oats.

...Just the facts

Quinoa (¾ cup cooked)
Calories: 127
Fat: 2 g
Saturated fat: 0 g
Cholesterol: 0 mg
Sodium: 7 mg
Total carbohydrates: 23 g
Dietary fiber: 2 g
Protein: 4 g
Vitamin E: 11% of Daily
    Value
Copper: 14%
Iron: 17%
Potassium: 18%

Quinoa's insoluble fiber stimulates bowel function, staving off constipation and diverticulosis. An array of research also shows that people who eat the most whole grain foods are less likely to have heart attacks or strokes, less likely to get cancer, and less likely to develop diabetes. The phytochemicals (natural plant chemicals) in whole grains appear to boost immune function, which not only fends off colds and flu but also fights serious stuff such as cancer. That's a lot of horsepower for such a tiny grain!

Good to Go

To prepare quinoa, put it in a fine-mesh strainer and rinse it under running water to remove the fine powder you see. Put 1 cup of quinoa and 2 cups of water in a 1½-quart saucepan and bring to a boil. Reduce the heat to low, cover, and simmer for about 15 minutes, or until all the water is absorbed.

SMALL BUT MIGHTY

Quinoa is a wee grain that starts out about the size of a sesame seed, then quadruples its bulk as it cooks. When you put 1 cup of grains and some water in a saucepan, then take off the lid—presto!—you have a whole potful! (It's almost as amazing as popping corn, but without the noise.)

Cooked, the grains turn into translucent mini pearls. Each has a tiny, yellowish "tail," formed when its outside germ spins away from the grain. Quinoa is amazingly light and fluffy rather than heavy and starchy like rice or barley. (Think of the difference between regular cooked rice and puffed rice cereal.) The flavor is very mild, maybe even bland, but that can be a plus for folks who are offended by the sturdy, slightly bitter taste of whole wheat.

What makes quinoa even better is that it's just brimming with nutrients. It packs more protein than any other grain, and

Here's a news flash for busy folks: Unlike other whole grains that take 45 to 60 minutes to cook, quinoa goes from package to table in just 15 minutes!

it stands out from the entire crowd of plant-based proteins because it delivers the full array of amino acids that make it as complete as meat. It's loaded with three times the vitamin E and twice the calcium, iron, magnesium, and potassium of other grains, and it even has a little more zinc. Its 2 grams of fat per ¾-cup serving are the heart-healthy monounsaturated and polyunsaturated kind.

FIND IT FRESH

You'll find quinoa at your local health food store or natural food store and in the health food section of many supermarkets. Look for small boxes that appear to be of recent vintage.

Here are some suggestions for adding quinoa to your weekly menu.

Replace rice. Use cooked quinoa in place of rice when you make stuffed peppers or cabbage rolls or to make "quinoa pudding."

Toss and turn. Blend cooked quinoa with sautéed vegetables.

Create a cool feast. Mix cold cooked quinoa with chopped fresh vegetables and your favorite dressing for a cool summer salad.

Make a better breakfast. Cook quinoa in fruit juice instead of water and serve it with chopped nuts for breakfast.

Improve your soup. Stir a tablespoon or two of dry quinoa into soup a few minutes before serving.

STOMACHACHE

That Settles It

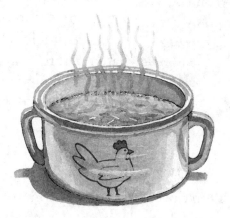

OKAY, IT'S TIME TO GET SOMETHING straight. Most stomachaches don't occur in your stomach at all, even though that's where the trouble usually begins. For various reasons, your stomach doesn't always do a great job of digesting its contents. When undigested food travels into the intestine, you're likely to experience cramps or painful gas. Thus, a stomachache is really an intestine ache—one that occurs when your bowel has to deal with your stomach's unfinished business.

A stomachache isn't always a routine problem. In fact, there's a long list of med-

FOOD NEWS

Troubled by a queasy tummy when you travel? Simply begin your journey with a cup of ginger tea. Not strong enough? Ginger capsules will deliver a more standardized dose. Need help along the way? Carry some candied ginger.

323

ical conditions that cause pain somewhere in the belly, and some of them are serious, so for those you should see your doctor. For ordinary stomachaches, though, here are a few things that are sure to help.

Add greens. Dandelion greens are a traditional remedy for stomach problems of all kinds. Eaten before a meal, the pleasantly bitter greens stimulate digestive secretions and reduce cramping.

Be sure to pick dandelions from an area that hasn't been treated with chemicals. The leaves are most tender when they're picked just before the flowers bloom. Don't overdo the dandelion, though, if you're taking diuretics or potassium supplements.

Subtract water. If you tend to get stomachaches after eating, you may want to give up drinking water or other liquids with your meals, because they dilute the stomach's acid secretions, says Andrew Parkinson, N.D., a naturopathic physician and faculty member at the Bastyr Center for Natural Health near Seattle. The acid, of course, helps you digest food.

Multiply bacteria. Your gut is loaded with beneficial bacteria that break down and digest food. Sometimes, these bacteria get depleted—if you've been taking antibiotics, for example—resulting in painful abdominal cramps.

A serving of yogurt is a great way to load your gut with more beneficial bacteria. Look for brands that contain live cultures. "It's not something you need on a daily basis, but it's a good idea to try to replenish those bacteria from time to time," says Dr. Parkinson.

Another easy way to boost their numbers back to healthful levels is to take supplements that contain acidophilus. One or two acidophilus capsules are often all you need to calm the upset feeling.

Drink to your health. If you're a wine lover, you may know this already: A glass of dry white wine before a meal is good for digestion. In fact, a trip to the liquor store will reveal many aperitifs and "bitters" traditionally used to jump-start the digestive process. These liquid appetizers contain natural chemicals that stimulate digestion.

Walk it off. An after-dinner stroll is a good idea, but you don't want to be too active after eating. If you are, your body won't have enough energy for proper digestion—and cramps and gas may result.

CINNAMON

The New Old Spice

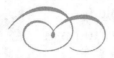

REMEMBER THE AROMA OF FRESH-FROM-THE-BAKERY cinnamon buns on Sunday mornings long, long ago? Back then, of course, they accompanied bacon and eggs—not exactly what we're touting in this book! Nowadays, we use the scent of cinnamon to lure hungry eaters to healthier foods, such as fruits, vegetables, and rice, but the most exciting news is that cinnamon is now being tested for its ability to knock out *Helicobacter pylori*, the bacteria that cause most stomach ulcers. Stay tuned for more on that front, but in the meantime, if you have an upset stomach, bloating, or gas, try a cup of cinnamon tea. The German Commission E, which studies herbal medicines in Europe, says it really works.

...Just the facts

Cinnamon (1 tsp ground)
Calories: 6
Fat: 0 g
Saturated fat: 0 g
Cholesterol: 0 mg
Sodium: 0 mg
Total carbohydrates: 2 g
Dietary fiber: 1 g
Protein: 0 g
Calcium: 3% of Daily Value
Iron: 5%
Manganese: 19%

ANCIENT WISDOM

Actually, the saga of cinnamon began with the birth of civilization. The Egyptian spice trade was booming in 2500 B.C. and included cinnamon, which came from Ceylon and eventually made its way to Greece and Rome. Citizens of the Eternal Empire developed a real "spice tooth," which they spread to all the territories they conquered. Not only did cinnamon and other spices taste good, but rumor has it that they also helped cover up the smell of rotting meat. But, hey, you shouldn't listen to rumors.

Researchers now think that cinnamon, along with cardamom, cloves, and other spices used in Asian cuisine, may actually prevent food spoilage. In one study, high doses of cinnamon bark oil stopped mold from growing in laboratory petri dishes. (Hmm...think this might work in our refrigerators?)

MODERN TWISTS

Cinnamon also seems to be as good for your heart as it is for your taste buds because it has some antioxidant activity. In one laboratory study, cinnamon and cloves turned out to be the nicest spices for preventing fatty acid oxidation. This chemical change turns cholesterol into the gunk that clogs your arteries, increasing heart disease risk. Other research suggests that cinnamon and cardamom may act by waking up antioxidant enzymes and sending them off to work.

If you're managing diabetes, add a little cinnamon to your oatmeal or brown rice. Research from the USDA shows that people with diabetes who use cinnamon regularly can reduce their blood sugar levels, triglycerides, total cholesterol, and LDL cholesterol. What a potent little powder!

STICK WITH THE BEST

Cinnamon is the dried inner bark of two trees in the laurel family that grow in Asia. One is true cinnamon and is pale tan, but most of the cinnamon in supermarkets comes from the other, and that's okay. This cinnamon is darker in color and has a stronger fragrance.

You can buy it ground or in sticks. When selecting cinnamon, look for a sealed container and check the freshness date. Store your cinnamon in a cool, dark place.

Then keep your cinnamon handy, because there are so many ways to use it. Try these.

Gussy up grains. Cinnamon delivers a wakeup call at breakfast. Stir it into hot whole grain cereal or sprinkle it on a whole grain waffle topped with fresh strawberries.

Tune up toast. Start with 100 percent whole wheat bread, spread with reduced-fat ricotta cheese, and sprinkle with ground cinnamon. Intense!

Streamline squash. Season winter squash, such as acorn or butternut, with ground cinnamon and toasted nuts, and you won't have to worry about whether butter or margarine is better.

Detail desserts. Dust deli custard, pudding, or rice pudding with ground cinnamon for a homemade touch.

Stir in flavor. Use a cinnamon stick to stir your hot chocolate or hot apple cider for a little fun and a lot of taste.

Spice up coffee. Toss in a piece of cinnamon stick when you grind your coffee beans. Exotic!

GINGER

Good for What "Ales" You

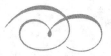

WHEN MY KIDS WERE LITTLE, WE SPENT A LOT OF TIME camping, and there was one treat we always brought from home: my famous gingerbread, a simple one-bowl cake that I could whip up just before we left for camp and allow to cool in the car. Little did the kids know that I stuffed the sweet treat with whole wheat flour and heart-healthy canola oil! They thought they were in cake heaven. What they also didn't know was that it was a powerful force against carsickness.

The secret, of course, was the pungent ginger that gave the cake its unforgettable flavor. That cake got all three kids addicted to its zingy taste, and now they can't get enough of Thai or Chinese cuisine, where the ancient flavor is essential to so many dishes.

...Just the facts

Ginger (1 tsp ground)
Calories: 7
Fat: 0 g
Saturated fat: 0 g
Cholesterol: 0 mg
Sodium: 0 mg
Total carbohydrates: 1 g
Dietary fiber: 0 g
Protein: 0 g
Iron: 2% of Daily Value

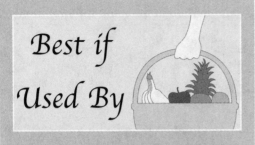

Best if Used By

You'll almost always buy more fresh ginger than you can use at one time, but that's okay. The leftovers will keep for months in your freezer, double-wrapped in plastic. Grating and slicing are actually easier when the ginger is frozen.

LOVIN' SPOONFUL

The good news is that ginger is more than just a potent flavor enhancer. Asians have long used it to tame troubled tummies, and now researchers are discovering that while ginger doesn't look very promising when you're weighing its vitamins and minerals, it's packed with a cool array of phytochemicals that protect just about every cell in your body.

• *Zingerone.* This phytochemical, for instance, protects polyunsaturated fat from being oxidized, so the fat can work its heart-protective magic.

• *Gingerol.* This ingredient fights cancer by preventing cancer cells from multiplying—and even by encouraging them to just drop dead. It also prevents platelets in your blood from clotting, which reduces your chance of a heart attack or stroke.

• *Glucosides.* These appear to have antioxidant activity that protects against cancer and heart disease.

• *Phenolic substances.* The pungent phenolic substances in ginger fight inflammation.

In addition, ginger appears to have mild antibacterial properties that may help prevent infection. What a spoonful—tasty and powerful!

A LIGHTER FORKFUL

With obesity becoming an increasingly bigger problem in the United States, many of us are looking for ways to keep our weight under control. One way to do it is to eat smaller portions of better-tasting food that's more satisfying. Another way is to eat big piles of highly seasoned vegetables, and that's where ginger can be a star player, spicing up stir-fries and even small portions of lean meat. It can also help reduce your weight-control woes when you use it to spice up your meals instead of burying them in tons of fat.

ZINGY GINGER

"Gingerroot" is a misnomer. Ginger is actually a rhizome, an underground stem that looks like a thick, lumpy root, but both new roots and new stems can grow out of it.

You'll find fresh ginger in the specialty section of the produce department of most supermarkets; look for ground ginger in the spice or baking aisle. You may find crystallized ginger there, too. It makes a tasty snack.

Use ginger to make your foods a little more exotic—and healthier! Here are some ideas.

Make snappier stir-fries. Finely chop fresh ginger and add it to the pan with the onions and garlic when you stir-fry.

Make zingier marinades. Add chopped fresh ginger or ground ginger to any marinade to perk up the flavor of lean beef, pork, or chicken.

Add sparkle to soups. Add ground ginger to carrot or squash soup to bring the soup to life.

Breathe easier. Add thin slices of fresh ginger to chicken soup when you're congested. It will help clear your nose.

MINT

Cool under Fire

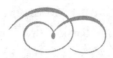

YOUR GRANDMA PROBABLY TOLD YOU THAT IF YOU HAD stomach cramps, peppermint would take care of them. She was a smart lady, because peppermint contains menthol, a substance that helps prevent spasms in your digestive tract, thus lessening cramps. What's more, a review of studies in the *Journal of Gastroenterology* suggested that peppermint oil may even help people who have irritable bowel syndrome, a condition that causes very frequent bowel movements.

Unfortunately, peppermint probably won't relieve heartburn—and, in fact, may even aggravate it—because it allows acid to flow more freely up into your esophagus. But two out of three isn't bad, right?

EXPERI-MINT

Mint is also growing a fine reputation for defending against another high-stakes

---

...Just the facts

Spearmint (2 Tbsp fresh)
Calories: 5
Fat: 0 g
Saturated fat: 0 g
Cholesterol: 0 mg
Sodium: 3 mg
Total carbohydrates: 1 g
Dietary fiber: 1 g
Protein: 0 g
Vitamin A: 9% of Daily Value

---

enemy. "Mint contains limonene, a powerful anticancer agent that studies suggest can block the development of breast tumors and can shrink them," points out Ritva Butrum, Ph.D., vice president of research at the American Institute for Cancer Research in Washington, D.C. Limonene hinders cancer cells from utilizing a protein that they need to survive. Mint also packs another breast cancer fighter, luteolin, which may inhibit the production of inflammatory compounds linked with the development of cancer.

At this point, scientists are testing these compounds to pinpoint the exact benefits they provide. In the meantime, Dr. Butrum says, "our best insurance is eating a wide variety of plant-based foods, including herbs such as mint."

DEMYSTIFYING MINT

If you have peppermint or spearmint growing in your house or garden, you won't have to shop for it, but if you do need to buy some, don't sweat it. Mint isn't hard to find—just head for the fresh herbs in the produce section of your local supermarket.

Look for a bunch that's evenly colored and shows no signs of wilting. Peppermint has bright green leaves and purple-tinged stems, while spearmint has gray-green or plain green leaves. If you have trouble distinguishing between the two, your nose should be able to detect the difference: Peppermint is more pungent than spearmint. (And it's not used in as many recipes.)

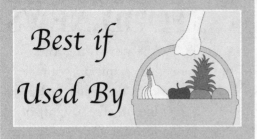

Best if Used By

After you take your mint home, shake it to remove grit and moisture, pack it loosely in paper towels, and keep it in the crisper drawer or a special produce storage container, such as the type made by Tupperware. It should stay fresh for about a week.

Here are some hot hints for using your cool mint.

Add zest to your salad. Toss a couple of tablespoons of chopped spearmint into your favorite fruit salad; it works particularly well with melons and berries. Or add it to a cucumber salad. I like to mix diced cucumber, diced tomato, parsley, garlic, lemon juice, olive oil, feta cheese, and, last but not least, spearmint.

Brighten up chicken. Turn ordinary grilled chicken into fireworks for the taste buds simply by topping it with creamy mint sauce. Don't worry—it only sounds fattening. Just mix ½ cup of low-fat plain yogurt, 1 tablespoon each of chopped spearmint and parsley, 1 teaspoon of lemon juice, 2 minced garlic cloves (you can add more if you like), and ¼ teaspoon of ground black pepper. Refrigerate for at least a few hours so the flavors blend. The sauce will keep for about five days, so it's a good way to jazz up leftover chicken, too.

Make over pesto. One of my favorite restaurants makes a delicious mint pesto, and you can easily substitute spearmint for basil in your own favorite pesto recipe.

Take a tea break. Ditch the coffee and soothe your nerves with a cup of peppermint tea. Simply steep a small handful of fresh peppermint in a cup of boiling water. If desired, sweeten with honey.

OLIVES

Sun-Kissed Protection

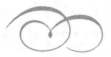

DOES SAILING MAKE YOU QUEASY OR FLYING TURN YOU green? The next time you launch yourself into major motion, take along some olives and, at the first sign of motion sickness, eat a couple. Olives contain tannins that dry your mouth, which reduces the excess saliva that can cause nausea.

Olives have been one of my dad's favorite foods ever since he was a little boy, and that turns out to be good news for him. It seems that because olives grow in searing sunlight, they produce a load of anthocyanins, flavonoids, and phenols—all of which are naturally occurring plant chemicals that protect the fruit against sun damage. Once they're inside you, these same phytochemicals (*phyto* is from the Greek language and simply means "plant") protect your cells from damage caused by pollution, illness, and even some natural

...Just the facts

Ripe olive (1 super-colossal)
Calories: 12
Fat: 1 g
Saturated fat: 0 g
Cholesterol: 0 mg
Sodium: 137 mg
Total carbohydrates: 1 g
Dietary fiber: Less than 1 g
Protein: 0 g
Vitamin E: 2% of Daily Value

body processes that can throw off substances that cause disease. In fact, olives seem to protect you from everything but the sun!

FATS FOR LIFE

Like the oil they produce, olives contain heart-healthy monounsaturated fat that can do the following.

• Help lower your cholesterol and triglyceride levels.

• Reduce blood clotting.

• Possibly offer some protection against breast cancer.

Don't get carried away, though; a little bit of good fat goes a long way. Three super-colossal-size, canned ripe olives deliver nearly 40 calories, so eating too many can make you gain weight.

The same three olives also pack more than 400 milligrams of sodium (about 17 percent of the Daily Value), and as you already know, a high-sodium diet increases blood pressure in some people. What you may not know is that lots of sodium may also drain calcium from your bones. The trick is to use a few olives here and there to accent the flavors of healthy foods.

FLAVORS GALORE

You're probably are most familiar with stuffed green Spanish olives or those jumbo ripe olives in a can. They will deliver the nutritional goods, but olive aficionados suggest that you broaden your horizons with other varieties, which are becoming more widely available.

One New York City restaurant boasts a complete olive

menu, while some local supermarkets offer "olive bars," where you can pack your own containers full of favorites such as Kalamatas, jumbo spiced green Italian olives, or even giant Cerignolas. Larger than a whole pecan in its shell, a ripe Cerignola is an inky black olive with thick, meaty flesh and a mild, less salty, less tart taste. Another exotic treat is the pistachio-size ripe French niçoise olive that is traditionally found in salade niçoise. These olives also make a beautiful garnish scattered over grilled salmon.

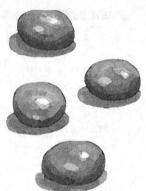

If you like your olives stuffed, you're in luck, because the creative juices are flowing at the olive-packing plant. Fabulous healthy fillings include almonds, garlic, mushrooms, onions, sun-dried tomatoes, jalapeño peppers, and for those who like things really hot, habanero chile peppers. You'll find them in the fancy foods section of larger supermarkets.

OLIVE ACCENTS

Your olive options are many—so experiment! When looking for new olive treats, check out either the deli or imported food section of your local store or try a natural food store. Investigate Italian and Greek food stores, which usually carry ethnic varieties and may let you taste before you buy. If you can't find olive novelties locally, visit the Santa Barbara Olive Company online at www.sbolive.com.

With an interesting array of

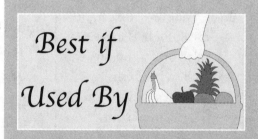

Best if Used By

There's no real trick to storing olives.

• You can store unopened cans or sealed jars of olives in a cool, dry pantry for up to one year. Refrigerate after opening.

• Refrigerate olives that are in unsealed deli containers, even though the olives have been both fermented and pickled.

FOOD NEWS

Entertaining? Have an olive-tasting party. Use a little red wine or some thinly shaved fresh Parmesan cheese for palate cleansing between bites, but keep the focus on the fancy fruit. Display 5 to 10 varieties, perhaps including slender green French Picholines, plump purple Italian Gaetas, and pea-size brown Spanish Arbequinas. Offer just enough so that each person eats about 10 olives. Follow with a light meal, such as a green salad and a dinner roll, with fresh berries and melon chunks for dessert.

olives on hand, try a few of these tasty ways to add sparkle to your meals.

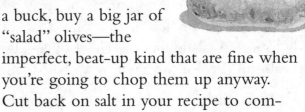

Make salads marvelous. Slice stuffed Spanish olives into potato salad, egg salad, or even tuna salad. To save a buck, buy a big jar of "salad" olives—the imperfect, beat-up kind that are fine when you're going to chop them up anyway. Cut back on salt in your recipe to compensate for the extra sodium in the olives.

Create greater grains. Rev up cold summer grain salads made with wheatberries, brown and wild rice, or tabbouleh with a few tangy chopped olives. Plump, smooth-flavored, oil-cured olives make your taste buds sing.

Spark up old standbys. Sliver a few Kalamata olives into that jar of store-bought spaghetti sauce for a piquant flavor that tastes homemade. *Molto bene!* Turn tacos into heart-healthy treats by wrapping lettuce, chopped tomatoes, chopped onions, ground turkey, reduced-fat cheese, and sliced olives in a soft corn tortilla. *Ai, Chihuahua!*

Tempt with tapenade. Whip out your blender and whirl up some tapenade, the Spanish olive spread. Served by little teaspoonfuls on thin crusts of toasted bread, it's an appetizer that makes your heart soar.

ULCERS

Fight Back

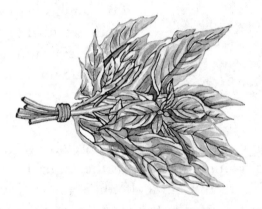

REMEMBER *THE ODD COUPLE*? ONE OF THE RECURRING themes of this classic 1970s sitcom was poor Oscar Madison's ongoing struggle with ulcers. He was always getting them, mainly (he thought) because of his terrible diet, constant cigar smoking, and the stress of living with his obsessively neat roommate, Felix Unger.

Funny as the show was, its ulcer premise is now obsolete. Today, Oscar would be treated with antibiotics to eradicate the true cause of his never-ending discomfort: tiny, screw-shaped organisms living in his digestive tract.

GUT LIKE A SIEVE

Here's the story. The digestive acids in your stomach are strong enough to dissolve the heaviest meal into a digestible

Most people with ulcers experience a burning sensation from time to time, usually between meals, when their stomachs are empty. Don't ignore the pain; see your doctor. Ulcers that aren't treated can bleed, and sometimes they bleed a lot. It's not uncommon, in fact, for people with ulcers to become anemic because of blood loss.

soup of nutrients. In fact, these acids are nearly as strong as battery acid, so why don't they digest your stomach just as efficiently as they break down a serving of your mother's pasta?

Nature, it turns out, designed the stomach to withstand constant acid onslaughts by giving it a thin, protective lining that prevents the acids from damaging the tender tissue underneath. Of course, this system works only if the protective barrier is intact.

That's where germs come in. *Helicobacter pylori*, a type of bacterium that commonly inhabits the stomach and intestine, digs into this protective lining. If you're infected with *H. pylori*, the lining may be pitted with tiny holes that permit stomach acid to leak through. The result: small, painful little sores known as ulcers. Ulcers can also be triggered by prolonged use of pain relievers, including aspirin and ibuprofen. You need to stay in touch with your doctor if you take these drugs on a regular basis.

HEAL THE HOLES

Most often, ulcers can be eliminated with a relatively simple, two-part treatment: antibiotics prescribed by your doctor to kill the bacteria and medications to lower levels of stomach acid. Along with treatment, however, there are a few lifestyle approaches that do make a difference.

Alter antacids. When the burning pain of ulcers flares, your natural instinct is probably to pop a few antacids. There's certainly nothing wrong with this approach in some cases, but some doctors suspect that quenching stomach acid with antacids may make ulcers worse in the long run.

"You need stomach acids to obliterate microorganisms," says Christie C. Yerby, N.D., a naturopathic physician in Sanford, North Carolina. "Lowering the acidity of the stomach makes it easier for ulcer-causing bacteria to survive."

If you're taking antacids but they don't seem to help, make an appointment to see your doctor. You may be doing yourself a lot more harm than good.

Eat onions. Having an ulcer is no reason to hold the onions. In fact, it's all the more reason to add them to salads, sandwiches, soups, and so forth. Onions contain compounds that seem to help eliminate ulcer-causing bacteria, so try to include them in at least one meal a day.

Skip sugar. Most of us love sugar—but we're not the only ones. The bacteria that cause ulcers are also extremely fond of sweets. "The more sugar you

Antioxidant Power

Here's how to boost your body's healing power with fruits and vegetables high in the antioxidant vitamins A, C, and E.

• Green peppers add crunch to your lunch and supply nearly a full day's supply of healing vitamin C.

• Replacing traditional iceberg lettuce with romaine gives you five times more vitamin A and C to heal those ulcers.

• Ounce for ounce, kiwifruit packs more vitamin C than oranges.

• Spinach doles out hefty doses of vitamins A, C, and E, along with lutein to protect your eyes and folate to protect your heart. Powerful!

• Ten grams of fat (preferably the healthy kind from olive or canola oil) are a must to help you absorb all the vitamin A from your fruits and vegetables.

Healing VITAMINS

If you don't eat a lot of fruit, vegetables, and other plant foods, you may not be getting enough of a few key nutrients—mainly vitamins A, C, and E—that are needed to repair damaged tissue throughout your body, including the stomach lining. If you have a history of ulcers, it's a good idea to take daily supplements that provide the recommended daily amounts of each of these important nutrients.

consume, the more you're feeding the bacteria that cause ulcers," says Dr. Yerby. Her advice: Give up sweets, or at least save them for very special occasions.

Down aloe. Aloe vera is one of nature's great healers, and it's especially good for ulcers because it coats irritated tissues and may promote faster healing. You can buy aloe juice at health food stores or, if you grow aloe at home to treat minor injuries, just break open a leaf and squeeze some juice into your mouth, Dr. Yerby suggests. You can take aloe up to a couple of times a day.

Get fish from a bottle. Doctors and nutritionists almost beg Americans to eat more fish, in part because it's such a rich source of essential fatty acids that help quell inflammation. If you have ulcers, however, eating too much fish may cause an increase in stomach acid—and pain, says Dr. Yerby. She recommends that instead of eating fish, people with ulcers take fish-oil supplements, which are available at drugstores and health food stores. Follow the directions on the label. You shouldn't take fish oil if you take aspirin regularly or are taking prescription blood-thinning medication.

Skip cocktails and smokes. Alcohol and tobacco tend to make ulcer pain worse, and they inhibit your body's ability to heal the damage. People who smoke and drink are also more likely to get ulcers than those who don't indulge.

Take a virtual vacation. Even though emotional stress

doesn't cause ulcers, it does increase levels of stomach acid, which can make the pain worse. Stress reduction should be part of every anti-ulcer strategy, says Dr. Yerby.

When you feel your stress level rising, close your eyes, breathe deeply, and visualize a peaceful scene from nature, she advises. Keep the scene in your mind for 15 to 20 minutes. You'll find that you feel a lot more relaxed afterward—and you'll have less discomfort.

Beat it with baking soda. For a handy way to neutralize acid that may be aggravating your ulcer, reach to the back of your fridge for that box of baking soda. Just dissolve a tablespoon in a glass of water and imbibe.

ASPARAGUS

Spear-ited Healing

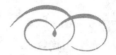

ASPARAGUS IS MY FAVORITE VEGETABLE. MY HUSBAND, Ted, can't stand it, so he eats cauliflower instead. Hooray! That leaves more for me!

...Just the facts

Asparagus (5 spears cooked)
Calories: 18
Fat: 0 g
Saturated fat: 0 g
Cholesterol: 0 mg
Sodium: 8 mg
Total carbohydrates: 3 g
Dietary fiber: 1 g
Protein: 2 g
Folate: 27% of Daily Value
Vitamin A: 8%
Vitamin C: 9%

Fresh asparagus is tops in taste and a good source of vitamin C, part of the nutrition arsenal that keeps your immune system in fighting trim and helps heal wounds, including ulcers. Ten spears provide about 20 percent of the new higher daily recommendation for vitamin C of 75 milligrams for women and 90 milligrams for men.

THE HEART-LOVING VITAMIN

There's more. Asparagus is a great source of folate, the B vitamin now thought to play an important role in preventing heart attacks.

For many years, research focused almost myopically on cholesterol as the culprit in heart disease. That research uncovered only part of the problem, so nutrition detectives had to start looking for other clues.

What they found was that many heart attacks are triggered by high blood levels of the amino acid homocysteine. Coincidentally, they noticed that folks with high homocysteine levels also tended to have low blood levels of folate and folic acid (the synthetic form of the B vitamin). Clinical trials have shown that eating more folate-rich foods and taking folic acid supplements can lower blood levels of homocysteine, and now scientists are trying to prove that lowering homocysteine reduces heart disease risk. Just 1 cup of cooked asparagus provides two-thirds of the Daily Value for folate, which is also critical for preventing certain birth defects.

TENDER TIPS

If you like your asparagus fresh, keep a lookout starting in January, when the first spears are hand cut in California. Midwestern and eastern crops keep fresh asparagus coming through July. When selecting fresh aspara-

Good to Go

When you're ready to use your asparagus, wash it under cool running water and snap off the tough part of each stem. Then simply steam, boil, or grill just until crisp-tender.

Fabulous Fill-In!

When fresh asparagus is out of season, you'll have to settle for frozen spears, which are still a good deal, in both taste and nutrition. In fact, there's nothing you can do with fresh asparagus that you can't do with frozen. Canned asparagus also packs plenty of nutrients, although it's higher in sodium.

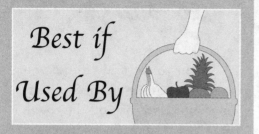

Best if Used By

Here's how to keep asparagus in tiptop condition.

- Wrap the stalks in wet paper towels or stand them in water, then cover with a plastic bag to prevent dehydration. Store them in the fridge.
- Eat your asparagus as soon as possible, because every day you wait wastes some of the folate and vitamin C—and that fresh-from-the-field taste.

gus, size doesn't matter. Just choose spears of similar diameter so they'll cook in the same amount of time. Look for clean, round, mostly green stalks and tightly closed purple tips. Avoid shriveled spears and those with dry, brown, or "sprouting" tips. These are signs of old age and declining quality. Avoid sandy spears; they're hard to clean, and the grit ends up in your teeth, ruining the pleasure of eating an otherwise elegant vegetable.

Here are some yummy ways to use fresh asparagus.

Add tips to stir-fries or pasta. Toss them in right before serving, since just 2 or 3 minutes of cooking time will turn them crisp-tender and add bright green color to the mix.

Grill or broil whole spears. Brush them lightly or mist with olive oil, then place them near the edge of the grill where they won't turn into charcoal, or broil at about 400°F for 4 or 5 minutes. Sprinkle with a few grains of Kosher salt. At a friend's party, I saw guests bypass the hot dogs and burgers and fight over the asparagus. They ate it with their fingers, too!

Boil tough stem ends. When they're tender, puree in a blender, then mix the puree with the cooking water and a little milk to make soup or a healthy "creamed" dish.

Top a salad with cooked tips. This makes a really artistic arrangement. (Remember, you feast with your eyes before you taste with your tongue.)

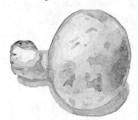

Chill cooked spears. Serve alone as a salad fit for a queen. Dress with sesame oil and rice wine vinegar; sweet, low-fat Catalina; or just a touch of creamy ranch.

Jazz up hot cooked spears. Drizzle with a squeeze of fresh lemon or lime juice instead of salt and butter.

Stuff a pita. Combine broiled or grilled asparagus spears, portobello mushroom strips, and eggplant slices for a very veggie lunch.

FOOD NEWS

You probably know that putting an apple in a brown paper bag with unripe fruits, such as peaches, speeds their ripening. That's because apples give off ethylene gas, the master synchronizer of chemical changes that cause fruits to ripen. Never keep apples near asparagus, though, because ethylene gas turns succulent stalks into tough, stringy spears.

BASIL

Aroma Therapy

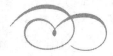

IT'S THE FRAGRANCE OF FRESH BASIL THAT GETS YOU. I grow it in my garden for cooking, yes, but also for the aroma. Lawn mowing suddenly turns from work to wonder when you brush by the basil, and its pungent perfume envelops you. There are only four tastes, you know—sweet, sour, bitter, and salty—but basil, a member of the mint family, has been hailed since ancient times for the way its aromatic compounds turn basic food tastes into gourmet flavors with just a snip of the scissors. Now, this traditional cooking herb is being hailed for its possible health effects as well.

SWEET SMELL OF SUCCESS

Researchers in India have been testing the oil from basil leaves on laboratory ani-

---

...Just the facts

Basil (½ cup fresh)
Calories: 6
Fat: 0 g
Saturated fat: 0 g
Cholesterol: 0 mg
Sodium: 0 mg
Total carbohydrates: 1 g
Dietary fiber: 1 g
Protein: 1 g
Vitamin A: 16% of Daily
    Value
Vitamin C: 4%
Calcium: 3%
Iron: 4%
Manganese: 15%

mals. According to their research, here's what basil can do.

• Dampen the ulcer-producing activity of aspirin and alcohol.

• Fight inflammation and swelling.

• Battle infection-causing bacteria.

It may also:

• Prevent colon cancer. Basil contains eugenol, a compound that increases production of antioxidants, at least in the intestines of lab animals. The antioxidants help get rid of toxic substances that may cause cancer, so there's a hint that basil may be helpful against colon cancer.

• Help build bones by doling out small quantities of the minerals calcium, copper, magnesium, and manganese, all of which seem to be important for a sturdy skeleton.

FOOD NEWS

Basil is easy to grow in your garden, on your deck, or even in a deep flowerpot on your windowsill. All you need is a lot of sun and warmth and a little rain. In fact, basil is perfect for those hot spots that scorch most normal plants.

Sow the seeds when the weather turns warm and let the soil dry out between waterings. After the plants have grown two sets of leaves, pinch off the tops so the plants will branch. Two or three plants will provide more leaves than you can ever use.

EPICUREAN DELIGHTS

If you don't grow your own, you can find fresh basil in most health food stores and many large supermarkets. Look for sturdy green leaves that aren't wilting or turning black.

Once you start using basil, you'll go gourmet often. Here are some ideas to get you started.

Toss spectacular salads. A handful of fresh basil tossed in with

You want your basil fresh and pungent, so here's how to store it.

• Store cut basil in the refrigerator. I especially like to use the Tupperware container with ventilation holes that allow the contents to breathe.

• Store basil bouquets in water either on your countertop or in the fridge. A bouquet—that's basil with the roots still attached—will stay alive for a week or two.

summer greens will have your guests asking, "Mmm, what's that?!"

Freshen up angel hair. For the best-dressed pasta when dining al fresco, stir together chopped fresh, ripe tomatoes; slivered fresh basil; some pressed garlic; and a little olive oil. Serve over hot pasta.

Savor the flavor. If you end up with too much basil (is that possible?), you can pulverize it in the food processor with just enough olive oil to make a smooth paste. Use the paste instead of butter or mayonnaise on sandwiches for a dash of heart-healthy unsaturated fat. Or freeze it in ice trays, then add it to soups, stews, and pasta dishes all year long.

Refill spice jars. Wash the leaves and pat dry, then place a small handful at a time on a paper towel. Microwave on high for about 5 minutes, or until bone-dry and brittle. Crumble the leaves, then store them in an airtight container in a cool, dark place. Add to chicken dishes, pasta sauce, salads, and all Italian fare.

ONIONS

A Slice for Life

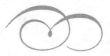

TRUE, KIDS DON'T USUALLY LIKE ONIONS, BUT WHEN I was little, my clever dad renamed them "mangles" and tricked me into eating them. I'm so glad! Now, I willingly add them to almost any savory dish—and that's a good thing. It seems the lowly onion is one of Mother Nature's truly power-packed veggies.

TEARS OF JOY

Onions boast several sulfur-containing compounds that are released when you slice into the bulb and break the cell walls. (Yes, they're real tearjerkers, but more about that later.) These sulfur compounds appear to help fight dangerous blood clotting as well as allergies, bacterial infections such as those associated with ulcers, and inflammation. In fact, if you run cold

...Just the facts

Onion (½ cup chopped)
Calories: 30
Fat: 0 g
Saturated fat: 0 g
Cholesterol: 0 mg
Sodium: 2 mg
Total carbohydrates: 7 g
Dietary fiber: 1 g
Protein: 0 g
Vitamin C: 13% of Daily
    Value
Calcium: 4%
Iron: 2%

water over a little kitchen burn, then apply a slice of onion, the same natural chemicals that usually make you cry also block the substances that make you feel pain. And here's a bonus: Onion juices have antibacterial properties that may help keep the wound from becoming infected.

DRY-EYED WONDER

Onions are also loaded with quercetin, a flavonoid also found in red wine, tea, and apples. The benefit? Quercetin has an antioxidant punch more powerful than vitamin E's for preventing "bad" low-density lipoprotein (LDL) cholesterol from gunking up your arteries.

One study showed that drinking several cups of tea (a big quercetin provider) daily was associated with lower risk of cataracts. Since the amount of quercetin absorbed from onions is double that from tea, eating onions frequently may help protect against cataracts, too. And since quercetin survives heat, you can enjoy your onions cooked or raw.

Other compounds in onions—adenosine and paraffinic polysulfides—keep blood platelets from clumping together and forming the clots that can trigger a heart attack or stroke. So eat your mangles!

ANTICANCER INGREDIENTS

A mound of evidence points to onions' components as important cancer fighters. In one study review, people who consumed the most quercetin had a 50 percent reduction in their risk of stomach and respiratory tract cancers.

Other studies suggest that onions' sulfur compounds put the brakes on colon and renal cancers by causing cancer cells to die. Additional research shows that piling on the onions may reduce the risk of lung, bladder, ovarian, and brain cancers.

BLOOD SUGAR BONUS

In one study, the blood sugar levels of diabetic rats that were fed a diet high in onions were managed as well as those of rats given insulin and other diabetes drugs. And the onion-eating rats got a bonus: They created less cholesterol than the rats on drugs. (Don't try this at home, though. Always check with your doctor before adjusting your medication.)

OH, THOSE ONIONS

There are two kinds of bulb onions. "Fresh" onions are the sweet, mild type that folks love to eat raw and are available in stores from March until August. These onions, which are grown in warmer climates, include Vidalias from Georgia, Walla Wallas from Washington, Mauis from Hawaii, and Super Sweets from Texas.

Fresh onions can be red, white, or yellow. All have thin, light-colored skins and a high water content that makes them tender and easily bruised. Handle them gently and use them quickly.

FOOD NEWS

One study showed that students who were fed a high-fat diet actually had a drop in triglyceride levels (but not in cholesterol) when they added big slices of onion to their burgers. So don't cry—just slice and dice!

The second kind of bulb onion is the "storage" onion. You'll find these from August until April. They are also red, white, or yellow. Storage onions have several layers of papery skin, less water than fresh onions, and a more intense flavor. Nothing is better for cooking. They turn a glorious brown when sautéed (with or without fat), and their pungent components turn to sugar and caramelize to create a unique, sweet, cooked-onion flavor.

Here are some savory ideas for cooking bulb onions.

Break a sweat. Instead of sautéing onions in a glob of fat, try "sweating" them. Here's how: Lightly coat a nonstick skillet with cooking spray. Add sliced storage onions and cook over medium heat, stirring occasionally, until they start to brown. Reduce the heat to low, cover, and cook until the onions sweat out their liquid and "melt down." If they start to stick or burn, add a little water. Serve over grilled chicken or pork tenderloin.

Slice paper thin. Use a serrated knife to shave thin slices of fresh red onions. Garnish your spinach salad with them or stuff them into a veggie pita.

Whack off a slab. Cut thick slices of fresh Vidalias or Walla Wallas for summer sandwiches. Try a thick slice on a grilled portobello mushroom sandwich on multigrain bread with sprouts and cheese.

Make onion soup. Sauté sliced yellow onions in a little olive oil until soft. Add a tablespoon of flour and cook for 5 minutes. Stir in a can of beef broth to create instant onion soup. Top with melba rounds dusted with freshly grated Parmesan cheese. Too cool!

PEACHES

Cling to the Benefits

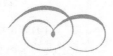

DURING THE DOG DAYS OF SUMMER, NOTHING BEATS THE heat like the taste of a plump, juicy peach. Sliced, diced, or even straight from the tree, peaches are lip-smackin' good— and good for you, too! Don't be fooled by all that great taste, though; peaches have a whole lot more to offer than just their fantastic flavor.

DOUBLE DUTY

For one thing, they're packed with vitamins A and C. Vitamin C heals cuts and wounds, such as ulcers, and helps produce the connective tissue collagen, which holds muscles, bones, and other groups of cells together. It also boosts your immune system, helps form and repair red blood cells, protects you from bruising, and even keeps your gums healthy.

...Just the facts

Peaches (2 medium)
Calories: 70
Fat: 0 g
Saturated fat: 0 g
Cholesterol: 0 mg
Sodium: 0 mg
Total carbohydrates: 19 g
Dietary fiber: 1 g
Protein: 1 g
Vitamin A: 20% of Daily
 Value
Vitamin C: 20%

When you're ready to enjoy your peaches:

- Wash them in cool water and dry with a paper towel.

- To peel peaches for a recipe, gently dip them in boiling water for 30 seconds, remove with a slotted spoon, and immerse in cold water. The skin should come off easily.

- To ditch the pit in freestone peaches (the type most commonly found in supermarkets), carefully use a sharp knife to cut on the seam around the peach, all the way down to the pit. Then twist each half in opposite directions. With clingstone peaches, which have pits that are even harder to remove, it's best to cut sections by slicing down to the pit and removing the desired amount.

Vitamin A helps you see normally in the dark and protects you from infection by keeping your skin and mucous membranes healthy. It also battles bad guys called free radicals that cause cell damage that may eventually lead to cancer and heart disease.

NEW ARRIVAL

That's not all that peaches offer. They're also a good source of glutathione, an antioxidant that may help prevent cancer, although it's still too early to tell for sure. A study published in the British medical journal *Lancet* found that older adults have lower levels of this compound than younger folks do. Consider it just one more reason among dozens to eat your peaches.

If you've come down with sinusitis, pick up a peach. A recent small study found that people with sinusitis are another group that may not be getting enough glutathione.

PEACHY CONFECTIONS

It's easy to pick a peck of perfect peaches! Narrow your search to those with a deep yellow or creamy background and avoid those with a green hue—they probably won't ripen. Then, depending on how quickly you'd like to eat them, choose peaches that are moderately hard (ready to eat in a few days) to slightly soft (ready now).

Now that you're the perfect peach picker, here's how you can prepare them—besides making a pie.

Slice and season. Sprinkle cold peach wedges with cinnamon and just pop them in your mouth for the ultimate low-cal, healthy snack.

Dare to cream. Mix bite-size peach pieces with low-fat whipped cream and a dash of nutmeg for a sinful-tasting—yet slim—dessert.

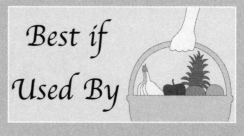

Best if Used By

All that wonderful, juicy flavor deserves to be preserved.
• Keep ripe peaches in the fridge, where they'll maintain their super taste for about a week. That allows plenty of time for you and your family to dig in.
• Place unripe peaches in a paper bag at room temperature for a day or two and transfer to the refrigerator when they're ripe.

Give cereal a wakeup call. Toss mini peach chunks into your ready-to-eat cereal or oatmeal. It'll perk you up—even at 6 A.M.

Sink into a salad. Combine peach wedges with basil and toasted almonds for the ultimate summer salad. Drizzle with your favorite vinaigrette.

Fire up the barbie. Brush peach wedges with vinaigrette and grill them for a few seconds—how long it will take depends on how hot the fire is. Serve them on top of grilled chicken.

Part Four

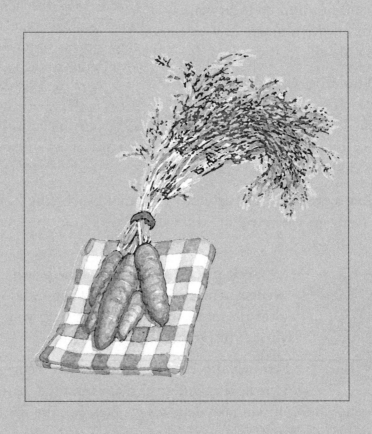

Face the Future
with a Smile

Let's face it, aging is not for sissies. As my friend Sandy once remarked, "After age 40, it's nothing but patch, patch, patch." Life's a lot more fun than that, but it does take a good bit of maintenance to keep an aging body in tiptop condition.

While most folks tend to focus on fending off cancer, heart disease, and diabetes, there are some other concerns that are all in your head. Almost everyone I know struggles with memory. "Is it Alzheimer's or just information overload?" they wonder. And hanging on to your pearly whites is nothing to sneeze at either, because healthy teeth and gums are key to eating well to fend off all those other diseases. Then, of course, there's eyesight, which we want to protect with all our might.

The next few chapters will help you get a head start on taking care of the old noggin and keep you head and shoulders above the crowd.

MEMORY LOSS

Build Total Recall

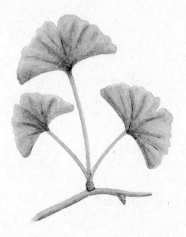

ON A RECENT STOP AT A LOCAL ATM, MY FRIEND Charlie completely forgot the access number he's had for a decade. He was panic-stricken that he might be in the early stages of Alzheimer's—a dreadful disease that his dad developed at an early age.

It's easy to fear the worst when you forget things. In most cases, however, forgetfulness isn't a symptom of disease but merely a by-product of being both distracted and depleted.

CONSIDER THE SOURCE

If you're a woman, you may be both distracted by dueling demands and experiencing a sharp decline in hormones that can occur following childbirth or a hysterectomy or as you near menopause. Estrogen enhances memory in a number of ways, helping nerve cells to grow in complexity and increasing connections between them. That's why when it nosedives, retrieving information may take longer.

Chronic stress also worsens brain fog. It depletes the adrenal glands, which take over the production of estrogen at menopause. If they're producing just a trickle of estrogen, you may have more obvious—and distressing—"senior moments." Worse, ongoing stress actually destroys neurons in the hippocampus, the brain's memory headquarters.

Other factors specific to memory loss in women include low levels of thyroid hormone and the tendency to skip meals. "When your blood sugar drops, thinking and remembering go out the window," says Elisa Lottor, N.D., Ph.D., a naturopathic physician and psychologist in Santa Monica, California.

FOOD NEWS

Cold-water fish, such as salmon and sardines, are the richest sources of docosahexaenoic acid (DHA), a type of omega-3 essential fatty acid that helps to promote cell-to-cell communication, improve focus, and possibly reverse memory loss. Not keen on fish? As long as you're not taking aspirin or blood-thinning medications, check your health food store for fish-oil capsules that contain DHA and take 1 to 3 grams daily.

BOOST YOUR BODACIOUS BRAIN

Some memory problems require a doctor's care. In many cases, however, forgetfulness can be reversed nonmedically by keeping your blood sugar levels stable. One way to do this is by grazing on several small meals featuring complex carbohydrates and protein, such as apple slices smeared with peanut butter. The following memory-enhancing methods will also help.

Arm yourself with antioxidants. Estrogen mops up

Studies have shown that deficiencies of iron and zinc can interfere with your concentration.

Boost your brain power by eating a serving of beans, lean meat, poultry, and fish a few times a week—they're loaded with both minerals.

oxygen damage to brain cells caused by free radical molecules, says Claire Warga, Ph.D., a midlife health psychologist in New York City. When your body's estrogen wanes, she suggests turning to plant estrogens that do double duty as natural antioxidants. "People with high levels of antioxidants tend to score better on memory tests," she says. To improve your memory, feast on antioxidant-rich fruits and veggies, such as oranges, grapefruit, broccoli, and carrots.

Count on choline. As estrogen dwindles, so does acetylcholine, a brain chemical used by memory cells to communicate with each other. To make up for the loss, stock your diet with lots of high-protein foods (such as soy foods, eggs, and lean meat) that contain choline, a component of lecithin used to make acetylcholine. Or opt for 2 tablespoons of lecithin (which you can find at health food stores) sprinkled on your cereal. By midday, you should notice the fog lifting and your recall becoming crystal clear. Still another choice is soy-extracted isoflavone tablets (55 milligrams) taken twice daily, which

9 1 1

If you have difficulty performing the steps of a familiar task, such as serving a meal; are confused about time and place; have forgotten the names of the president or close family members; or your memory lapses are getting worse, ask your doctor for an evaluation. You may need tests to determine your thyroid levels and/or detect circulatory disorders.

research from the University of California, San Diego, has shown to help verbal recall. If you're at risk for breast cancer, however, check with your doctor before supplementing, since isoflavones may have an estrogenic effect on tissues.

Grab the ginkgo. This herb helps to clear the cobwebs because it shunts more blood to the brain. As long as you're not taking other medications, take 120 to 240 milligrams a day of a standardized product. Better yet, check your health food store for ginkgo in formulas that include huperzine A, an herbal extract of Chinese moss that appears to help maintain healthy levels of neurotransmitters, the brain chemicals that help memory cells communicate with each other.

Shop for PS. Phosphatidylserine (PS) is a fatty substance made from soybean oil that researchers at the Memory Assessment Clinics in Bethesda, Maryland, believe may resemble the nutrient in the brain that helps sharpen focus and enhance recall. "The only known side effect is a positive one—improved mood—and PS seems to work especially well when combined with ginkgo," says Dr. Lottor. Check your health food store for both. The suggested dose of PS is 100 milligrams three times daily, and you'll need to give it several weeks to work, she adds.

Dance or play tennis. While any physical exercise

According to early animal studies at Tufts University in Boston, eating ½ cup of antioxidant-rich blueberries a day may help sharpen memory. Is your market fresh out of blueberries? Go for strawberries and spinach, both of which have nearly the same memory-restoring effects.

Folks over 50 need a multivitamin that serves up a full day's supply of three critical brain-boosting nutrients that are absorbed better from supplements than from food. They are vitamin B$_{12}$ (2.4 micrograms), folic acid (400 micrograms), and vitamin D (400 IU), according to the National Academy of Sciences, which sets the Recommended Dietary Allowances.

enhances blood circulation and therefore memory, studies show that activities such as tennis that require moving in sync with a partner and responding to each other's movements are the best way to keep your brain on its toes. Regular dancing, in fact, lowered the risk of Alzheimer's among older people by a whopping 76 percent in one study.

Chew gum. Chomp some Doublemint, and you'll ace that real estate exam! British researchers have found that chewing gum improves memory, possibly because it raises the heart rate, which in turn boosts the delivery of glucose and oxygen to the brain and creates a surge in insulin, which may be key to recall.

Treat your feet. Tense, distracted…and can't remember where you parked the car? Take several deep breaths, then get yourself a foot massage, suggests Vasant Lad, M.A.Sc., director of the Ayurvedic Institute in Albuquerque. The soles of your feet correspond to the area of the brain that activates memory, he explains. In fact, using a type of massage oil called brahmi (commonly known as gotu kola) is recommended if "you freeze up and can't recall things," Dr. Lad adds.

BLUEBERRIES

A Jog Down Memory Lane

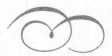

RESEARCHERS AT TUFTS UNIVERSITY IN BOSTON HAVE uncovered the first hint that blueberries may help reverse short-term memory loss. They divided older rats into four groups. One group received their usual diet, while the others got supplements of either blueberry, strawberry, or spinach extract. By far, the blueberry group out-performed all the others on memory tests. What's this all about?

Your brain sucks up a ton of oxygen while tending to its daily chores. Just rest-ing, it takes about 20 percent of your body's total supply, and thinking can hog 40 to 50 percent of all the oxygen your heart and lungs can pump out. Processing oxygen is necessary for life, but it comes with a high price tag. It produces free rad-ical garbage that can clutter up your brain or damage its delicate structures. Add that

...Just the facts

Blueberries (1 cup fresh)
Calories: 81
Fat: 0 g
Saturated fat: 0 g
Cholesterol: 0 mg
Sodium: 9 mg
Total carbohydrates: 21 g
Dietary fiber: 4 g
Protein: 1 g
Vitamin C: 30% of Daily
  Value

Blueberries are bursting with tannins, compounds that boot out the bacteria responsible for urinary tract infections. Researchers at Rutgers University in Chatsworth, New Jersey, found that these tannins prevent the germs from attaching to the wall of your bladder, where they thrive. How many blueberries should you eat? Researchers aren't sure—but if you have frequent urinary tract infections, you may want to think about tossing a handful in your mouth whenever you're in the kitchen!

to chronic diseases that can pile up, magnifying each other's effects, and down you go into the swirling vortex of memory loss. So it's blueberries to the rescue.

THE SMART BERRY

In another study at Tufts, blueberries outranked more than 50 other fruits and vegetables in amount of antioxidants—compounds that protect you against memory loss, cancer, heart disease, and even wrinkles. It turns out that the health-promoting bounty comes from the very pigment, called anthocyanin, that gives these berries such a cool color. This pigment gobbles up the free radicals that cause cell damage in your brain and body.

"If you'd eat just ½ cup of blueberries daily, you'd double the antioxidants you get for the entire day," says study leader Ronald Prior, Ph.D., who admits that he hardly ever ate blueberries until he conducted this research. Now he has a ½-pint-a-day habit.

Scientists are now working to isolate the memory-boosting compounds in blueberries and test them on humans. In the meantime, eat blueberries so you'll remember . . . to eat blueberries!

GO WILD WITH BLUEBERRIES

Ounce for ounce, wild blueberries pack double the antioxidants of their plumper cultivated cousins, so if you spot them at the supermarket, snatch them up. Wyman's, the largest wild-blueberry marketer, sells them fresh, frozen, and canned.

If the only blueberries you can locate are the cultivated kind, don't pass them by. You've still found a blue-ribbon winner! Look for berries that are dry, firm, and uniformly colored.

You've bought the best. Now put your blueberries to the test in the kitchen with these tasty treats.

Color your salads healthy. Leave the iceberg lettuce at the supermarket, because it offers very few nutrients. (Think of it as crunchy water!) Instead, buy dark greens, such as spinach or romaine lettuce, then top them with fresh blueberries, feta cheese, and low-fat balsamic vinaigrette.

Paint your desserts, too. Instead of topping your frozen yogurt with sprinkles, try blueberries, or frost a cake and then coat it with blueberries. For a dessert that's super-easy, just fill a dish with blueberries and top them with a dollop of whipped cream.

Brighten your mornings. Add fresh blueberries to cold cereal or stir frozen blueberries into oatmeal.

Best if Used By

Here's what to do when you get your blueberries home.

• Store them in the refrigerator, where they'll last for at least a week—if you don't devour them immediately.

• If you've picked a boatload at a local farm, place them in a single layer on a baking sheet or tray and freeze them for a few hours. When you're sure they're frozen, transfer them to airtight containers and store them in the freezer until you need them. They'll keep for at least a year.

BROCCOLI

The Green for Your Gray Matter

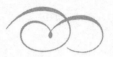

RESEARCH ON THE WAY FOOD AFFECTS YOUR BRAIN IS SO new that no one knows for sure all the ways food protects your gray matter, but some amazing trends are emerging. The most surprising is that just about anything that's good for your heart is good for your brain. Take lowering your cholesterol. If your arteries are clogged with sludge, the blood carrying needed oxygen has trouble flowing to your brain, so you can't think as well, and that's a setup for memory loss, says Jim Joseph, Ph.D., chief of the neuroscience laboratory at Tufts University in Boston.

Researchers recently found that women who ate broccoli just once a week had half the risk of heart disease compared with those who didn't pile any on their plates. The connection isn't clear yet, but

---

...Just the facts

Broccoli (1 medium stalk)
Calories: 45
Fat: less than 1 g
Saturated fat: 0 g
Cholesterol: 0 mg
Sodium: 55 mg
Total carbohydrates: 8 g
Dietary fiber: 5 g
Protein: 5 g
Vitamin A: 15% of Daily
    Value
Vitamin C: 220%
Calcium: 6%
Iron: 6%

---

broccoli ranks high on the list of fruits and veggies loaded with the most antioxidants, known to fight memory loss.

THE MEGA-VEGGIE

Good to Go

Right before you're ready to eat or cook your broccoli, wash it in cold water. Soak it for a few minutes if you have trouble removing all the dirt.

Like the Brady Bunch, broccoli comprises at least six do-gooders: vitamin A, vitamin C, vitamin K, fiber, and the plant compounds lutein and sulforaphane. Scientists believe that many of these elements work together to provide its health benefits, including its chief perk, preventing cancer. Specifically, here's what broccoli can do.

• *Protect your prostate.* A study at the Fred Hutchinson Cancer Research Center in Seattle found that eating three servings of vegetables daily can lower the risk of prostate cancer by an amazing 45 percent! "If some of those vegetables are the cruciferous kind like broccoli, men could drop their risk even further," says study coauthor Alan Kristal, Dr.P.H.

• *Shield your bladder.* Another investigation, which looked at 50,000 men, determined that those who ate a ½-cup serving of broccoli just twice a week reduced their chance of developing bladder cancer—the fourth leading cancer—by half.

• *Guard your colon.* Research at the University of Utah Medical School in Salt Lake City suggests that broccoli may cut the risk of colon cancer.

Beyond the cancer front, studies have shown that broccoli may be just what the doctor ordered for these health problems.

• *Hip fractures.* The vitamin K in broccoli may help lower the chance of fracturing a hip when you get older, according to a study at Tufts.

• *Cataracts.* In a Harvard study of more than 36,000 men, scientists discovered that eating foods high in lutein—specifically, broccoli and spinach—may reduce the risk of developing cataracts.

Now, you could load up on broccoli every day to ensure that you receive all its benefits, but you probably don't have to. Researchers do say, however, that you should try to eat at least a ½-cup serving of cruciferous veggies daily. These include not only broccoli but also bok choy, brussels sprouts, cabbage, cauliflower, and kale.

SHADES OF GREEN

In the market for some fresh broccoli? Choose carefully! Look for uniformly dark green or purplish blue-green florets. They're richer in vitamins A and C than paler florets. Check out the color of the stalks and stems, too. They should be green and rich looking. Avoid broccoli with yellowing florets, because it's past its prime and won't taste good no matter how you prepare it.

No time to clean broccoli? Look for packaged washed florets, such as Mann's Broccoli Wokly (cute, huh?), in the produce sec-

Best if Used By

Once you buy broccoli, baby it.
• Store it in a plastic bag in the crisper of your fridge to protect its vitamins.
• Ideally, you should use it within a day or two. It'll keep for no longer than four to five days.
• Don't wash broccoli before storing it, because that will speed the growth of mold.

tion next to bagged salad mixes.

Once you've chosen your broccoli, use it to whip up these tempting dishes.

Surprise your pasta. Stir broccoli into tomato sauce or toss pasta with garlic, olive oil, broccoli, and a few tablespoons of the hot water you used to cook the pasta.

Say cheese. Most prepackaged broccoli with cheese sauce is loaded with saturated fat. I like to make my own, mixing steamed broccoli with warmed D. L. Jardine's Queso Loco Cheese Salsa. Log on to jardinesfoods.com to find out where to buy the salsa. You can also stir cooked broccoli into low-fat mac and cheese, such as Lean Cuisine.

Go for a slam dunk. Snack on raw broccoli florets with low fat ranch dressing, honey mustard, or Catalina dip.

Toss a salad. Every once in a while, lose the lettuce and instead combine broccoli and orange slices in a light citrus vinaigrette.

EGGS

Memory Jump-Starters

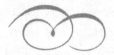

WANT A BABY WITH A GREAT MEMORY THAT LASTS FOR-
ever? Be a good mom while you're pregnant and nursing, and
eat some eggs. Their yolks are the top
source of choline, a recently recognized
essential nutrient for brain development.

Here's what we know: Rats whose
moms chowed down on choline during
pregnancy and lactation learn mazes faster
and with fewer mistakes. Getting choline
early, while its brain is developing, permanently changes and enlarges a rat's hippocampus, where memory resides. Even in
old age, rats raised on choline have better
memories.

FOOD FOR THE AGES

So, do human brains work the same
way? We don't know yet, but changes in

...Just the facts

Egg (1 medium)
Calories: 68
Fat: 5 g
Saturated fat: 1 g
Cholesterol: 186 mg
Sodium: 55 mg
Total carbohydrates: 0 g
Dietary fiber: 0 g
Protein: 6 g
Vitamin A: 9% of Daily Value
Vitamin B$_{12}$: 13%
Vitamin D: 11%
Calcium: 2%
Iron: 3%

---

blood levels of choline in human and rat moms during pregnancy and breastfeeding are similar, suggesting that it's possible, so studies are under way. Meanwhile, get cracking. A two-egg meal doubles blood choline levels. Milk is another good source.

Here are some other folks who thrive on eggs.

• Athletes in heavy training should shake a leg and hard-boil some eggs, too. Recent research has shown that blood choline can drop by 40 percent after heavy exercise. Also, choline supplements boosted performance in marathon runners and helped maintain blood choline levels in triathletes.

Why not just take a supplement? "It takes several grams of choline supplements to cross the blood-brain barrier, and that much makes you smell like fish!" says Jim Joseph, Ph.D., chief of the neuroscience laboratory at Tufts University in Boston. So break an egg, and you'll get other benefits, too, such as high-quality protein.

• Older adults need more protein, B vitamins, vitamin D, calcium, and zinc than younger people do, yet many don't even meet the Daily Values,

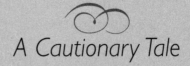

A Cautionary Tale

In recent years, the risk of salmonella poisoning from eating raw eggs has risen dramatically. Although most healthy people can withstand the onslaught, some risk death by dehydration from prolonged diarrhea. Fortunately, thorough cooking makes eggs perfectly safe.

If you're in one of the following high-risk groups, avoid eggs with runny yolks, raw cookie dough, real Caesar salad (which is made with raw eggs), and traditional eggnog.
  • Pregnant women
  • Young children
  • The elderly
  • People whose immune systems are compromised by chemotherapy or HIV infection.

much less get bonus amounts. What's more, they probably need more choline for memory, says the Institute of Medicine in Washington, D.C.

Why are they falling short? Older people require fewer calories, which means every bite has to be jam-packed with nutrients—so it's eggs to the rescue! They come in single-serving packages (no leftovers!) stuffed with easy-to-digest protein for maintaining muscle and building immunity against pneumonia and flu.

THE YOLK'S ON US

Years ago, Woody Allen made one of his funniest movies, called *Sleeper*, in which he awoke from a coma to find that everything that was "bad for you" when he fell asleep was now "good for you." Well, things aren't quite that bad in the nutrition world, but sometimes it seems as if it is, especially when we start to talk about eggs.

The yolks (the part that you've been throwing away!) are loaded with these important nutrients.

• *B vitamins.* These vitamins boost germ-fighting immunity, maintain memory, and prevent heart attack and stroke.

• *Vitamin D.* It builds bone and boosts memory and clear thinking.

• *Lutein and zeaxanthin.* These two carotenoids are critical for preventing age-related macular

Best if Used By

Once you've chosen the perfect eggs, store them right.
• Stash them deep in the fridge (not in the door!), where they'll stay plenty cold and be good for about two weeks.
• If you hard-boil a batch of eggs, cool them under running water and then put them right back in the fridge. Use them within a week.

degeneration, the major cause of blindness in adults. These sight-saving nutrients are absorbed more easily from eggs than from green vegetables.

UNSCRAMBLED SCIENCE

Thirty years ago, when the drive to defeat heart disease went into high gear, we were told to limit cholesterol intake to 300 milligrams a day. Since an egg yolk packs 186 milligrams, it might have seemed reasonable to just ditch eggs, but even the American Heart Association said that folks on a cholesterol-lowering diet may eat two or three eggs (with yolks) a week.

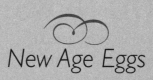

New Age Eggs

In defense of nutritionists, I'd like to say that no one ever advised the nation to stop eating eggs entirely. Cut down? Yes. Change their accompaniments? Definitely! Forget fried eggs with bacon and sausage and white toast slathered with butter. All that saturated fat could send your cholesterol soaring. But if you boil or poach your egg, for example, serve it with whole wheat toast spread with peanut butter, and wash it down with a glass of orange juice, your heart will jump for joy!

After years of research, we've learned that it's not the cholesterol in foods but the saturated fat oozing from bacon, burgers, and ice cream that raises our blood cholesterol. In fact, most people (except for those with diabetes or very high cholesterol) can eat an egg a day with no problem.

Egg studies abound, but you may find two of particular interest. One followed 38,000 men for 8 years, and the other tracked 80,000 women for 14 years. Both studies found that—except for people with diabetes—those who ate an egg a day were no more likely to have heart attacks or strokes than those who ate less than one a week. So don't be hard-boiled—enjoy an egg now and then!

FOOD NEWS

If you've been avoiding eggs, you may have missed these new arrivals.

• *Eggland's Best.* These patented eggs come from chickens fed a vegetarian diet, canola oil, and extra vitamin E. As a result, two eggs deliver 50 percent of the Daily Value for vitamin E (important for heart health and immune function), about six times more than standard eggs.

• *EggsPlus.* The chickens producing these eggs are fed vitamin E and flaxseed, pushing vitamin E content for two eggs to 50 percent of the Daily Value and providing 200 milligrams of omega-3 essential fatty acids (the kind you usually get only from fatty fish). Omega-3's have been shown to reduce the risk of heart disease and stroke.

EGGS-ACTLY RIGHT

Eggs are available in sizes from small to jumbo. Medium eggs, however, are the size called for in most recipes, and they are the most economical. To prevent salmonella poisoning, buy only eggs that have been kept cold in the dairy case. Check each egg in the carton, and don't buy any that are cracked or dirty.

You probably know just what to do with an egg, but here are a few more suggestions.

Make a meal in a bowl. Peel and slice a hard-boiled egg to add protein to your salad. Add some low-fat cheese and croutons made from whole grain bread.

Eye-light spinach. Chop a hard-boiled egg, then scatter the pieces on cooked spinach for eye appeal and lutein-rich eye protection.

Crown a waffle. Toast a whole grain waffle and top it with a poached egg.

Make veggie egg salad. To your chopped hard-boiled egg and mayo, add sliced radishes, cubed cucumber, and shredded carrots. Pile everything on a whole grain roll along with a dark green lettuce leaf.

RED WINE

Mind-Body Elixir

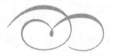

HEALTH ORGANIZATIONS ARE ALWAYS RELUCTANT TO ENcourage people to drink alcohol, because it opens the door to so many other problems. The more research they do, though, the more it becomes clear that, for adults who aren't pregnant or coping with alcoholism, enjoying moderate amounts of alcohol with meals adds to the joy and length of life. It also improves your mind, fends off diabetes, builds bone, and protects your heart.

...Just the facts

Red wine (5 fl oz)
Calories: 106
Fat: 0 g
Saturated fat: 0 g
Cholesterol: 0 mg
Sodium: 0 mg
Total carbohydrates: 3 g
Protein: Less than 1 g
Vitamin B$_6$: 3% of Daily
   Value
Iron: 4%
Magnesium: 5%
Potassium: 4%

GIFT OF THE GODS

Research has found many benefits from moderate indulgence.

• One study of Japanese-American men living in Hawaii, for instance, showed that those who had about one drink a day

Good to Go

Drink your wine with meals. Food slows alcohol absorption, and wine may have greater benefits when it interacts with food. It also enhances the flavor of food, which is the very best reason to enjoy it.

while in their forties and fifties ended up 26 years later performing better on tests of thinking and reasoning than either those who didn't drink at all or those who drank more heavily.

• Two other studies, one of male doctors in the United States and the other of female nurses, showed that compared with people who never drank, moderate drinking (four to seven drinks per week) reduced their risk of developing type 2 diabetes.

• A study of women over age 65 showed that those who drank moderately had greater bone density than those who didn't drink. Scientists think that the benefit accrues because alcohol affects parathyroid hormone levels in a way that decreases bone loss.

THE HEART OF THE MATTER

A while back, researchers wondered how it could be that Americans who stuff down burgers, ribs, and fries keel over from heart disease, while the French get just as much fat dining on foie gras, creamy sauces, and pastry, but their hearts never skip a beat.

Could it be? *Mais oui!* The French, like the long-lived Italians and Spaniards, often drink wine in the normal course of dining. Scientists already knew that wine was a natural antioxidant, so the research was on.

It's also known that any kind of alcohol can have its benefits, but wine seems to be special. Take a look at this: The people of Belgium and Czechoslovakia drink as much alcohol as the French do, but they drink it in the form of beer—and they have more heart disease.

In searching for the heart answer, scientists stumbled onto resveratrol and quercetin, the two compounds in wine that seem to work along with the alcohol to create a kind of synergy that prevents "bad" low-density lipoprotein (LDL) from turning into sludge on your artery walls and setting you up for a heart attack.

What's more, resveratrol appears to be a potent cancer fighter. It can block an enzyme that cancer cells need in order to grow, and it appears able to detoxify mutagens—invaders that coax healthy cells to change into cancerous ones.

PERMISSION TO BE WILDLY MODERATE

Now here's the bad news: Red wine's benefits arrive through a very small window of opportunity. Study after study has shown that moderate drinking (one drink a day for women, two drinks a day for men) is all it takes to get the goods. More is not better.

In fact, it's much worse. Drinking more than one or two glasses of wine—or any other form of alcohol—a day actually increases the risk of some cancers as well as high blood pres-

FOOD NEWS

Several years ago, a friend of mine started making his own wine, and from time to time, he would give me a peek at the process. In his basement winery, I learned that the difference between red and white wines is how long the crushed grapes are allowed to "sit on the skins." White wine is removed quickly, while red wine is allowed to linger so it can pick up the red color.

Now, scientists have discovered that along with the color, red wine also soaks up resveratrol, a natural compound that protects the grapes from fungi. It turns out that resveratrol also appears to protect the human heart from cholesterol and other vital organs from cancer.

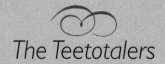

The Teetotalers

The 2000 Dietary Guidelines for Americans acknowledge that moderate alcohol intake may be beneficial for your heart, but they quickly point out that if you don't want to drink, you can get similar benefits by eating a healthy diet, controlling your weight, exercising regularly, and not smoking. The guidelines also point out that certain people should not drink at all.

- Children and teenagers.
- Pregnant women and those who could become pregnant.
- Problem drinkers, alcoholics, recovering alcoholics, and relatives of alcoholics.
- Anyone who plans to drive, operate machinery, or participate in any activity that requires attention, skill, or coordination. (Remnants of a single drink can remain in your blood for 2 to 3 hours.)
- Anyone taking prescription or over-the-counter drugs that can interact with alcohol. (Check with your pharmacist or health care provider.)

sure, stroke, birth defects, alcoholism, violence, suicide, and automobile accidents. There is also a high level of concern about the fact that older adults are increasingly at risk for late-onset alcoholism. Get the message straight: The benefits of red wine are not a green light for overindulgence.

RED RULES

Remember the old rule about red wine with red meat, white wine with chicken and fish? Well, what do you serve with minestrone, crusty bread, and a salad? The "rules" for choosing wine are way too complicated to include in this book, so we'll keep it simple.

Some experts suggest that wines containing the most tannins (the chemicals that make wine "dry") also contain the most healthy ingredients, so enjoy the big reds: cabernet, merlot, and port.

GET IN THE SPIRIT

Make your wine a spritzer. Mix it with seltzer water for a sparkling, light, refreshing drink. Or cook with it. Poach your salmon in red wine. By the time you finish simmering the salmon, it'll be rich with the wine's flavor and packed with its antioxidants.

A SIMPLE SOLUTION

Cut yourself? If you've packed a loaf of bread and a jug of wine for your picnic, pour some wine into the cut. Its polyphenols kill bacteria and prevent infection.

SPINACH

A Green Light for Mind and Sight

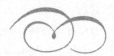

...Just the facts

Spinach (1 cup frozen, cooked)
Calories: 53
Fat: 0 g
Saturated fat: 0 g
Cholesterol: 0 mg
Sodium: 163 mg
Total carbohydrates: 10 g
Dietary fiber: 6 g
Protein: 6 g
Folate: 51% of Daily Value
Vitamin A: 296%
Vitamin C: 26%
Copper: 13%
Magnesium: 16%
Manganese: 89%

REMEMBER THOSE BLUEBERRIES THAT were so good for boosting memory in old rats? Well, a diet high in spinach works just as well for memory. Spinach, like blueberries and other intensely colored vegetables, is packed with antioxidants that neutralize cell damage and help clear the way for more focused thinking and better memory in rats—and probably in humans, too. What's more, spinach improves motor learning, which is necessary for stroke recovery.

In nutritional analysis, spinach looks as though it's loaded with calcium and iron—and it is. Unfortunately, it's also full of oxalates that bind those minerals so your body can't absorb them. That's okay, though, because spinach comes fully loaded with plenty of other nutrients to recommend it. True, carrots pack a little more beta-carotene, and yes, kale serves up more lutein and zeaxanthin. Surely, oranges deliver a tad more vitamin C. But only spinach supplies big doses of all four.

VISIONARY VEGGIE

Nothing beats spinach for fending off three major eye problems: age-related macular degeneration (AMD), cataracts, and night blindness.

• AMD is a sight stealer—and the number one cause of incurable blindness in folks over 65. The reason? The macula of the eye, a tiny spot on the retina, begins to fail, and along with it goes central vision, the kind you need for reading and for seeing straight ahead.

Until recently, no treatment seemed to work. Now, though, there's the great green hope—spinach. The macula, it turns out, is packed with two sight-protecting carotenoids, lutein and zeaxanthin. So is spinach.

In a small pilot study of 14 men with AMD who ate ½ cup of cooked spinach four to seven times a week, 13 had improvements in night vision, con-

Fabulous Fill-In!

Feel free to use convenient frozen spinach whenever the mood strikes. A food chemistry researcher found that after one year, frozen spinach retained two times more vitamin C than fresh spinach that had spent just seven days in refrigeration. And what about canned spinach? Cup for cup, it's equal to or better than frozen for amounts of almost every vitamin and mineral. What could be easier?

trast, and adjustment to bright light. Seven of 8 with distorted vision had improvement or complete remission of symptoms.

While nobody's quite sure how it all works, researchers think that lutein protects the macula by absorbing harmful blue light and defending against any light that does penetrate the macula. Other high-lutein greens include kale, collards, and turnip greens.

• On the cataract scene, a Harvard study of 36,000 male health professionals found that those who ate the most foods high in lutein and zeaxanthin had a 19 percent lower risk of cataracts that were severe enough to require surgical removal. The men's top vegetable picks: spinach and broccoli.

• In a parallel study of 50,000 female nurses, those who most frequently ate foods high in lutein and zeaxanthin had a 22 percent decreased risk of severe cataracts. Their top veggie picks were spinach and kale. Is there an echo in here?

A MULTITASKING VEGGIE

Now that women can remember to eat their spinach, they'll reap some other benefits, too.

• Researchers at the University of Minnesota found that women who ate the greatest amount of green leafy vegetables had the lowest risk of developing ovarian cancer. Wondering why? In

Good to Go

When you're ready to eat your spinach, start this way:

• No matter what the bag says about the spinach being prewashed, rinse, rinse, rinse it until the water is free of superfine sand. The curlier the spinach, the harder it is to get the sand out.

• Remove the heavy stems, including the midribs running up the backs of the leaves, so the leaves will be tender and delicious raw or will cook quickly and evenly.

German studies, spinach turned out to be one of the top veggies tested for their ability to prevent cells from turning cancerous.

• On the quality-of-life front, Italian researchers found that the women who ate less meat and more green vegetables were least likely to have painful benign uterine fibroids.

START SMART

Fresh spinach is available all year long and comes in three styles. You'll find dark green, curly Savoy both loose and in 10-ounce bags. Flat, smooth-leaf spinach, which is the kind used for frozen and canned spinach, is now showing up in fresh bunches in health food stores. There's also a semi-Savoy, which is halfway between curly and flat.

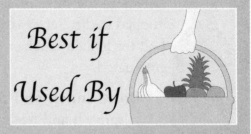

Best if Used By

Here's how to keep those lovely leaves crisp and tasty.

• If you buy spinach in a bag, just toss it in the vegetable crisper in your fridge until you're ready to use it.

• Don't wash spinach until you're ready to use it. Wet spinach disintegrates faster than dry spinach, which should hold up well for three or four days in the fridge.

When selecting fresh spinach, look for dark green, crisp spinach with no yellow spots and medium-size leaves with thin stems. Avoid spinach that looks limp or pale.

Now you're ready to make spinach the highlight of your day. Try these ideas.

Crank up soups. Add leftover cooked or fresh spinach to any canned or homemade soup for a giant-size burst of nutrition.

Follow Popeye's lead. Popeye loves spinach, and he loves Olive Oyl. So will you. Simply sauté fresh spinach leaves in a little olive oil and some finely chopped garlic. Serve as a side dish or as a bed for grilled chicken or fish. You'll be infatuated.

Boost lunch and dinner. Stuff fresh spinach and feta cheese into whole wheat pita pockets for a dazzling and delicious lunch. Use cooked spinach as stuffing for rolled chicken breasts or appetizer pinwheels.

Indulge yourself. Buy a bag of baby spinach. It's the hot new version that requires no stemming, so you just rinse and eat. Also keep an eye out for the microwavable cellophane bag. Just slit the bag so steam can escape, then toss the whole thing into the microwave. No dishes required!

GUM PAIN

Clean Up Your Act

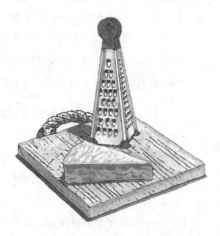

My friend Rick says there's one aspect of dentist visits that always gives him the willies. It's the poster that shows, in full color, the horrible progression of gum disease. The first pictures show nice, healthy gums, and the last ones illustrate what happens when you don't take care of them—they look like something from *Night of the Living Dead*.

SNEAK ATTACK

Unfortunately, gum disease can sneak up on you. The stuff that causes it, a toxin-filled, sticky film called plaque, is nearly invisible.

Good to Go

Toothpaste with baking soda and peroxide kills the germs that cause gum disease and keeps plaque from forming. It's a double whammy that prevents gum problems in the first place, so use it early and often.

387

Good overall nutrition keeps your gums healthy, but there are a few nutrients that help even more.

• *Vitamin C.* This all-purpose nutrient is essential for gum health, so making sure you get enough will help keep your gums in good shape, especially when they're recovering from gingivitis. Have some oranges or a few servings of pineapple, grapefruit, or other fruits and vegetables that are rich in vitamin C.

• *Folate.* One of the B vitamins, folate helps repair and replenish gum cells that have been damaged by gingivitis. The best way to get enough is to take a daily multivitamin that supplies 400 micrograms of folic acid (the synthetic version of folate). You can also get plenty by eating lots of plant foods, along with folate-fortified breakfast cereals.

It's produced by bacteria in your mouth, and every day, it clings to the surfaces of your teeth and underneath your gums. If you don't keep plaque under control with daily brushing and flossing, it proliferates like mold gone mad in a science experiment. Over time, chemicals and bacteria in plaque irritate your gums. If it's not stopped, your gums become red and swollen. They shrink and pull away from your teeth, and eventually, they can get so weak that your teeth loosen or fall out.

There's some good news and some bad news about gum pain. The bad news first: Once you have pain, you probably already have gum disease. If your gums bleed easily and are red and swollen, you're probably in the early stage, called gingivitis.

BUILD YOUR DEFENSES

Now, here's the good news. Gum pain caused by gingivitis is entirely reversible. All you have to do is be more diligent about flossing and brushing. Severe gum disease always requires a dentist's care, but there is no reason at all to let things go that far. If you follow these tips, you'll keep your gums in the pink—and totally free of pain.

Brush up your technique. Regular brushing is the best way to reverse—and prevent—gum pain. But don't make the mistake of using too much elbow grease. You're not trying to sandblast the sides of a building, just break up the thin layers of plaque that may have formed. To be sure you get it all, move the brush in little circles rather than up and down, says Emily A. Kane, N.D., a naturopathic physician in Juneau, Alaska. If you've only recently started having problems, a week or two of gentle brushing is often enough to erase the pain.

Go for a trade-in. Don't forget to change your toothbrush a few times a year. Old brushes are often full of bacteria, which means you could actually be causing more problems. You can also clean your brush periodically. "From time to time, I soak my toothbrush in hydrogen peroxide overnight to kill bacteria," says Dr. Kane.

Chill the pain. One of the most effective treatments for aching gums is also one of the easiest: Just wrap some ice in a washcloth or small towel and place it against the outside of your mouth for about 20 minutes. Cold acts as a local anesthetic, quickly numbing the pain.

Swirl with salt. Here's a nearly instant way to take away gum pain: Mix ½ teaspoon of salt in a cup of warm water. Take a mouthful of the solution, swirl it around in your mouth, then spit it out. The soreness will disappear like magic, and it probably won't come back for at least an hour or two.

You can repeat the saltwater rinse as often as necessary to get relief.

Pop a pill. Aspirin, ibuprofen, and other over-the-counter pain relievers work very quickly when you need relief from gum pain. Unless you're sensitive to these drugs, take one every 4 hours or as directed on the label.

Press on. Pressing the acupressure point for headaches, the web of skin between your index finger and thumb, is often effective for gum pain. Give the area a firm squeeze, hold it for a moment, then release. Do this several times in a row to see if it helps.

Rub away the pain. Massage is good for all sorts of aches and pains, including gum pain. It also speeds healing because it increases circulation and promotes better blood flow. Using the tip of your finger, rub your gum firmly where it hurts, then massage all the way around your upper and lower gums. If you do this every day, your gums will feel better—and they'll heal more quickly, too!

A SIMPLE SOLUTION

Clove oil is a natural painkiller that works well for just about any kind of oral pain. Dip a cotton swab in the oil, which you can find at a health food store, and dab a little on the sore areas of your gums. Don't have clove oil? Open the spice rack, take out a whole clove, and tuck it between your teeth and gums. It's not as effective as the concentrated oil, but it will turn the throbbing down a notch.

Bark up the right tree. Two herbal tinctures, prickly ash bark and Jamaican dogwood, are traditional favorites for reducing gum pain. Pick up a tincture of either at a health food store, then moisten a cotton ball or swab and apply it where it hurts two or three times a day.

Try tea and see. A swish of chamomile tea will bring soothing relief to sore gums. Steep a tea bag in hot water for 10 to 20 minutes, then let the tea cool. Take a mouthful, swirl it around for about 30 seconds, and swallow it or spit it out. Continue the process until you've used all the tea. Avoid using chamomile if you are allergic to ragweed.

FOOD NEWS

Cinnamic aldehyde, an essential plant oil used to flavor chewing gums such as Wrigley's Big Red, does more than cover up breath odor, according to research from the University of Illinois at Chicago. It's also a natural antibacterial agent that crushes the bacteria responsible for bad breath, cavities, and gum infections.

CANTALOUPE

The Now-and-Later Healer

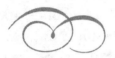

RIPE, JUICY CANTALOUPES ARE JUST WHAT THE DOCTOR ordered if you have gum pain, both immediately and in the long run. Right now, your tender gums will really appreciate the soft, tender texture of this exquisitely delicious fruit. Later, the nutritional wonders of cantaloupe will help heal those tender tissues and brighten your smile again.

...Just the facts

Cantaloupe (¼ melon; about 1 cup cubed)
Calories: 48
Fat: 0 g
Saturated fat: 0 g
Cholesterol: 0 mg
Sodium: 12 mg
Total carbohydrates: 12 g
Dietary fiber: 1 g
Protein: 1 g
Vitamin A: 90% of Daily Value
Vitamin C: 65%

BETA YOUR SMILE ON IT

Cantaloupe is so much more than just good eating. It's also one of the best natural sources of beta-carotene, whose main function is to act as the raw material from which your body creates vitamin A. And one of vitamin A's top jobs is to take care of your body's surfaces, inside and out, which are lined with epithelial cells that protect your body against germ warfare.

Outside, vitamin A makes epithelial cells tough, to create skin. Inside, it makes them tender, to create the mucous membranes that line the nose, mouth, lungs, stomach, intestines, bladder, urethra, uterus, and vagina, forming a barrier against invading germs. Vitamin A also creates the mucus itself. This sticky fluid is essential because it prevents your stomach lining from being digested along with your food, and in your lungs, it traps debris and hauls it out of your airways before it can hurt your body.

Vitamin A is also vital for maintaining vision, forming bones, and building healthy babies. Plus, researchers suspect that it beefs up sensors that notice cancer cells and warn your immune system to take action.

Best if Used By

Get the best from your cantaloupe by following these tips.

• If it's still too firm, leave it on your kitchen counter for a few days, until it begins to soften and its greenish color turns golden.

• Refrigerate a whole ripe melon until you're ready to use it, up to a week.

• Once you cut the melon, use it within four or five days.

CAN'T-FAIL CANTALOUPE

Cantaloupe connoisseurs know just how to find the sweetest, juiciest melons, and you can easily do the same. Look for an evenly shaped melon without dents, bruises, cuts, or discoloration. It should be smooth and well rounded at the stem end. Check the color of the skin under the netting—it should be glowing golden. Unlike other ripe melons, which often have a bit of vine attached, mature cantaloupes dehisce, smoothly slipping free of the stem attachment. Choose a melon that's heavy for its size—the sign of juiciness—and be sure it's intoxicatingly fragrant.

Once you've found the perfect cantaloupe, turn it into some luscious treats.

Make an edi-bowl. Cut the cantaloupe in half and load it up with blueberries, raspberries, 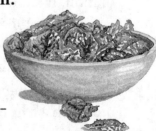 and a little vanilla yogurt for a berry-nice breakfast. Or fill it with high-calcium cottage cheese and serve it with a piece of thinly sliced and rolled lean ham for lunch. For special events, carve a melon basket and fill it with honeydew and watermelon balls drizzled with honey and dusted lightly with cinnamon.

Slice it nice. Nothing beats an ice-cold wedge of cantaloupe for instant refreshment after a long, hot run or your daily workout. To be sure it's ready when you are, cut the cantaloupe into wedges, carve off the rind, and store the pieces in an airtight container in the fridge.

Toss and turn. Toss red leaf lettuce, thinly sliced red onion, fresh cilantro, sliced water chest-

A SIMPLE SOLUTION

Several salmonella outbreaks caused by cantaloupe triggered fever, cramps, and diarrhea in more than 400 people. Children, older folks, and people with compromised immune systems due to chemotherapy or HIV infection are especially at risk for this type of food poisoning.

What's cantaloupe got to do with it? It can carry salmonella bacteria, and you'll drag those germs through the melon with the very first cut. Before slicing a melon, wash your hands and then the outside of the melon with soap and hot running water. Cut the melon in half and scrape out the seeds, then clean up thoroughly. Wash your hands and the cutting board and utensils so that you don't transfer the germs to other fruits and vegetables.

nuts, and cantaloupe chunks with light Catalina dressing for a distinctive and summery side salad.

Mix 'n match. Use a large melon baller to make cantaloupe, honeydew, and watermelon balls, then thread them on bamboo skewers.

Jazz up your pasta. Mix cooked chicken chunks, cantaloupe balls, low-fat mayo, and a few chopped cashews with your favorite cooked pasta shape for light luncheon fare.

Chill a melon cooler. Freeze cantaloupe chunks, then whirl a cupful in your blender with ½ cup of fat-free milk and ¼ teaspoon of mint flavoring for an instant slushy cooler. Or freeze cantaloupe balls to use as never-melt ice cubes for beverages.

FOOD NEWS

Beef liver, fish-liver oils, eggs, fortified milk, butter, and margarine deliver fully active, preformed vitamin A, which is stored in your liver until you need it. That sounds good, but too much vitamin A can be toxic. Fortunately, however, vitamin A can also be created from carotenoids—mostly beta-carotene, which is never toxic, because your body doesn't store it the same way.

CHEESE

Plaque Buster

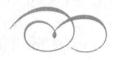

WHEN YOU SMILE FOR THE CAMERA, YOU SHOW OFF sparkling teeth and healthy gums, right? If not, it's time to just say "Cheese!" Here's why. When you munch on crackers or other starchy foods, their carbohydrates turn into the sugars that feed the organisms that live in plaque. The well-fed bugs celebrate by spewing out acids that eat holes in your teeth.

MILK IT FOR ALL IT'S WORTH

Dairy foods, such as low-fat milk, yogurt, and cheese, protect your teeth in several ways.

• Casein, the protein in dairy food, prevents plaque from sticking to your teeth and actually makes sugary foods (like those cookies you love) less likely to cause decay.

...Just the facts

Parmesan cheese (2 Tbsp grated)
Calories: 57
Fat: 4 g
Saturated fat: 2 g
Cholesterol: 10 mg
Sodium: 233 mg
Total carbohydrates: 0 g
Dietary fiber: 0 g
Protein: 5 g
Calcium: 17% of Daily Value

• Cheese eaten alone increases the calcium and phosphate in plaque, which protects your teeth.

• Cheese contains tyramine, which helps increase saliva to rinse your teeth clean.

• The fat in a small amount of cheese eaten as part of an otherwise low-fat diet can help clear out problem starches before they cause plaque problems.

So when it's time for a snack or dessert, just say "Cheese!"

Good to Go ➡

Here's how to handle "golden moldies."

• If you notice mold on fresh or soft cheese, discard the cheese.

• If you see a single spot of mold on hard cheese, cut off the spot to ½ inch beneath the mold and eat the rest as soon as possible.

• Throw out any hard cheese that has more than two spots of mold.

CHEESY HELP FOR THE REST OF YOUR BODY

Cheese, like other dairy foods, delivers plenty of calcium. Once it gets past your teeth and gums, the magical mineral goes to work protecting all your body parts. Most of your body's calcium is stored in your bones, where it gives them the strength to support you, protect your internal organs, and work with your muscles so you can move. About 1 percent of your calcium resides in your bloodstream, where it regulates cell walls and sends messages between cells.

It's crucial that you meet your calcium requirements because if you fall short, your bones sacrifice some of their stores of the mineral and give it to your bloodstream. If your bones are continually called upon to make up your dietary deficit, they become weak and

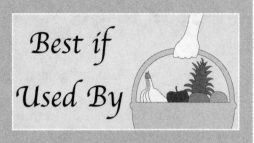

Best if Used By

To preserve your purchase, refrigerate it as soon as possible in its original wrapper or an airtight container. Hard cheeses, such as Cheddar, should keep for several months, while fresh or soft cheeses, such as ricotta, may last for only one to three weeks.

prone to fractures. Unfortunately, research shows that one in two women has an osteoporosis-related fracture sometime in her life.

Before you hit the big five-o, you need about 1,000 milligrams of calcium daily. After that, your quota increases to 1,200 milligrams a day. Most 1-ounce servings of cheese provide about 170 to 210 milligrams of calcium, a good chunk of what you require daily. And lovers of Italian food, rejoice: Parmesan cheese offers a whopping 330 milligrams!

Unfortunately, many women have cut cheese out of their diets—or trimmed it back considerably—because they're being fat conscious. While some cheeses, especially soft varieties such as Havarti, pack 10 grams of fat per ounce, others, such as part-skim mozzarella and part-skim ricotta, contain a more reasonable 5 grams, so read labels carefully. Plus, many manufacturers have come out with reduced-fat versions of popular cheeses. For everyday meals, focus on low-fat types and save the high-fat baked Brie for holidays and other special occasions.

BREAKING NEWS

The latest research suggests that while you're striving to come up with enough calcium to protect your bones, you may be helping your body in other ways. Consider this.

• A study of more than 400 women found that getting 1,200 milligrams of calcium daily reduced symptoms of premenstrual syndrome, such as irritability and bloating, by half.

← *Calcium Best Buys* →

Sure, cheese is loaded with calcium. Trouble is, some types contain a lot of calories, too. To determine which cheeses are calcium bargains—and which are busts—we divided the calcium content by the number of calories to get a calcium quotient. Of course, the higher the quotient, the better.

Cheese	Calcium Quotient
Cream cheese, fat-free	3.4
Parmesan	3.0
Ricotta, part-skim	2.9
Swiss	2.7
Mozzarella, part-skim	2.6
Romano	2.6
Edam	2.3
Gouda	2.1
Asiago	2.0
Monterey Jack	2.0
Feta	1.9
Muenster	1.9
Cheddar	1.8
Colby	1.7
American	1.5
Blue cheese	1.5
Goat cheese	0.5
Cream cheese, regular	0.2

• Another study suggests that calcium may lower the risk of colon polyps, which can lead to cancer.

• A clinical trial of 32 obese patients showed that those who got 1,200 milligrams of calcium daily from dairy foods lost more weight, more body fat, and more dangerous abdomi-

FOOD NEWS

Serving tip: Most cheese aficionados prefer to leave hard cheeses at room temperature for about an hour before serving, which gives them a chance to warm up and "breathe," thus heightening their flavor. Don't do the same with fresh, unripened cheeses, such as ricotta or cottage cheese, though, because they may spoil.

nal fat than those who ate the same number of calories but got only 400 milligrams of calcium from food or 800 milligrams from supplements.

• If you're plagued by muscle cramps every time you do something strenuous, research suggests that you may not be getting enough calcium. Make sure you get more of the mineral—and ditch those annoying cramps—by eating a few bites of cheese every day.

All that research is really something to smile about—so just say "Cheese!"

CHEESY CHOICES

Ahh, don't you love the aroma in a cheese store? It's as if you can taste the Parmesan with your nose! When selecting cheese, check the expiration date on the package before buying. Be sure the packaging is intact and look for surface mold and dried-out spots.

Here's how to get creative with cheese.

Get your goat. Instead of mayo, spread a thin layer of goat cheese on your deli sandwich.

Make your soup snazzy. Sprinkle reduced-fat Cheddar in the center of your bowl of tomato soup.

Use your noodle with spaghetti. Make your pasta taste more like lasagna without all the extra fuss and calories simply by adding ½ cup of part-skim ricotta cheese to your tomato sauce.

GRAPEFRUIT

Good for Gum Repair

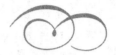

THE GRAPEFRUIT MAY PLAY SECOND FIDDLE TO THE orange in some houses, but not in ours! That's because grapefruit—especially the red and pink varieties—is teeming with antioxidants that fend off health problems large and small. And if your gums need repair, grapefruit's team of nutrients is just what the doctor (or dentist) ordered.

COLLABORATION'S THE THING

The antioxidants in grapefruit work both alone and in tandem to fight disease, so eat your grapefruit and enjoy these advantages.

• *A carload of C.* The bigwig of these antioxidants, as you undoubtedly know, is vitamin C. Just half a grapefruit guarantees you all the vitamin C you need for the

> ## ...Just the facts
>
> Pink grapefruit (½ medium)
> Calories: 60
> Fat: 0 g
> Saturated fat: 0 g
> Cholesterol: 0 mg
> Sodium: 5 mg
> Total carbohydrates: 16 g
> Dietary fiber: 6 g
> Protein: 1 g
> Vitamin A: 15% of Daily
>   Value
> Vitamin C: 110%

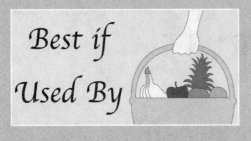

Best if Used By

Store your beautiful bounty on the kitchen counter if you're planning to eat it within a few days. If not, put it the fridge, where it will keep for as long as six weeks.

entire day! In addition to clobbering free radicals, substances that cause cell damage, vitamin C helps repair and maintain collagen, your body's connective tissue, including your tender gums.

• *Buckets of beta.* Pink and red grapefruits are also packed with beta-carotene, crucial for healthy gums. Studies have shown that this antioxidant may also play a valuable role in fending off cancer and heart disease when it's consumed in foods (but not in vitamin supplements).

• *Lots of lycopene.* Both of these colorful grapefruit varieties, but especially red, are loaded with lycopene, an antioxidant that seems promising in the prevention of prostate cancer.

• *Spoonfuls of fiber.* All grapefruit varieties supply a lot of fiber, mostly the soluble type. This kind of fiber helps lower levels of low-density lipoprotein (LDL) cholesterol—the bad kind—thus protecting your heart. To get the most fiber, don't skip the walls that separate the grapefruit segments—they contribute at least half of the total amount.

• *An answer to asthma.* Preliminary studies suggest that adding grapefruit to your daily diet can help reduce asthma symptoms.

• *Full cooperation.* The antioxidants in grapefruit may team up to stave off strokes. A Harvard study found that drinking a glass of grapefruit juice or orange juice daily lowered the risk of a common type of stroke by 25 percent.

HEFTY CHOICES

For the most cancer-fighting beta-carotene and lycopene, choose pink, or better yet, red, grapefruit. When selecting it, heft the fruit. The heavier it feels for its size, the more yummy juice it contains. Avoid rough-looking fruit that has puffy skin and protruding ends, a sign that it's old and will probably be fairly dry.

Once you check out these ideas, you'll never have grapefruit hanging around for very long.

Add zing to your salad. Toss Ruby Red grapefruit wedges into green salads for an extra boost of color, fiber, and flavor. Drizzle with citrus vinaigrette.

Add colors galore. Combine segments from white, pink, and red grapefruits in a fruit salad. It'll light up your eyes.

Add zip to your fish. Sprinkle shrimp with grapefruit juice instead of lemon juice, or stir-fry shrimp and grapefruit pieces. Top broiled or grilled fish fillets, such as salmon or flounder, with grapefruit pieces.

Add honey. If fresh grapefruit isn't sweet enough for you, drizzle it with a little maple syrup or honey.

KIWIFRUIT

Mighty Midget

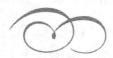

WHEN YOUR GUMS HAVE RUN AMOK AND YOU NEED A little extra vitamin C, reach for kiwi! True, having an orange would be a big help with its 70 milligrams of C, but one kiwifruit, at just 45 calories, delivers 75 milligrams of vitamin C—5 milligrams more than an orange twice its weight. A bonus: A kiwifruit offers three times more vitamin E than an orange does.

ANTIOXIDANT FEAST AND FAMINE

By now, you know that vitamins C and E act as powerful antioxidants in your body, gobbling up substances that can cause the cell damage responsible for cancer, heart attack, stroke, diabetes, and even cataracts. But USDA data shows that many Americans don't meet the minimum

...Just the facts

Kiwifruit (1 medium)
Calories: 45
Fat: 0 g
Saturated fat: 0 g
Cholesterol: 0 mg
Sodium: 5 mg
Total carbohydrates: 12 g
Dietary fiber: 2.5 g
Protein: 1 g
Folate: 7% of Daily Value
Vitamin C: 100%
Copper: 6%
Magnesium: 6%
Potassium: 7%

requirements for these nutrients—especially vitamin E. The numbers are startling: A whopping 71 percent of women over age 20 and more than 60 percent of men over age 50 fall short of the recommended daily amount of vitamin E.

The unfortunate consequence is that you tremendously raise your risk of getting some of the most-feared diseases. For instance, research reported in the *Journal of the National Cancer Institute* showed that women who didn't eat a lot of foods rich in vitamin E and beta-carotene had a 21 percent increased risk of developing breast cancer. Likewise, a study of more than 1,600 men, published in the *British Medical Journal*, found that those with the lowest intake of vitamin C were at the highest risk for heart attacks.

FOOD NEWS

Want a sweeter kiwi? In late summer, check out gourmet stores for golden kiwi. This variety has smoother skin, a more oval shape, and yellow flesh that's sweeter than green.

KEEP YOUR EYE ON THE PRIZE

In addition to its powerful antioxidant vitamins, kiwifruit holds another disease-fighting weapon: lutein, a powerful carotenoid that's also found in your eyes. In one study, kiwifruit ranked higher in lutein content than spinach and all other produce except yellow corn.

Recent research suggests that lutein may protect your eye tissues from damage that leads to age-related macular degeneration, the leading cause of blindness in older Americans. Unfortunately, a study published in the *Journal of the American Dietetic Association* found that lutein intake is decreasing among Americans, particularly among Caucasian women.

With lutein and oodles of vitamins C and E, you'd think there wouldn't be room for anything more in one little kiwifruit—but there is! The fuzzy fruit also offers these nutrients.

- *Folate.* This B vitamin is important for preventing birth defects and may protect against heart attacks.

- *Copper.* It's essential for a strong immune system.

- *Magnesium.* Bone formation and regulation of heart rhythm are two body functions that rely on magnesium.

- *Potassium.* It's critical for blood pressure control.

And, oh, yeah, two kiwifruits supply 5 grams of fiber, about 20 percent of what you need daily. So what are you waiting for? Go ahead and dig in!

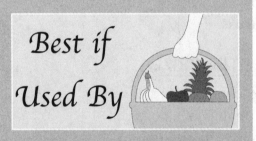

Best if Used By

Here's how to keep your kiwi at its peak.

- Place ripe kiwi in the fridge, where it'll keep for up to a month—far longer than most other fruits.

- Put hard, unripe kiwi in a vented plastic bag with an apple or a banana and leave the bag on your kitchen counter for a day or two.

EVERY DAY IS KIWI DAY

It used to be that finding good kiwifruit year-round was as hard as finding a pair of jeans that really fit. Now, though, with imports from Chile and New Zealand plus California's crop, you can buy kiwifruit 365 days a year. Look for a firm, unblemished kiwi that yields slightly to your touch.

If you try these mouthwatering creations, your kiwifruit will never be in cold storage for very long.

Pile them on pancakes. Instead of drowning your pancakes in maple syrup (1 tablespoon alone packs 52 calories, and who stops there?), top them with chopped kiwifruit and other favorite fruits.

Mix and match. Strawberries and kiwifruit make a great team. To enjoy this winning combination, mix 1 cup of sliced strawberries, 1 cup of sliced kiwi, 1 cup of low-fat milk, and 1 cup of low-fat plain yogurt in a blender until smooth.

Be a star. Slice kiwifruit lengthwise in ¼- to ⅓-inch pieces and then use a small cookie cutter to make star shapes. It's an excellent—and easy—appetizer for a 4th of July picnic.

Sauce up your fish. Puree kiwifruit with a tad of lemon juice and serve with salmon, shrimp, or any other fish for a great taste.

STRAWBERRIES

Rehab Your Gums

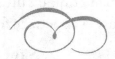

LOOKING FOR MORE TASTY WAYS TO KEEP YOUR GUMS healthy? Consider strawberries. They're loaded with so much antioxidant vitamin C that a single medium berry boasts 19 milligrams—about 25 percent of the recommended daily intake for women and 17 percent of the quota for men. And who can stop at eating just one? Vitamin C is touted for boosting immunity, making wounds heal faster (some dentists recommend it to their patients before gum surgery), and fending off heart disease and cancer. Those are big jobs for a little berry!

THE ANTIOXIDANT HARVEST

Vitamin C isn't the only antioxidant do-gooder found in strawberries. They also contain cancer-fighting ellagic acid and anthocyanin, the pigment that gives

---

...Just the facts

Strawberries (8 medium)
Calories: 50
Fat: 0 g
Saturated fat: 0 g
Cholesterol: 0 mg
Sodium: 0 mg
Total carbohydrates: 15 g
Dietary fiber: 4 g
Protein: 1 g
Folate: 20% of Daily Value
Vitamin C: 140%

---

the berries their beautiful red hue.

When researchers at Tufts University in Boston measured the total amount of antioxidants in more than 50 fresh fruits and vegetables, strawberries ranked sixth, nudged out by blueberries, blackberries, kale, garlic, and cranberries. The point? Of these top six foods, strawberries are the easiest to eat every day.

Good to Go →

When you're ready to use your berries, wash them with the caps attached so they don't absorb a lot of extra water, then remove the caps with a paring knife.

Eating a food that has a lot of antioxidants is one thing, but how well do they work together? Better than a Fortune 500 company. Here are the latest scientific findings.

• A study at Ohio State University in Columbus found that the antioxidants in strawberries may be able to inhibit cancer of the esophagus.

• A Harvard study of more than 1,200 people concluded that strawberry lovers were 70 percent less likely to develop cancer than those who rarely ate the fruit.

• A project at Tufts suggests that eating strawberries may help slow down age-related memory loss.

PROTECTING YOUR BABY

If you're a mom-to-be or are trying to conceive, think strawberries! One serving (about eight berries) supplies about 20 percent of the folate that expectant moms need to help ward off neural tube birth defects, such as spina bifida.

Because these birth defects occur early in the first trimester, the National Academy of Sciences in Washington, D.C., actually recommends that all women of childbearing age seek out plenty of folate from foods and take a 400-microgram supplement of folic acid (folate's synthetic counterpart) daily.

Why should you load up on folate if you aren't planning a pregnancy? More than half of all pregnancies are—how shall we put it?—unscheduled.

After the first trimester, though, don't ditch the strawberries. They offer 4 grams of fiber per serving, plenty to help ward off the constipation that so often comes with pregnancy.

Best if Used By

Here's how to baby those beautiful berries.

• Carefully inspect them, discarding any smashed or moldy ones. You can return the good berries to the original carton, but the California Strawberry Commission suggests that you transfer them to a large container lined with a paper towel. Layer the berries in the container, using additional paper towels between layers.

• Store your berries in the fridge immediately, then use them within two or three days.

RED AND READY

Picking strawberries is as easy as pie! Look for berries that are dry, bright red, and fully ripe. Berries don't ripen after being picked, so what you buy is what you get. Choose those that are still sporting their cute little green caps, since. removing the cap activates an enzyme that begins to destroy the vitamin C in the berry.

Enjoy your berry bounty in these wonderful ways.

Sweeten salads. Add strawberry slices to spinach salad for a touch of sweetness. A side benefit: The vitamin C in the berries will help you better absorb the energy-boosting iron in the spinach.

Go Italian. In Italy, cooks commonly drizzle some high-quality balsamic vinaigrette on a bowl of sliced strawberries.

Escape the cold. Even in the winter, you can whip up this refreshing drink, put a mini umbrella in it, and pretend you're on a sunny beach. In a blender, process 1 cup of sliced strawberries, 1 cup of sliced pineapple, 1 cup of pineapple juice, and 1 cup of low-fat strawberry yogurt until smooth. Sip away your worries.

Beat shortcake. For a change of pace, fill cantaloupe halves with sliced strawberries and top with a scoop of vanilla sorbet (Häagen-Dazs makes a great one!) or frozen yogurt.

Make naturally pink lemonade. In a blender, mix a quart of lemonade (either homemade or store-bought) with 1 cup of fresh or thawed frozen strawberries.

VISION LOSS

Read the Writing on the Wall

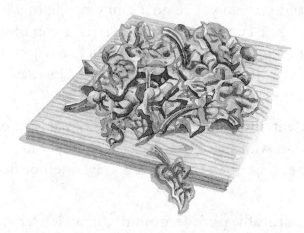

EVERY CHANCE I GET, I TRY TO SNEAK SOME GREEN leafy vegetables into my husband, Ted. It's more than just that age-old admonition to eat something green every day. It's also because Ted's eye doctor has hinted that he may have the beginnings of cataracts. In addition, his mother developed age-related macular degeneration (AMD) late in life, and I'm worried that Ted may be at risk, too. So I've embarked on a vision mission, and I'm pretty excited about it. When he's not

Fabulous Fill-In!

Dark green, leafy vegetables deliver the most eye-protective lutein and zeaxanthin, but egg yolks, green peas, pumpkin, celery, yellow corn, cucumbers, and green beans also deliver modest amounts to help you get your fill.

looking, I sneak in a little spinach, broc-coli, kale, or collard or mustard greens—whatever is dark and green—because of two amazing compounds that protect sight.

SEE CLEARLY NOW

Although we've long been helpless in the face of fading eyesight, new research sheds light on some diet strategies that appear to keep us looking good and seeing straight. Here are easy things you can do to focus your menus.

Go for the green. Dark green vegeta-bles are bursting with some beta-carotene relatives called lutein and zeaxanthin. These same two nutrients show up in megadoses in a spot in the center of your eye. Called the macula, that little spot is what lets you see straight ahead, such as when you're reading, driving, or just looking at the face of someone you love. If the macula degenerates, central vision fades.

Now here's a surprise: People who eat the most vegetables rich in these nutrients tend to have the most of both in the macula of their eyes. Furthermore—and here's where it gets good—they have a 40 percent lower risk of AMD.

What's the connection? Researchers suspect that lutein and zeaxanthin filter out and protect against some harmful light that can damage the macula and lead to vision loss.

Eat to keep your peepers clear. There's a second good reason to make dark, leafy greens absolutely irresistible. It looks as if they also help slow cataracts, and not just because of lutein

Healing VITAMINS

If you're at risk for macular degeneration, talk to your doctor about sup-plementing with vitamin C, vitamin E, beta-carotene, zinc, and copper. These vitamins and minerals have been shown to reduce the odds of disease progression by 25 percent. Your doctor can determine which amounts are right for you.

If your friends and family are resistant to eating green vegetables, make it easy for them by:

• Mixing them with salad greens

• Tossing them into soups and stews

• Slivering them into pasta dishes

• Shredding them into mashed potatoes

and zeaxanthin. The green foods your mother harped on are also exploding with antioxidant vitamins C and E. Along with all the other ways these vitamins protect your body, they appear to help the lenses of your eyes fend off the cell damage that becomes cataracts. This green cuisine is serious stuff!

Choose high-C fruits. When it comes to vitamin C, the greens don't have to go it alone. Citrus fruits such as oranges, grapefruit, and tangerines are stuffed with C, too. And don't forget berries, kiwi, and melons.

Eat natural E. To increase your food sources of vitamin E, switch from processed white bread and pasta to brands made from whole grains. And bring on the nuts. Eating a small handful (about an ounce) four or five times a week will increase E without breaking your calorie bank. Almond butter and peanut butter deliver the goods, too.

Trade bad fat for good. Eating less sunflower and corn oil—the fats that ooze out of junk food—and more of the healthy fats from fish, walnuts, and flaxseed appears to lower the risk of AMD.

FOOD NEWS

Ten grams of healthy fat per meal (such as that from olive or canola oil, nuts, seeds, and peanut butter) are a must to help you absorb the carotenes that are so important for your eyes.

BELL PEPPERS

A Sight for Sore Eyes

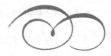

BELL PEPPERS, ESPECIALLY THE RED TYPE, PACK A POWER-ful punch of lutein and zeaxanthin, two key plant compounds that appear to play a role in preventing age-related macular degeneration (AMD). This condition affects the macula in the center of the retina, causing loss of central vision, and is the most common cause of irreversible blindness in people over age 65.

Now here's where bell peppers come in: Lutein and zeaxanthin are common pigments found in the macula, and studies have shown that people with AMD have fewer of these pigments than those who don't have the disease.

You can take supplements to boost your body's levels of lutein and zeaxan-thin, but most eye doctors recommend

...Just the facts

Red bell pepper (1 raw,
    about 3½ ounces)
Calories: 20
Fat: 0 g
Saturated fat: 0 g
Cholesterol: 0 mg
Sodium: 1 mg
Total carbohydrates: 5 g
Dietary fiber: 1 g
Protein: 1 g
Vitamin A: 8% of Daily Value
Vitamin C: 186%

Not sure which color bell pepper to buy? See why you should head for red.

Pepper (1 cup chopped)	Vitamin C (mg)	Beta-carotene (units)	Lutein (mcg)
Red	191	2,379	6,800
Yellow	184	120	770
Green	89	198	700

getting these compounds from foods because they may work synergistically with other nutrients not found in a pill. So open your eyes to bell peppers as well as beets, kale, spinach, and other veggies that are rich in these compounds.

BOOST YOUR C LEVEL

For just a third of the calories in an orange, a red bell pepper packs twice as much vitamin C, a whopping 141 milligrams! A green one is on par with an orange, delivering about 66 milligrams of C, which appears to play a part in fending off cataracts.

Two Good!

Along with a three-day supply of vitamin C to protect your vision, red bell peppers deliver cancer-fighting red pigments. That's double the bang for your calories!

In your body, vitamin C acts as an antioxidant, gobbling up free radicals. These molecular troublemakers cause the cell damage that eventually leads to heart disease and cancer.

Based on promising research, the U.S. government recently raised the suggested daily intake of vitamin C from 60 milligrams to 75 milligrams for women and

90 milligrams for men. Smokers, the government suggested, should take in an additional 35 milligrams, for a total of 110 milligrams for women and 125 milligrams for men who smoke. Nicotine apparently leads to both cell damage and depletion of vitamin C.

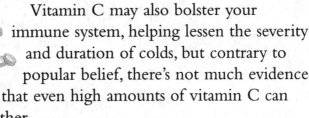

Good to Go

When you're ready to use your peppers, wash them just before eating or cooking. Scrub any that have a waxy coating.

Vitamin C may also bolster your immune system, helping lessen the severity and duration of colds, but contrary to popular belief, there's not much evidence that even high amounts of vitamin C can stop sniffles altogether.

SEASONS IN THE SUN

Summertime is pepper time, when you easily can find all colors of fresh bell peppers at a reasonable price. Look for peppers that are firm and glossy, with unwrinkled skins and green stems. Avoid any with soft or sunken areas, cracks, slashes, or black spots.

Here are ways to use peppers that even Peter Piper never considered.

Upgrade bruschetta. Instead of spreading Italian bread with the traditional tomato topping, cover it with roasted red bell pep-

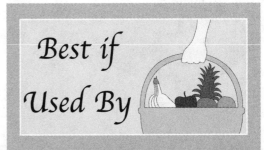

Best if Used By

Store peppers in a plastic bag or container in the fridge. Green and yellow peppers generally last a week, while red ones stay fresh for just three or four days.

pers and fresh mozzarella cheese.

Create pepper spread. In a blender, puree 1 cup of roasted red bell peppers, peeled and cut into strips. Add 1 cup of fat-free cheese and 2 cloves of garlic and puree until smooth. Stir in 1 tablespoon of chopped fresh basil.

Brighten green beans. Add pieces of chopped red pepper to fresh, frozen, or canned green beans. The green-red color scheme is perfect for holiday parties.

Wake up your nachos. Melt reduced-fat Cheddar cheese on baked tortilla chips. Top with chopped red pepper pieces for extra crunch.

Fabulous Fill-In!

If fresh bell peppers are too pricey for your pocketbook (in the winter, it almost takes Bill Gates's bank account to afford them), buy a jar of roasted red peppers for sandwiches and salads or frozen pepper strips for stir-fries. You'll save a bundle and still reap all the nutrition.

CORN

Look Sharp

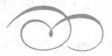

LET'S FACE IT: A LOT OF MEN DON'T LIKE MANY VEGE-tables. Corn and potatoes are pretty much all they'll eat, so many cooks end up making a lot of corn, despite the fact that it doesn't offer much in the way of traditional vitamins and minerals. Fortunately, however, new research shows that corn packs a wad of antioxidants that are essential for eye health, and that's good news for everyone!

SEE THE LIGHT

Fresh yellow corn contains lutein and zeaxanthin, antioxidants that eye doctors are raving about, and we're talking about more than just a kernel of them. Corn is one of the best nongreen sources of these plant compounds. Even canned corn has them, although it offers only about half

...Just the facts

Corn on the cob (1 medium ear)
Calories: 75
Fat: 1 g
Saturated fat: 0 g
Cholesterol: 0 mg
Sodium: 15 mg
Total carbohydrates: 17 g
Dietary fiber: 1 g
Protein: 3 g
Folate: 9% of Daily Value
Vitamin A: 5%
Vitamin C: 10%
Iron: 3%

the amount found in fresh yellow kernels.

What's the fuss about? Here's what these nutrients can do for your eyes.

• *Shut out macular degeneration.* Researchers have found that people with low levels of lutein and zeaxanthin in their diets are more likely to develop age-related macular degeneration (AMD)—the leading cause of blindness in older Americans—than those with higher levels. A study at Harvard showed that consuming 6 milligrams of lutein per day reduced the risk of AMD by 43 percent! (One ear of corn provides about 1 milligram.)

• *Cut out cataracts.* Corn may also help protect your peepers by warding off cataracts. Another Harvard study concluded that men and women who ate a lot of lutein-rich foods cut their risk of cataracts by about one-fifth.

NEWS FROM THE LAB

Scientists in other areas of medicine are also exploring the health benefits of these antioxidants. And their results are pretty amazing, as well.

• Preliminary research suggests that lutein and zeaxanthin may help protect against the sun damage that leads to skin cancer.

• Another study found that men and women with the highest amounts of lutein in their diets had a 17 percent lower risk of colon cancer than those with the lowest levels.

The bottom line? The ears have it!

BE A COB SNOB

Want to find the freshest, sweetest corn? Skip the supermarket and buy it directly from a farmer. Because corn begins to lose its sweetness after it's picked, much of what you find at the supermarket is already past its prime. Instead, head to the country or a local farmers' market—and take a cooler with you.

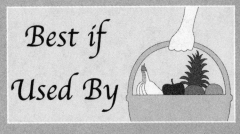

Ideally, you should cook corn the same day you buy it, but you can put the unhusked ears in a plastic bag and store them in the fridge for up to three days.

When selecting corn, look for tight, bright green husks, then strip back part of the husks to check the kernels. Be sure the kernels at the tip are smaller than those in the middle. If not, it's a sign that the corn may not be as sweet as you'd like. Once you purchase the perfect ears, stash them in a cooler if you have a long trip home, because heat saps corn's sweetness.

Now here are a couple of cooking ideas.

Ban the butter. Instead of blasting corn with butter, which isn't exactly heart friendly, season it with herb vinaigrette.

Upgrade salsa. Sure, you could pay $5 a jar for salsa, but it's not necessary. Instead, buy one of the buck-a-bottle brands and mix in corn that's fresh from the cob or straight from the can. We won't tell.

Tuck into tacos. Mix corn with chicken pieces, tomatoes, lettuce, and cheese for a special taco filling.

Toss into salad. Add canned, frozen, or fresh-cut corn to summer salads for a dash of sunshine.

KALE

Eyes Right!

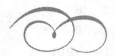

KALE IS MY FAVORITE VEGETABLE, AN idiosyncrasy passed down from my mom and on to my daughter Bobbi. Thus, I'm always surprised when the supermarket cashier asks, "Now what is this?"

Unless you're from the Deep South, you may not know, either—but you should, because kale is king when it comes to providing carotenoids, substances that protect your eyes against cataracts and age-related macular degeneration (AMD), the leading cause of blindness among older Americans.

HITS THE SPOT

Your eyes may be the windows to your soul, but they're also important for seeing

...Just the facts

Kale (½ cup cooked)
Calories: 17
Fat: 0 g
Saturated fat: 0 g
Cholesterol: 0 mg
Sodium: 15 mg
Total carbohydrates: 4 g
Dietary fiber: 1 g
Protein: 1 g
Vitamin A: 120% of Daily
   Value
Vitamin C: 44%
Vitamin K: 400%
Calcium: 5%
Iron: 4%

the light. Unfortunately, seeing the light has its downside. The very act of "looking" produces dangerous, unpaired free-radical oxygen molecules. While seeking an oxygen mate, these free radicals can damage the macula of your eye. This tiny spot in the center of your retina, which is critical for seeing straight ahead, is packed with the antioxidant pigments lutein and zeaxanthin, which scavenge free radicals before they can harm vision.

Early studies suggest that eating foods such as kale and spinach, which are rich in these carotenoids, makes the macular pigments denser, protecting against AMD, which fortunately takes decades to develop. Start now to get to know and love kale.

You may have to hold your nose when you're cooking it, though, and turn on the exhaust fan before the pot begins to boil. Otherwise, the cabbage-like smell may dampen your enthusiasm for this sweet, tender, powerhouse vegetable.

A GIANT KILLER

Cruciferous (cabbage family) vegetables, such as kale, have long been known to reduce the risk of cancer, and now scientists are beginning to understand a little of the "why." Kale is packed with phytochemicals, naturally occurring elements in

Careful!

Kale's vitamin K helps your blood clot so you don't bleed to death, but if you're taking Coumadin (warfarin), beware. Since this prescription medicine is designed to reduce clotting to prevent heart attacks and stroke, your diet and the drug could work against each other. Talk to your doctor about adjusting your medication to suit your new, healthier food choices before you start eating more kale or other dark green, leafy vegetables.

When your allergies to air-borne pollens act up, eat some kale. It's rich in quercetin, a natural antihistamine—and it doesn't cost as much as those drugstore antihistamines!

plants that help your body fight disease and infection.

Additionally, despite all the progress being made in reducing deaths from heart disease, it remains the number one killer of both women and men in the United States. The big problem stems from excess cholesterol in your bloodstream, which clings to the walls of your arteries and blocks the flow of blood.

Cholesterol can't latch on unless it's combined with dangerous free-radical oxygen—formed in a process called oxidation—and that's where kale comes to the rescue. In laboratory tests, kale outranked all other vegetables in its ability to prevent this process from getting started.

A BONE BUILDER

Recent research at Tufts University in Boston suggests that you may need 110 micrograms of vitamin K daily to activate a protein called osteocalcin, which is needed to make bones strong. With 274 micrograms of vitamin K, a ½-cup serving of raw kale provides more than double that dose.

Two Good!

Kale delivers a double benefit for your bones: It's one of the green leafy vegetables that add to your calcium quotient, and it serves up a huge dose of vitamin K, needed for bone health.

SHOOT THE CURL

You can buy kale frozen in blocks or loose in bags, but it's definitely best when it's fresh. When selecting fresh kale, look for very curly, small leaves that are medium to dark green. They'll be far more tender and delicately flavored than those big, tough, leathery leaves, and they'll cook a whole lot faster. Avoid any leaves that look moldy or have yellow spots.

You can substitute kale for spinach anytime, or try these ideas.

Make a bed. Use kale as a bed for grilled chicken with mango salsa.

Make it Italian. Shred kale and add it to baked lasagna.

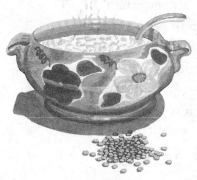

Make super soup. Toss leftover cold, cooked kale into steamy bean, lentil, or vegetable soup.

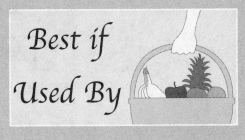

Best if Used By

Here's how to store your kale.

• Rinse it, shake off the excess water, wrap it in paper towels, and put it in a plastic bag. Stash it in a cold, dark area of your refrigerator to protect its fragile vitamins.

• Cook kale within three to four days, because it can turn bitter if it's stored any longer.

MANGOES

Magic for Your Eyes

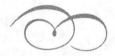

ONE OF THE MOST COMMONLY EATEN FRUITS IN THE world, mangoes originated in southeast Asia more than 4,000 years ago and have been used in folk remedies ever since. Now, modern science has jumped on the bandwagon, touting not just its tropical taste sensations but also its power to protect vision.

THE EYES HAVE IT

Mangoes contain lutein and zeaxanthin, antioxidants that help protect vision by warding off age-related macular degeneration. They also offer a healthy dollop of vitamin C, which is important for fending off cataracts. What's more, mangoes are loaded with 40 percent of the vitamin A that you need for the entire day.

...Just the facts

Mango (½)
Calories: 70
Fat: less than 1 g
Saturated fat: 0 g
Cholesterol: 0 mg
Sodium: 0 mg
Total carbohydrates: 17 g
Dietary fiber: 3 g
Protein: 1–3 g
Vitamin A: 40% of Daily
   Value
Vitamin C: 15%

Since mangoes are so rich in antioxidants, it's a sure bet they're potent cancer fighters, too. To test the mango's anticancer potential, researchers from the University of Florida in Gainesville dropped either mango extracts or water on mouse cells. The mango was 10 times more effective at inhibiting the development of cancerous cells than the water.

In humans, study after study has shown that vitamins A and C gobble up free radicals, substances that may contribute to cancer and heart disease, so it's safe to say that adding mangoes to your day is a smart move for better health.

MAGNIFICENT MANGOES

Chances are, you've never bought a mango. If you have, you can skip this lesson for the beginners. Mangoes are most plentiful from February through September (although you may be able to find them in some supermarkets around Christmastime). They come in several varieties that don't resemble each other very much (see "All in the Family" on page 428). For that reason, you can never really judge a mango by its color. Fortunately, there are

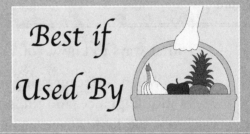

Best if Used By

Store your mangoes right to keep them delectable and guard their nutritional bounty.

• Place ripe mangoes in the refrigerator, where they'll keep for two to five days.

• Put unripe mangoes in a paper bag on your kitchen counter for a couple of days, then transfer them to the fridge.

← All in the Family →

There are four common varieties of mangoes. Each differs in size, appearance, flavor, and fiber content from the other three. They are so different, in fact, they don't even look like they're related.

Mango	Color When Ripe	Flavor	Fiber Content	Availability
Harden	Yellow with a red-orange blush	Mild	Medium	February–June
Keitt	Green; may have a slight yellow blush	Rich	Low	July–September
Kent	Green-yellow; may have a red blush	Very sweet	Low	June–August
Tommy Atkins	Red	Mild	High	April–July

other ways to know you're getting the best fruit.

When selecting mangoes, use your nose. A good mango has a lush fragrance, and the better it smells, the better it will taste. Press the flesh; a ripe mango yields slightly to gentle pressure (like a peach). Avoid fruits with lots of black spots. Some black specks on the skin are normal, but too many of them may indicate damage to the flesh underneath. Pass up any mangoes that have loose or shriveled skin.

Now that you have your supply of this tropical treasure, treat yourself to some healthy fun.

Shake up chicken or pork. Marinate either meat (in the fridge, of course) in mango juice for about an hour, then grill or broil it—and serve with mango slices. You'll think you've died and gone to a tropical paradise.

Pick a peach replacement.
Mangoes have so much in common with peaches that you can substitute an equal amount of them in most of your recipes.

Enjoy brighter breakfasts.
You can incorporate mango into almost any breakfast. Stir small pieces into plain yogurt, top pancakes or waffles with mango slices instead of syrup, or stir chopped dried mango into your muffin or quick bread mixes.

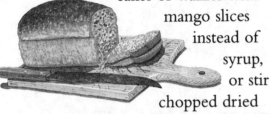

End on the right note. Think no dinner is complete without dessert but still want to fit into your jeans? Keep it simple. Drizzle mango slices with a teaspoon of melted chocolate or chocolate syrup. Top low-fat vanilla frozen yogurt with mango slices and a dollop of whipped cream. Or pick up a pint of Häagen-Dazs mango sorbet—it tastes incredible and delivers a big scoop of vitamin A.

Good to Go

Ready to dig in? Here's how.

• Most mango flesh clings to a large, flat pit. Your best bet is to begin by slicing off both ends of the fruit with a good, sharp, thin-bladed knife.

• Set the mango on one of the flat ends and cut the peel from top to bottom along the curvature of the fruit (never eat the peel).

• Slice away the fruit by carving lengthwise along the pit.

PUMPKIN

The Vision Veggie

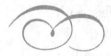

PUMPKIN IS AS POTENT A VEGETABLE AS YOU'LL FIND anywhere. Its deep orange color is a sure sign that it's just crazy with carotenoids, which fight both heart disease and cancer, and it's the equal of yellow corn in the amount of lutein it can serve up. Lutein pumps up the macula of your eye (critical for reading, watching the speedometer, and noticing stop signs), protecting it against harmful blue light and thus fending off age-related macular degeneration.

BETA BOOSTER

Cup for cup, pumpkin ranks with cantaloupe and cooked carrots as a top beta-carotene carrier, and it delivers twice as much alpha-carotene as any other fruit or vegetable. Both beta- and alpha-carotene

...Just the facts

Pumpkin (½ cup canned)
Calories: 42
Fat: 0 g
Saturated fat: 0 g
Cholesterol: 0 mg
Sodium: 6 mg
Total carbohydrates: 9 g
Dietary fiber: 3 g
Protein: 1 g
Vitamin A: 338% of Daily
   Value
Vitamin C: 6%
Vitamin E: 9%
Calcium: 3%
Iron: 9%

Give Thanks for Breakfast

Early one Thanksgiving morning, just as the pumpkin pies were coming out of the oven, my mother-in-law called to remind me that my dinner contribution that year was to be celery and olives, not pie. Oops! Now what?

Without a moment's hesitation, I seized the day and called my family down to breakfast. I served them each a piece of warm pumpkin pie with a glass of ice-cold fat-free milk. Never before and never since has a piece of pie been so appreciated! The kitchen was still warm, and that heavenly spicy fragrance was wafting about. Everybody was hungry, and eating pie for breakfast was just so...decadent!

Fortunately, it was nutritious, too. That's because the canned pumpkin we all use to make pie is just packed with carotenoids (three whole days' worth!), vitamin E, copper, iron, magnesium, and potassium.

I used fat-free evaporated milk instead of cream in the filling, so it was low in fat, and since it also included eggs, each slice had as much protein as an ounce of meat. Instead of lard or shortening in the crust, I used heart-healthy canola oil, so my family started the day with an extra dose of vitamin E, plenty of B vitamins (including folate), and half of their heart-healthy monounsaturated fat for the day. Truly, not all pies are created equal, and this one was head and shoulders above the crowd.

can become vitamin A, with all its power to protect your night vision and build skin and mucous membrane barriers against bacteria and viruses.

Beta-carotene alone can supercharge your immune system. It's been shown to jump-start natural killer cell activity in older men. It makes bacteria-munching monocytes work more

To get your perfect pumpkin ready to eat:

• Wash off all the dirt under running water.

• Place the pumpkin on a sturdy cutting board and use a large, sharp knife to cut it in half.

• Scoop out the seeds and set them aside. (Toast them later if you like—they're yummy.)

• Cut the pumpkin into chunks and do either of the following.

1. Put the chunks on a well-greased baking sheet and bake at 325°F for about an hour, or until the pulp is soft. Scrape the pulp from the shell, then toss it into your food processor and puree.

2. Peel the chunks and place them in a saucepan. Add about ½ cup of water, cover, and simmer until tender, about 25 minutes.

effectively, and it highlights troublemaking antigens so that helper T cells can make the right antibodies to neutralize the antigens.

Pumpkin is a powerful vegetable. It's time we all ate more of it!

PUMPKIN PICKOVER

Beyond pie, when was the last time you ate pumpkin as a vegetable? You could be missing a lot, and using pumpkin in a meal is really pretty simple. When selecting pumpkin, check out farmers' markets and roadside stands. Find one of those small, flat, red-orange pumpkins if you can, because it will be sweetest, or select a small, bright orange, jack-o'-lantern- type pumpkin. Pass up large pumpkins, which tend to be tough and stringy—and harder to work with. The last thing you need is a wrestling match! No matter what kind of pumpkin you buy, get one that's unblemished, evenly shaped, and fresh smelling.

With plenty of fresh pumpkin on hand, you're ready to enjoy it in these smashing ways.

Mash it like potatoes. Top warm, pureed pumpkin with a little margarine,

ground cinnamon, and fat-free milk and serve like mashed sweet potatoes.

Make surprising sauce. Add a little salt and pepper to pureed pumpkin, then use it as "gravy" for lean pot roast.

Serve as a side dish. Reheat pumpkin chunks in the microwave, then sprinkle with pumpkin pie spice and chopped toasted pecans. It's great with pork tenderloin.

Heat up super soup. Stir pumpkin chunks into canned soup for a flavor and nutrient boost.

Can it. Take the shortcut and get your pumpkin from a can. Season with ground ginger, stir in some raisins or dried cherries, and microwave until warm. It's great with baked chicken.

Part Five

GIRL TALK

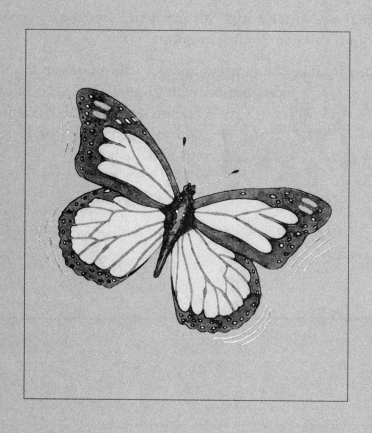

Harness Your Raging Hormones

I hate to whine, but being a woman, and thus subject to estrogen's whims, does have its drawbacks. Fortunately, we know now that diet can turn down the volume on our hormone-related gripes, so let's skip the whining and just pour a cup of tea, grab a chunk of chocolate, and talk about the food facts of a woman's life.

Two problems that most of us experience at one time or another are menstrual woes and urinary tract infections. In the following chapters, we're going to take a closer look at these two "female problems" and follow each with chapters on foods that are sure to ease your difficulties—and help you enjoy being a girl!

Reset Your Cycle

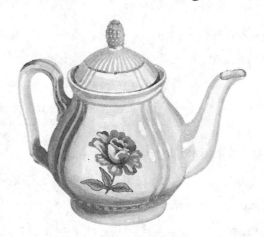

MOST PEOPLE DON'T CALL PERIODS THE CURSE ANY-more, but many women often do feel as if they're under a wicked spell each month. One woman I know has viselike cramps that keep her couch-bound for a day or two every month, while another has periods that arrive cramp-free but with a flow so heavy that it gushes straight through super tampons and jumbo napkins—and ruins her best slacks.

PERIOD OF ADJUSTMENT

It's actually quite common for periods to go haywire, especially once you hit

FOOD NEWS

Studies show that ¼ cup of soy nuts or a table-spoon of flaxseed (both available at health food stores) can help regulate the menstrual cycle if you're skipping periods. Just be sure to "go nuts" every day, perhaps by swirling some into a smoothie.

your forties—the perimenopausal years—when your hormones themselves go haywire. During this time, you may start producing too much estrogen, which builds up uterine tissue, or too little progesterone, which keeps this buildup in check and controls ovulation, the main period regulator. You may also have excessive levels of prolactin, a hormone that prevents the liver from clearing excess estrogen. All of this can turn a previously light flow into a deluge.

Flooding and cramps can also occur if you're overproducing a hormone called prostaglandin F2 alpha. Some women naturally produce an excess of this hormone, but a high-fat, low-nutrient diet can raise levels, too.

A SIMPLE SOLUTION

Cold-water fish, such as salmon and tuna, contain essential fatty acids that help lower levels of prostaglandin F2, which contributes to flooding and cramps, and boost levels of prostaglandin F3, which relaxes the uterine muscle. Not big on fish? Take 1 to 3 grams of fish oil (available at health food stores) daily. Studies show that it can cut cramps—and ibuprofen use—by half, but don't use it if you take aspirin regularly or are taking prescription blood-thinning medication.

Finally, underlying medical conditions can trigger period problems. A leading cause of flooding is fibroids, noncancerous uterine tumors that plague up to 40 percent of women over age 35 and disrupt the uterine contractions that expel menstrual flow. There are also others, including endometriosis, a condition that occurs when uterine tissue migrates outside the uterus.

MANAGE THE MONTHLIES

These gentle remedies—not one of which will upset your stomach—will help you break the spell of monthly misery.

Go with the flow. Vitex, also known as chasteberry, is an herb that helps regulate periods, lightening a very heavy flow, says Tori Hudson, N.D., a naturopathic physician and director of A Woman's Time clinic in Portland, Oregon. Take 30 to 60 drops of chasteberry tincture (which you can find at health food stores) daily. You should start to see results within four to six months.

Stem the tide. Red raspberry leaf is a highly prized uterine tonic that helps to stem heavy bleeding, spotting between periods, and cramps, possibly because it's a great source of calcium, magnesium, and other minerals that enhance muscle contraction. As long as there's no possibility that you're pregnant, Carole Leonard, a certified nurse-midwife and chair of the New Hampshire Council of Midwifery in Hopkinton, suggests drinking at least two cups of raspberry leaf tea daily. Look for prepackaged tea at a health food store and prepare it according to the package directions.

Two Good!

Gamble (or gambol!) on lamb for a two-fisted punch: plenty of protein and a quarter of your day's iron quota in the form that's absorbed better than iron from plants. Getting enough of this mineral from foods helps replace what's lost during heavy periods.

Relax your cramps. Folks in Jamaica use a West Indian herb called Jamaican dogwood to poison fish. When used in humans, however, this muscle relaxant/sedative kills cramps "better than any remedy I know," says Judy Lyn Patrick, N.D., a naturopathic physician who specializes in women's health in Tucson. She recommends taking Jamaican dogwood in capsule form (available at health food stores) according to the label directions.

Sip ginger tea. This tangy root dampens production of troublemaking prostaglandin F2 and lightens menstrual flow. Stir ¼ to ½ teaspoon of powdered ginger into a cup of hot water and drink it daily, suggests Dr. Hudson.

Rub in relief. Natural progesterone creams such as ProGest help block excess estrogen and can lighten menstrual flow in some women, says Christiane Northrup, M.D., director of the Women to Women clinic in Yarmouth, Maine. Apply ¼ to ½ teaspoon of cream (which you can find at drugstores and health food stores) to smooth, hairless skin twice a day for three weeks prior to menstruation. Stop during the week of your period.

Keep in touch. Pressing on the center of your top lip just under your nose for 1 minute every 15 minutes several times a day can help stanch a heavy flow, says Leonard.

Let your little light shine. According to a small study con-

Fabulous Fill-In!

Dandelion is brimming with iron, which you may be lacking if you're flooding every month. Ironically, iron deficiency may actually open the floodgates, while eating iron-rich foods may help to close them. To be sure you're getting plenty (and unless you're taking diuretics or potassium supplements), mix 20 drops of dandelion tincture, available at health food stores, into a glass of orange juice and sip it throughout the day, every day. The vitamin C in the juice will enhance absorption of the iron. You can also try eating edamame (green soybeans), another rich source of iron.

ducted at the University of California, San Diego, women with irregular menstrual cycles who sleep with a light shining in their eyes have shorter cycles. If your periods are irregular, get a timer for your bedside lamp and set it to go on after you're snoozing.

Cloak yourself in kindness. To help regulate heavy flow, chop up a tablespoon of lady's mantle leaves (their folds resemble a pleated coat), steep them in a cup of boiling water for 10 minutes, and strain. Drink one or two cups a day for two weeks prior to your period. Or take lady's mantle tincture according to the label directions for two weeks prior to menstruation, and your period may be lighter when it arrives.

It may take two months or more to see benefits. Both forms of the herb are available at health food stores.

BEEF

The Iron Chef

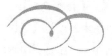

CONSIDER IRON THE FEDEX OF nutrients: It delivers oxygen to cells, where it is used to produce energy. And consider beef the truck that does the delivery.

Women with heavy menstrual periods lose lots of iron every month, and without enough iron, you can become anemic, a condition that leaves you exhausted, irritable, and weak. Although most of the foods in your fridge contain iron, meat is your best bet because the iron from meat is absorbed six to nine times better than the iron from most nonmeat sources. For instance, to obtain the same amount of iron found in a 3-ounce serving of beef, you would have to eat at least 3 cups of spinach. Even then, you wouldn't be able to absorb it as well as the iron in beef.

...Just the facts

Eye round (3 oz roasted)
Calories: 149
Fat: 5 g
Saturated fat: 2 g
Cholesterol: 59 mg
Sodium: 53 mg
Total carbohydrates: 0 g
Dietary fiber: 0 g
Protein: 25 g
Niacin (vitamin B_3): 16% of Daily Value
Vitamin B_6: 16%
Vitamin B_{12}: 31%
Iron: 10%
Selenium: 33%
Zinc: 27%

Unfortunately, 7.8 million American women don't get enough iron, making it the top nutritional deficiency in the United States. The good news is that the problem is deliciously easy to fix.

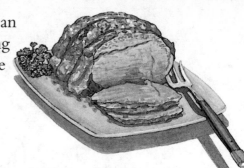

LEAN CUISINE

Beef? In a health book? But of course! While greasy hamburgers are loaded with the saturated fat that can send your cholesterol through the Golden Arches, some cuts of beef are almost as low in fat as chicken. Plus, beef is loaded with disease-fighting nutrients that are hard to come by in even the healthiest diet. So get out your knife and fork while we fill you in on the good news.

Beef got a bad rep because, compared with other meats, it has a lot of saturated fat. Study after study has linked a diet high in saturated fat to heart disease. But not all cuts of beef are unacceptable. In fact, eight cuts of beef meet the USDA's standards for being considered lean: eye of the round, top round, round tip, top sirloin, bottom round, top loin, tenderloin, and flank steak.

A 3-ounce serving of most of these cuts contains 6 grams of total fat and 2 grams of saturated fat. When you choose one of these lean cuts, your cholesterol levels will respond the same way that they do to chicken.

In a study of 145 men and women with mild to moderately high cholesterol,

FOOD NEWS

What about ground beef? We recommend that you don't buy it very often. Even the leanest ground beef is still pretty high in fat.

Most supermarkets carry ground beef that ranges from 80 percent lean (that's 210 calories and 14 grams of fat for 3 ounces) to 93 percent lean (170 calories and 9 grams of fat). Occasionally, you'll see 96 percent lean beef.

Your best bet: If you must buy ground beef, choose the leanest you can find and mix it with skinless ground turkey.

researchers at three major medical centers compared the effects of lean white meat with those of lean red meat on the participants' cholesterol levels. For about nine months, half of the participants derived 80 percent of their meat intake from lean red meat. The other half of the group ate lean white meat. After a four-week break, the groups switched the types of meat they were eating. During the entire study, the participants were instructed to follow a healthy eating plan that was recommended by the American Heart Association.

The result: Whether they were eating red or white meat, the participants lowered their levels of "bad" low-density lipoprotein (LDL) cholesterol and improved their levels of "good" high-density lipoprotein (HDL) cholesterol. "A heart-healthy diet containing up to 6 ounces of lean red meat daily can positively impact blood cholesterol levels," says lead researcher Michael H. Davidson, M.D.

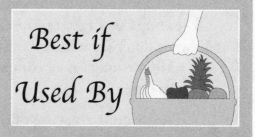

Best if Used By

Once you've bought the beef you want, here's how to keep it fresh.

• Tuck the package into a plastic bag so that any bacteria on the wrapper won't contaminate other foods in your shopping cart. Then head home right away—especially in the summer.

• Store beef in the coldest part of your fridge—usually the meat drawer. Fresh beef is safe to eat until the "sell-by" date.

• Alternatively, you can freeze it. Roasts and steaks will keep for 6 to 12 months, and ground beef is fine in the freezer for 3 to 4 months.

MORE BEEF BODY BUILDERS

Okay, so now you know that eating lean beef boosts your blood and loves your heart, but it has other perks, too. Beef supplies these other vitamins and minerals that may be in short supply in your diet.

• *Zinc.* Yes, indeed, that's the same nutrient found in those lozenges you take to zap colds. Nearly 75 percent of Americans don't meet the recommended zinc requirements, and not getting enough may compromise your immune system or even cause memory loss.

A 3-ounce serving of beef supplies more than 25 percent of the Daily Value for zinc (chicken breast provides just 6 percent). *Note:* Since too much zinc can be as detrimental to the immune system as too little, you should hover around the daily requirement, which has been set at 12 milligrams for women.

• *Selenium.* A serving of beef provides about one-third of your daily requirement for selenium. A powerful antioxidant, selenium may lower the risk of cancer (especially skin cancer), fight heart disease, and ward off infections.

• *B vitamins.* Beef boasts vitamin B_6 (a deficiency can cause depression), vitamin B_{12} (not getting enough could lead to fatigue or even nerve damage), and niacin (a severe deficiency can trigger disorientation and skin problems).

TRIM YOUR TUMMY

In addition to vitamins and minerals, beef contains a compound called conjugated linoleic acid (CLA). Studies on animals have found that CLA may inhibit tumors in the breasts, ovaries, lungs, and colon; decrease bad cholesterol levels; normalize reduced blood glucose levels; and—get this—decrease body fat.

We know this sounds like an infomercial, but this research is really happening. Scientists are now conducting human studies to see if the benefits hold true. In the meantime, keep your fingers crossed.

MAKING THE CUT

Unless your brother's a butcher, figuring out how to select the best-tasting and best-for-you beef can be a puzzle, so I'll walk you through it.

When selecting beef, consider freshness first. Choose meat that has the most distant "sell-by" date on its label—a tip-off that it has recently been put on the shelf. If you can't locate a sell-by date, look at the color of the fat and the meat. The fat should always be white; yellow fat is a sign of age. Unpackaged meat should look cherry red, and vacuum-packed meat should be dark purple. Notice brown or gray areas? That means the meat is on the old side—not necessarily spoiled, but not the freshest you can buy.

Select the leanest cuts. Look for beef that has only a little marbling or external fat. Remember, you can always ask the butcher to trim away excess fat. Once you find the cut you like, check what grades are available. "Select" offers the least fat, followed by "choice" and then "prime."

You probably have zillions of recipes for beef, but think about the following suggestions, because they use beef more as an accent than a main course, which means smaller portions and less saturated fat to clog your arteries.

Add muscle to soup. Toss a little leftover steak or roast into vegetable soup for the next day's lunch or dinner.

Stack it up. Have a sandwich with a slice of roast beef and a slice of turkey, or tuck a little bit of beef, a little bit of chicken, and a lot of vegetables into tacos or fajitas.

Pump up salad. Add cold roast beef strips to your lunchtime salad to keep you going until dinner.

CHICKEN

Health Wizard

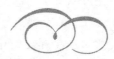

...Just the facts

Chicken breast (3 oz roasted, no skin)
Calories: 140
Fat: 3 g
Saturated fat: 1 g
Cholesterol: 72 mg
Sodium: 63 mg
Total carbohydrates: 0 g
Dietary fiber: 0 g
Protein: 26 g
Riboflavin (vitamin B$_2$): 7% of Daily Value
Niacin (vitamin B$_3$): 59%
Vitamin B$_6$: 20%
Vitamin B$_{12}$: 5%
Iron: 5%

VERSATILITY IS THE BEAUTY OF chicken—not only in cooking but also in the nutrition it provides. A 3-ounce piece of chicken contains at least 5 percent of the Daily Value for eight different vitamins and minerals that are crucial to maintaining good health, including the easy-to-absorb form of iron (called heme iron) that helps replace menstrual losses, pumps up your blood, and energizes your body so you can keep up with your busy schedule. Even better news is that chicken's heme iron helps you absorb more iron from the grains and vegetables you eat along with it.

Chicken—unlike many other foods—can taste incredibly different, depending on the recipe. Think about it: If you season steamed asparagus with Italian herbs or top it with hollandaise sauce, it still tastes like, well, asparagus. If you grill chicken and toss it into a warm flour tortilla with salsa, peppers, and onions, it takes on an entirely different flavor than if you roast it with rosemary and garlic.

WING YOUR WAY TO HEART HEALTH

The most abundant nutrient in chicken is niacin. Just a single chicken breast packs nearly 60 percent of what you need for the entire day. Studies suggest that niacin may lower cholesterol and drop your risk of heart disease.

If you're substituting chicken for beef, your heart will appreciate that, too. Three ounces of roasted chicken has just a single gram of saturated fat, while the same amount of ground beef is brimming with 6 grams or more! When you slice the saturated fat in your diet, you also slice your risk of ticker trouble. Swapping beef for chicken breast also saves calories. A serving of roasted chicken breast sans the skin contains about 100 fewer calories than a portion of ground beef and about 50 fewer than steak. Over time, the calorie cutting will add up, and you'll lose weight—another bit of good news for your heart.

Good to Go

When you make those fabulous chicken dishes:

• Thaw frozen chicken in the fridge (never on the countertop!) or by immersing it in cold water.

• Remove the skin either before or after cooking. Leaving the skin on while cooking doesn't increase the calorie or fat content of the meat, but it helps keep moisture in.

• Use a meat thermometer to check for doneness. Whole chickens should reach 180°F, bone-in chicken parts should reach 170°F, and boneless parts need to register 165°F. Immediately refrigerate any extra chicken.

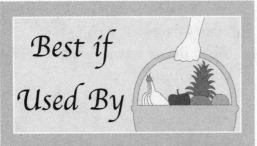

Best if Used By

At home, unpack chicken and other meats first and immediately store them in the coldest part of the fridge. If you're not planning to use the chicken for two days or more, freeze it in the store package.

Chicken is also peppered with vitamin B_6, vitamin B_{12}, and zinc—a trio that keeps your immune system strong so you're less likely to catch the virus of the week. And if you're coming down with a cold, whip up a batch of chicken soup—or better yet, get a loved one to do it. Chicken contains the amino acid cysteine, which is chemically similar to the bronchitis drug acetylcysteine. Plus, research suggests that chicken soup helps block the production of neutrophils, white blood cells that contribute to upper respiratory cold symptoms.

GET A LEG UP ON CHICKEN

It's important to handle chicken with care to keep your family healthy. To begin with, pick up the chicken last so it won't be unrefrigerated while you check out the magazines, look for a new lipstick, compare nutrition labels on crackers, and do other time-consuming stuff. When you choose your package, put it into a plastic bag (many supermarkets have bags in the meat department. If yours doesn't, snag some from the produce section). If the outside of the package is contaminated with salmonella or another type of bacteria, the plastic bag will keep the bugs from spreading to your other groceries. Also, when you check out, ask the cashier to bag your meat separately. Finally, if you're driving home in warm weather, put your groceries in the car (not the trunk) to keep them as cool as possible.

Since you probably have plenty of recipes for chicken, we

won't bore you with the basics, but here are some ways that you can get creative with this wonderfully adaptable food. C'mon, don't be chicken!

Poultri-fy pizza. Top a pizza crust with tomato sauce, roasted peppers, grilled chicken pieces, and a sprinkling of Parmesan and smoked mozzarella cheeses. This version of pizza—minus the usual coating of high-fat cheese and pepperoni—becomes a healthy meal.

Chicken out on tacos. Replace ground beef with shredded chicken breast; your taco will taste every bit as good.

Wing it with spaghetti. Stir grilled chicken pieces into pasta dishes. No one will miss the meatballs.

PORK

The Meat Factor-y

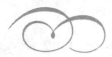

...Just the facts

Pork tenderloin (3 oz cooked)
Calories: 139
Fat: 4 g
Saturated fat: 1 g
Cholesterol: 67 mg
Sodium: 48 mg
Total carbohydrates: 0 g
Protein: 23 g
Thiamin (vitamin B_1): 53% of Daily Value
Riboflavin (vitamin B_2): 19%
Niacin (vitamin B_3): 20%
Vitamin B_6: 30%
Vitamin B_{12}: 8%
Iron: 7%
Potassium: 11%

MADE IN THE KITCHEN OF THE RIGHT person, pork can rival any gourmet food, and it really can be as lean as chicken! This is good news for young children, teens, and menstruating or pregnant women, who are most likely to be affected by iron deficiency, because pork is another proud producer of heme iron, the kind your body soaks up like a sponge to rebuild your iron stores. In addition, pork, along with chicken and beef, delivers the "meat factor," known to increase your body's absorption of iron from plant foods by as much as two to four times!

EAT HIGH ON THE HOG

When it comes to vitamins and minerals, pork is, well, a hog. It offers major amounts of 10 nutrients in just a 3-ounce serving. Here are some of pork's nutritional highlights.

• *Thiamin.* Pork packs 53 percent of your daily requirement for this vitamin, which is essential for metabolizing carbohydrates, protein, and fat.

• *Vitamin B$_{12}$.* When you eat a serving of pork, you soak up about 8 percent of your daily requirement this vitamin, which builds red blood cells.

• *Phosphorus.* Pork kicks in about one-quarter of your requirement for this bone-strengthening mineral.

• *Potassium.* You probably think that only fruits and veggies offer potassium, a mineral that helps maintain normal blood pressure. Pork offers 11 percent of your daily quota.

Now, I bet you're probably thinking, "Sure, pork's leaner than it used to be, but can I substitute it for chicken in my diet?" In a word: Yes. A study at Duke University Medical Center in Durham, North Carolina, found that substituting lean pork for fattier meats in the diets of people with high cholesterol dropped their levels by about 7 percent— the same amount as for a group

Best if Used By

Fresh pork will keep for four or five days in the fridge.

Good to Go

When you're ready to use your pork:

• Trim off any visible fat.

• Use a meat thermometer to ensure that the meat cooks to 160°F. Food safety experts used to recommend cooking pork to 170°F, but they've reduced the recommendation because the parasite that causes trichinosis—a disease that pork could transport—is killed at 137°F. Cooking to 160°F gives you a big margin of error, and the meat should still be juicy and a little pink in the center.

that ate skinless chicken. Thus, if your family is complaining about having chicken again, add some pork to your weekly menu. The bottom line is that they're both healthy for your heart. Mix and match them in your diet to beat boredom.

NO PIG IN A POKE

When it comes to pork, you can choose from a lot of cuts, including tenderloin, boneless sirloin chop, boneless loin roast, boneless top loin chop, loin chop. and rib chop. Each has from 4 to 9 grams of fat in a 3-ounce serving. You can go that one better by looking for Smithfield Lean Generation Pork, sold by a company that has specially bred its hogs to be leaner.

When selecting pork, for freshness' sake, make sure the meat is pink to pinkish gray, except for pork tenderloin, which should be deep red. Always check the "sell-by" date.

There are so many ways to dine on swine. Here are just a few.

Make over fajitas. You don't have to limit yourself to beef or chicken fajitas, since pork gives them awesome flavor, too.

Try a saucy trio. When you're grilling at home, try brushing a variety of sauces on different parts of your chops or tenderloin for scintillating taste treats.

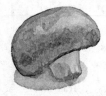

Go crazy with kebobs. Both kids and adults get a kick out of kebobs. Thread pieces of pork on a skewer along with your favorite veggies.

RAISINS

Energizer Buddies

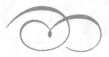

WHAT'S NOT TO LIKE ABOUT RAISINS? YOU HAVE TO ADMIT that their ad campaign—raisins rocking to "Heard It through the Grapevine"—was pretty cute, but if that didn't make you want to reach for a box and start munching, this will: Raisins are rife with the nutrients that will keep you groovin' for years and years! To start with, they kick in a good deal of energizing iron, considering that they're a nonmeat food.

While most men get plenty of this nutrient, 15 percent of women under age 50 are either iron deficient or anemic—two conditions that sap your energy. Snacking on raisins really may help you dance, so if you're feeling exhausted all the time, try a few days of raisin munching. If your fatigue is due to low iron levels—and if you're a menstruating woman,

---

...Just the facts

Raisins (about ¼ cup)
Calories: 130
Fat: 0 g
Saturated fat: 0 g
Cholesterol: 0 mg
Sodium: 10 mg
Total carbohydrates: 8 g
Dietary fiber: 2 g
Protein: 1 g
Iron: 6% of Daily Value

When you get home with your raisins, store them in the fridge. That way, they'll retain their nutritional value and their great taste for up to five months. If you prefer eating raisins at room temperature, just take them out of the fridge shortly before eating. They'll quickly warm up.

there's a good chance it is—then the iron in raisins will zip up your iron levels and reenergize your life.

MORE RAISIN THERAPY

What else do raisins have to offer?

• *Antioxidants.* Abundant in raisins and other fruits, antioxidants are substances that protect you from free radicals, which cause the cell damage that can lead to cancer, heart disease, and lots of other health problems. For optimal protection, researchers suggest that you get about 3,000 to 5,000 units of antioxidants daily. Just one itty-bitty 1½-ounce box of raisins kicks in 1,400 units!

Your memory benefits, too. A study on animals at Tufts University in Boston suggests that the antioxidants in grapes—which are fresh raisins—may help ward off memory loss and improve motor skills.

• *Fiber.* Raisins contain a hefty dose of inulin, a type of fiber that may reduce the risk of colon cancer. Studies suggest that inulin retards the growth of abnormal cells, which may lead to cancer.

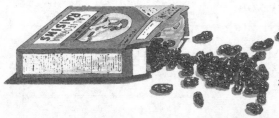

The fiber in raisins, plus tartaric acid (another unique compound found in high amounts in grapes), also helps prevent constipation. When researchers gave people who were eating low-fiber diets (as most of us are) three 1½-ounce boxes of raisins daily, the average time that it took waste to move through their gastrointestinal tracts was cut in half.

Granted, three boxes of raisins are a lot, but the researchers speculate that substituting even one box of raisins for another food in your diet (such as potato chips) may keep you from singing those bathroom blues.

GRAPEVINE SECRETS

The different types of raisins don't vary much in nutrients, so sample all of them to see what you like best. One caveat: If you're allergic to sulfur, pass up golden raisins (sultanas), because they're usually treated with sulfur to preserve their color. When selecting raisins, look for a box or a bag that's tightly sealed. Squeeze the package to see if the fruit is soft. If you purchase raisins in bulk, look for covered bins, and make sure the raisins appear moist and clean.

Now you're ready to rock 'n roll with these raisin recipes.

Rock on. Most cereals that come with raisins are also loaded with extra sugar. Instead, stir a handful of raisins into your own favorite healthy brand of cereal.

Roll 'em. For another breakfast treat, roll raisins into pancake or muffin batter.

Snack on. Take a 1½-ounce box of plain raisins or the cinnamon-topped kind to work with you and eat them when the vending machine calls.

Replace 'em. Whenever a recipe calls for chocolate chips, use half the chips and substitute raisins for the rest.

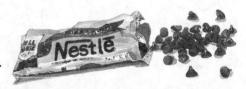

SHELLFISH

Seaside Treasures

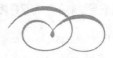

KICK OFF YOUR SHOES, ROLL UP YOUR PANTS LEGS, AND let the surf tickle your toes while your clambake sizzles in the sand. Then stroll on over to a sumptuous feast of shellfish—clams, crabs, lobster, mussels, oysters, scallops, and shrimp—so packed with minerals that they'll boost your blood, build your bones, and rev up your immune system to fight everything from the sniffles to heart disease and cancer.

LEGAL BOOTY

Clams, mussels, oysters, and shrimp are treasure troves of iron, needed for fending off anemia and recently shown to be crucial for your brain to achieve maximum reasoning power. Kids need it, teens need it, and all women who are pregnant or menstruating need it by the sand-pail full.

...Just the facts

Steamed clams (3 oz)
Calories: 119
Fat: 6 g
Saturated fat: 1 g
Cholesterol: 34 mg
Sodium: 115 mg
Total carbohydrates: 3 g
Dietary fiber: 0 g
Protein: 13 g
Vitamin C: 21%
Calcium: 5%
Iron: 78%

Clams flood your body with 78 percent of your daily needs, while other shellfish deliver 15 to 30 percent.

Shellfish are also an outstanding low-calorie source of protein, which is needed to maintain every cell in your body (including blood cells) and to keep your immune system in top fighting condition. Some research also suggests that protein satisfies your hunger so you feel satisfied sooner and don't keep on eating. In other words, eating protein may help you control your weight.

Good to Go

When it's time to cook your shellfish:

• Boil or steam mollusks in a small pot, watching for the shells to open.

• After they open, continue boiling for 3 to 5 minutes or steaming for 4 to 9 minutes to ensure that they're completely cooked. Discard any that haven't opened.

• Simmer shucked shellfish for at least 3 minutes.

Also, since shellfish contain almost no saturated fat, you don't have to worry about them raising your cholesterol levels, as you do with fatty meats. True, some shellfish, especially shrimp, pack more cholesterol than beef does, but research tells us that for most people, it's the saturated fat you eat, not the cholesterol in your food, that makes your cholesterol skyrocket. So relax and enjoy!

BONE-A-FIED BENEFITS

Shellfish can help strengthen your bones, too, but that's not because of their calcium, which is only in the shell! Their real secret is an array of trace minerals, such as magnesium

← *Iron Mollusks* →

Shellfish dish out low-fat protein and more concentrated nutrients than beef or poultry. Catch up with them, and you'll improve your nutritional net worth!

Shellfish (3 oz)	Calories	Fat (g)	Notable Nutrients (% DV)
Clams	125	2	Iron: 78 Vitamin B_{12}: 784 Copper: 17 Riboflavin (vitamin B_2): 10 Manganese: 2
Lobster	98	3	Iron: 2 Copper: 80 Zinc: 16 Vitamin E: 4
Mussels	146	4	Iron: 32 Vitamin B_{12}: 340 Manganese: 165 Riboflavin (vitamin B_2): 21 Thiamin (vitamin B_1): 17
Oysters	117	4	Iron: 20 Vitamin B_{12}: 394 Vitamin D: 273 Zinc: 417
Scallops	113	3	Iron: 20 Vitamin B_{12}: 25 Vitamin E: 7
Shrimp	84	1	Iron: 15 Niacin (vitamin B_3): 11 Zinc: 9
Beef round	169	4	Vitamin B_{12}: 96 Zinc: 32 Niacin (vitamin B_3): 23 Iron: 19

and manganese, that your bones need in small but critical quantities. These trace minerals may be missing from your diet if you eat a lot of processed foods, such as white bread, crackers, pretzels, and cookies.

All shellfish are not created equal when it comes to minerals (and vitamins), so mix and match varieties for best nutrition (see "Iron Mollusks"). For bone strength, here are some noteworthy choices.

• Scallops are a good source of magnesium, which may prevent unusual formations that make bones brittle and more likely to break.

• Mussels are so loaded with manganese that only six steamed mussels pack a whole day's worth. This mineral is especially important to women because it may help reduce the loss of calcium in bone after menopause.

• Oysters are one of the few food sources of vitamin D, and without this nutrient, you just can't get calcium into your bones.

UNDERWATER RICHES

Oysters may grow on river bottoms, but they're tops when it comes to delivering zinc. In fact, one little oyster delivers 15 milligrams—a whole day's worth!

Zinc is a mineral that's involved in at least 60 different enzymes that interact along complex pathways to affect your appetite, taste, and night vision, as well as your body's ability to fight invaders ranging from viruses that trigger colds and flu to carcinogens that cause cancer. In the United States, half of all people over age 50 fail to get enough zinc from their diets.

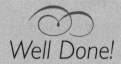
Prefer to eat your shellfish raw? Consider this: Raw mollusks may carry Norwalk viruses, which can cause severe diarrhea. Worse yet, they may harbor the bacterium *Vibrio vulnificus*, which, in up to half of all cases, triggers deadly blood poisoning in just two days.

People with diabetes, gastrointestinal problems, liver disease, or compromised immune systems due to HIV infection, cancer, or other conditions are most at risk for getting sick from eating raw seafood—although even the healthiest person can fall victim. So cook your seafood to wipe out any bacteria. Remember: That raw seafood bar can be a raw deal!

If you ever get one of those colds that seems to hang around forever, check with your doctor to be sure it's nothing serious, then try adding a serving of shellfish to your diet once a day. The increased zinc may give your immune system enough of a boost to get it—and you—back on track. Don't overdo it, though. Over many months, getting an average of more than 15 milligrams of zinc daily can have the opposite effect and slow your immune system.

FRESHNESS ON THE HALF-SHELL

It's very important to buy shellfish that are fresh and healthy. One sign of freshness is their smell, which should be more like a fresh ocean breeze than a fishy odor. Mollusks (clams, mussels, oysters, and scallops) in the shell should be alive, so choose only those that are tightly closed or that close quickly when you tap on the shell.

Try these quick-as-a-wink ways to get more shellfish into your daily fare.

Soup it up. Stir canned clams into leftover vegetable soup to boost flavor, protein, and minerals.

Cut the fat. Top your next spinach salad with crabmeat instead of bacon, and you'll eliminate a ton of saturated fat.

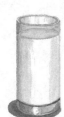

Warm it up. Ward off winter chill by simmering shucked oysters with fat-free milk and a little celery seed.

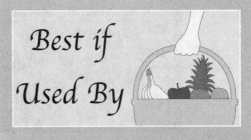

Best if Used By

Store live shellfish in a container covered loosely with a clean, damp cloth. Don't store them in airtight containers or in water.

Cool it down. Grill peeled, deveined shrimp on a skewer with pineapple chunks, bite-size pieces of green bell pepper, and cherry tomatoes for an easy summer meal.

URINARY TRACT INFECTIONS

Flush Naturally

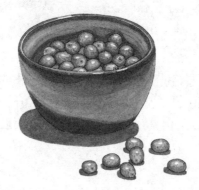

URINARY TRACT INFECTIONS ARE AMONG THE MOST common—and the most annoying—health issues that women deal with. About a third of American women will get a urinary tract infection (UTI) at some point in their lives, and some women get them over and over again. The infections can occur anywhere in the urinary tract, but they usually affect the urethra, the tube through which urine leaves the body, or the bladder. The main symptom is a burning sensation, along with urinary urgency—the sudden, overwhelming need to go to the bathroom.

"I used to have five or six infections a year," says Crystal Abernathy, N.D., a naturopathic physician in Charlotte, North Carolina. "It's a very irritating thing to deal with."

Although it took some time, Dr. Abernathy eventually discovered how to keep the pesky infections under control. She hasn't had an infection in years—and the advice she shares here will work just as well for you.

TRADING PLACES

Most UTIs occur when bacteria that normally live in the area surrounding the anus make their way inside the urethra. Once they get into that warm, moist environment, they quickly multiply, and sometimes they even work their way up to the bladder. Men sometimes get UTIs, but their extra inches of anatomy make it harder for bacteria to get inside. Women don't have that protection, so they're a lot more vulnerable.

9 1 1

Call your doctor immediately if you have a urinary tract infection accompanied by fever, blood in the urine, or back pain. These are signs that you may be developing a kidney infection, which can be life-threatening without prompt treatment.

ATTACK!

With quick treatment, most UTIs disappear after a course of antibiotics. You usually have to take the drugs for a week, although shorter treatments are available. In the meantime, now's the time to think about ways to prevent future infections and take steps to keep your current discomfort to a minimum. Here's what you need to do.

Skip your just desserts. Sweets can be a real problem if you get frequent UTIs. Sugar encourages the growth of bacteria, and it reduces the ability of your immune system to battle infection. "It's sort of a double whammy," says Dr. Abernathy.

And remember, it's not just sweets like candy that cause problems, but all sources of sugar, including the sugar in pack-

"Vitamin C is helpful because it supports the immune system," says Crystal Abernathy, N.D. When you have a UTI, plan on taking 500 milligrams of vitamin C every 2 hours, she suggests.

Vitamin C in large amounts may cause diarrhea. If you're having problems, cut back on the dose until you find a level that works for you. If you have kidney disease or stomach problems, discuss vitamin C with your doctor before giving it a try.

aged foods. Read labels so you know what you're getting.

Be a teetotaler. The bacterial colonies that cause UTIs love alcohol because it's converted into sugar in your body. Give up the drinks until the infection is gone.

Down an herbal cocktail. "I use a combination of four different herbs to treat urinary tract infections," Dr. Abernathy says. "It tends to be pretty effective; people usually start getting relief in 1 to 4 hours."

The herbs she uses are uva-ursi (sometimes called bearberry), buchu, echinacea, and goldenseal, which are all available at health food stores. Take 200 milligrams of each three times daily for a week, she advises.

Muscle up on protein. You need plenty of protein to keep your immune system healthy. To make sure you're getting enough, divide your weight by 2.2 to get your weight in kilograms, then eat 1 gram of protein daily for each kilogram of body weight.

As long as you eat a healthy diet that includes plenty of whole grains, legumes, and lean meat and fish, you're almost guaranteed to get enough protein to boost your defenses against UTIs.

Fill up on cranberry juice. One cure for UTIs that both folk healers and mainstream medical practitioners agree on is cranberry juice. The natural chemicals in the juice make it harder for bacteria to attach to the inside walls of your bladder. Rather than sticking around and causing trouble, they're more likely to be washed out of your body in urine. Stock up on sugar-free cranberry juice, then drink at least three glasses a day when you have a UTI.

Pour on the water. The more water you drink, the more bacteria will be flushed from your bladder. "Drink at least 2 quarts of water a day," Dr. Abernathy suggests.

That may seem like a lot of H_2O, but if you carry water with you and sip it throughout the day, you won't even realize how much you're drinking.

Tidy up. It's an unfortunate fact of anatomy—the proximity of the anus and urethra—that makes women vulnerable to bacterial invasions. If you always wipe from front to back after using the toilet, you'll be less likely to push bacteria somewhere where they can cause problems.

Some women find that they get UTIs after sex because intercourse can push bacteria where they shouldn't go. Urinating after intercourse can flush out any germs that may have worked their way into the urinary tract.

Answer nature's call. When your body tells you that it's time to find a restroom, do it. Holding urine in the bladder for too long gives bacteria a chance to multiply.

Two Good!

Blueberries and cranberries (even the dried ones) are double trouble for urinary tract infections, since both pack enough condensed tannins to wash bugs away. Both also fight memory loss.

Choose supplements carefully. If you take supplemental magnesium or calcium, be sure to get the citrate form, says Dr. Abernathy. Citrates are easier for your body to absorb, and they make the urine more alkaline, which can help prevent UTIs.

Warm away pain. To quickly ease the localized discomfort of a UTI, apply a warm compress to the urethral opening and the surrounding area, suggests Dr. Abernathy. Moist warmth can reduce muscle spasms that result in pain, she explains. A long soak in a warm bath will have similar soothing effects.

Hunt for magic mushrooms. Most supermarkets offer several tasty varieties of gourmet mushrooms. You should definitely stock up on them when you have a UTI, because they boost the ability of your immune system to combat infections. "Different mushrooms stimulate different aspects of the immune system, so it's good to combine them and get a broad spectrum of effects," says Dr. Abernathy. The types to look for include shiitake, reishi, and maitake.

CRANBERRIES

Drink to Your Health

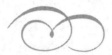

ARE YOU SICK AND TIRED OF THOSE UTIs—YOU KNOW, what your doctor calls urinary tract infections? Well, if you're ready for relief, it's time to start juicing up with cranberries.

Maybe you think that the stories about the protective power of cranberries are just old wives' tales. They're not! Research done at Harvard Medical School showed that elderly women who drank 1¼ cups of cranberry juice every day for a month were only 42 percent as likely to have UTIs as women who didn't drink the juice. What's more, if they continued drinking the tangy thirst quencher, their chances dropped even further.

Now, researchers at Rutgers University's blueberry and cranberry research center in Chatsworth, New Jersey, think they've

...Just the facts

Light cranberry juice cocktail with Splenda (1 cup)
Calories: 40
Fat: 0 g
Saturated fat: 0 g
Cholesterol: 0 mg
Sodium: 7 mg
Total carbohydrates: 10 g
Dietary fiber: 0 g
Protein: 0 g
Vitamin C: 88% of Daily Value

When you bring your ruby berries home, here's how to keep them in tiptop shape.

• Store them in their original bag in the refrigerator. They'll keep for up to two weeks.

• Alternatively, freeze them in the original bag wrapped in extra plastic (to protect against freezer burn and dehydration), then use them all year long.

• Just before eating refrigerated or frozen berries, rinse and under running water and sort them.

found the reason. *E. coli* bacteria (the usual cause of UTIs) grow little hooks, like Velcro, that latch onto urinary tract walls. Instead of being washed away by the water you drink, they hang around and multiply, causing a massive infection. Fortunately, cranberry juice packs a powerful antidote, called condensed tannins, that appears to detach the hooks so bacteria can be washed away.

To get enough condensed tannins, you'll need a drink that's 27 percent cranberry juice. Although the cranberry juice you find in the supermarket measures up, it has added sugar. Usually, sweetened juice wouldn't be considered a healthy food, but cranberry juice is an exception. In its natural state, this juice is so sour that you can't drink it straight.

Unfortunately, the sweetened variety also packs 175 calories in the 10 ounces you'll need each day to flush the bugs. If you're calorie conscious, switch to Ocean Spray Light Cranberry Juice Cocktail, which is sweetened with Splenda (sucralose) and weighs in at just 50 calories per 10-ounce serving.

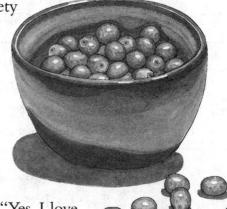

By now you're probably thinking, "Yes, I love

that tart, refreshing taste, but every day?" Cheer up—you have other choices.

• A quarter cup of Craisins (dried cranberries infused with cranberry concentrate and sugar) also packs enough tannins to get the job done.

• One cup of fresh or frozen blueberries also works.

• Ten ounces of cranberry/blueberry cocktail provides the same bacteria-squelching power as straight cranberry juice.

Don't go too far astray, though. Mixing peach, kiwi, or other nonberry juices with cranberry tastes delicious but waters down the tannins' power, leaving you unprotected.

BERRY GOOD NEWS

Cranberries also contain ellagic acid, now being explored as a colon cancer fighter. Also, in laboratory petri dishes, cranberry extract prevents cholesterol from becoming sticky enough to clog arteries. Since cranberries are low in the ingredients now known to fight arterial gunk, researchers are still playing "Name That Antioxidant," but a rose (or antioxidant) by any other name still gets the job done. Just call it all cranberry magic—and enjoy!

Cranberries are rich in quercetin, a natural antihistamine that can help cut down on the sneezing that comes with airborne allergens.

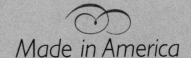

Made in America

Cranberries are an all-American fruit that Native Americans used for food and medicine long before the *Mayflower* landed. The Pilgrims, however, did invent the name we use today.

As ships sailed between the Old World and the New, American sailors packed a couple of buckets of vitamin C–rich cranberries to prevent scurvy. British sailors relied on limes, hence the nickname "limey."

DON'T GET BOGGED DOWN

Fresh cranberries are available from September through December, just in time to make your own cranberry sauce for Thanksgiving. Look for berries that are plump, firm, and dark red. As with most fruits and vegetables, the darker the color, the more antioxidants they contain.

Use cranberries in these tasty ways.

Hit the sauce. Spread cranberry sauce on your turkey sandwich. It's a deliciously fat-free way to enjoy Thanksgiving leftovers as well as a pretty good way to dress up deli sandwiches year-round. Try it on pork chops, too. They're leaner and drier now, and zesty cranberry sauce keeps them juicy and flavorful.

Pick pilaf. Cook up a batch of wild rice and toss in some chopped celery, chopped dried apricots, and fresh or frozen cranberries. If company is already knocking at your door, use a white rice–wild rice quick mix.

Drink peach melba. Whip up some fat-free frozen yogurt, a cup of fresh peaches, and a cup of cranberry juice cocktail.

Give in to your Craisin craving. Once you taste them, you'll wonder how you did without them! Toss a few tart, tangy tidbits into your trail mix, vegetable salads, and savory pasta dishes. Stir them into couscous and decorate with pine nuts, or mix them into wheatberries with a few oil-cured olives and a tablespoon of chopped walnuts.

Replace half the raisins. In muffin and quick bread recipes, you can replace half or all the raisins with cranberries for color contrast and sweet-tart taste.

INDEX

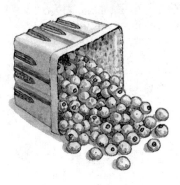

kiwifruit and, 404
peaches and, 355
strawberries and, 408
treatments for, 388–90
Gymnema, 96

H

Hand washing, 283
Harvest Mornings cereals,
    118
Hawthorn, 132
Heartburn, 71, 111, 332
Heart disease. *See also*
        Angina
    apples and, 307
    apricots and, 29
    artichokes and, 285
    asparagus and, 344–45
    avocados and, 200–202
    bananas and, 289
    beans and, 207–8
    beef and, 444
    beets and, 103
    bell peppers and, 416
    blackberries and, 33
    broccoli and, 368
    brown rice and, 106–7
    brussels sprouts and, 42
    cabbage and, 46
    canola oil and, 211
    cauliflower and, 55
    cherries and, 9
    chicken and, 447
    cinnamon and, 327
    fennel and, 224
    figs and, 261
    garlic and, 58
    ginger and, 330
    grapefruit and, 402
    green beans and, 314
    kiwifruit and, 405, 406
    lentils and, 264
    margarine and, 227–28
    nuts and, 232
    onions and, 352
    papaya and, 68

parsley and, 237
peaches and, 356
pineapple and, 70–71
potatoes and, 184
prunes and, 270
pumpkin and, 430
quinoa and, 321
raisins and, 454
soy and, 247
sweet potatoes and, 80
tea and, 17
turkey and, 295
wheatberries and, 278
wheat germ and, 193
whole wheat bread and,
    120
wine and, 378–79
yogurt and, 301
Heat compress, 466
Helicobacter pylori, 340
Hemorrhoids, 121, 276
Herpesvirus, 58
Hiccups, 68
High blood pressure
    apricots and, 29
    bananas and, 289
    barley and, 99
    bok choy and, 164–66
    brussels sprouts and, 42
    causes of, 159–60
    celery and, 167–69
    cucumbers and, 171
    green beans and, 314
    kiwifruit and, 406
    milk and, 179
    mushrooms and, 61
    oats and, 117–18
    olive oil and, 143
    papaya and, 68
    pork and, 451
    potatoes and, 183–84
    readings, 160
    squash and, 187
    treatments for, 160–63
    watermelon and, 88–89
    wine and, 379–80

High cholesterol, 196–99.
        See also Cholesterol
        levels
Hip fractures, 370
Hives, 117
Honey, 281
Horseradish, 291–93
Hot peppers, 309–12
Hot-tub therapy, 95
Hydration
    celery and, 169
    constipation and, 258
    cucumbers and, 171
    diarrhea and, 282
    stomachache and, 324
    UTIs and, 464

I

IBS. *See* Irritable bowel
        syndrome
Immune function
    asparagus and, 344
    bell peppers and, 417
    brussels sprouts and, 42
    canola oil and, 210
    chicken and, 448
    eggs and, 374
    garlic and, 58
    kiwifruit and, 406
    mushrooms and, 61
    nectarines and, 267
    papaya and, 66
    peaches and, 355
    pineapple and, 71
    pumpkin and, 431–32
    pumpkin seeds and, 157
    quinoa and, 321
    raspberries and, 273
    shellfish and, 460
    squash and, 189
    sweet potatoes and, 80
    turkey and, 295
    yogurt and, 299
Indoles, 45
Infections
    basil and, 349
    beef and, 444